ESSENTIALS FOR NATURAL HEALING

Healing for the Whole Body: Emotional, Mental, Physical, Spirit and Soul

Instructor & Holistic Practitioner
KIMBERLEY ANNE BUCKLER

Essentials for Natural Healing
Copyright © 2017 by Kimberley Anne Buckler

No part of this publication may be reproduced, distributed, or transmitted in any form or by any means, including photocopying, recording, or other electronic or mechanical methods, without the prior written permission of the author, except in the case of brief quotations embodied in critical reviews and certain other non-commercial uses permitted by copyright law.

Photos by: BlindDrop Design Inc.

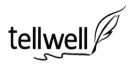

Tellwell Talent
www.tellwell.ca

ISBN
978-1-77370-101-1 (Paperback)
978-1-77370-102-8 (eBook)

TABLE OF CONTENTS

INTRODUCTION V
    Holistic Healing: The process of healing the body naturally: emotionally, mentally, physically and spiritually.

DEDICATION..VII

CHAPTER 1 1
    Holistic Healing Techniques

CHAPTER 2 15
    Energy Healing

CHAPTER 3 23
    Healing Property Terms

CHAPTER 4 27
    Proper Nutrition Essentials: Minerals, Vitamins, Oils, Enzymes, Proteins and Antioxidants

CHAPTER 5 67
    Mother Earth's Foods and Medicines

CHAPTER 6 71
    Dairy

CHAPTER 7 79
    Fruits

CHAPTER 8 101
    Grains

CHAPTER 9 109
  Herbs and Other Healing Plants

CHAPTER 10 243
  Legumes

CHAPTER 11. 253
  Meats

CHAPTER 12 263
  Nuts, Oils & Seeds

CHAPTER 13 281
  Vegetables

CHAPTER 14 303
  Essential Oils

CHAPTER 15 319
  Ailments and Alternative Options

CHAPTER 16 437
  Safe and Natural Ways to Keep a Healthy Home

CHAPTER 17 465
  Food Preservation

CHAPTER 18 487
  Gardening for Health

CHAPTER 19 497
  A Recipe or Two, Tasty and Healthy

REFERENCES 501

INTRODUCTION

Holistic Healing: The process of healing the body naturally: emotionally, mentally, physically and spiritually.

MANY TIMES WHEN A PERSON IS PRESCRIBED CHEMICALS, THE PERSON IS GIVEN A MASK to cover what is happening to the body. Not many of the holistic options have side effects. The holistic options can provide a stronger and longer lasting healing foundation.

This journey to holistic healing and healthly living started when I was around sixteen years old. A friendship with a very down to earth friend brought forth information as to why I was not feeling good physically and how my eating habits needed to change. Even today, I still enjoy those home baked cookies, but I am not near that weight I was at 16. I slimmed down, and my overall health is very good.

While I was becoming aware of the foods that I was consuming, I began to learn about the different effects that the products on the store shelves have on our bodies. I also realized that many work environments are toxic and how I needed to protect myself better when I was there.

Our food, the environment and our thinking patterns create an effect on how our human bodies react on a daily basis. When any one of these factors is not being looked after, we experience ill health and discomfort on many levels. This can be physically, emotionally, mentally and spiritually. My body and mind have been a walking testament of how I am living. From having a bunion on my foot that was very painful to migraines that had me taking painkillers, I realized that I needed to make some more changes in my life.

Today, after years of finding alternative resources and healthier options, I am headache free, have a much higher vibrational level and am very happy. I am no longer scared to travel due to discomforts or fears of getting sick. I hope this book will help you out, the same way the information helped me out over the years. With this, I have so much gratitude for being able to live on such an amazing planet that can provide our bodies with so many healthy options and healing tools.

PLEASE TAKE NOTE: **I am not a doctor, herbalist or a naturopath. I cannot personally advise anyone of what they should take or what therapies they need.** My background is the practising of Reiki and other forms of energy work. I will not take any personal responsibility for your health and well-being. You are the one that is stepping forward and seeking amazing ways of healing naturally. I suggest that you use this as a handbook to further your research to find out what can be used naturally to assist in enhancing your life in all areas of well-being: emotionally, mentally, physically and spiritually. I had a lot of fun finding out what everything did for my body, including the vitamins, minerals, omega oils and more.

WARNING: If you are on any prescribed medication or therapies, you need to get confirmation from your licensed practitioner or naturopath first before taking any additional vitamins, minerals, herbs or oils.

This book was prepared to get you interested in what you are placing on the table and what can enhance your health at the same time as pleasing your taste buds. Along with healthy eating to heal the body, we can have fun preparing safe cleansers and body products to use with a lot of the herbs and fruits listed in the book.

Have fun discovering the blessings of Mother Earth.

Blessing to you on your journey to a healthier lifestyle and well-being.

DEDICATION

I WOULD LOVE TO DEDICATE THIS BOOK TO MY TEENAGE FRIEND ROCCO, MY CHILDREN, grandchildren, Cousin Shelley and Mother Earth.

When I was about sixteen years old, I met an amazing young lady named Rocco. She got me thinking about what I was eating and how it was affecting my health and weight. I started to slim down and feel a lot more energetic.

My children's sensitivities to food, chemicals in cleaning products and processed foods opened another door of experiences. When they came home after eating food laced with food dyes or sugar, I knew I had to be patient till it wore off.

My grandchildren also showed signs of sensitivities to flowers, food colouring and materials used in clothing. We had to be careful what one was wearing and what food they were consuming.

My cousin, Shelley, was the one that really introduced me to the power of herbal medicine. I still remember the day she gave me a herbal combination to help my stomach. It took me about two months before I finally tried the herbs. This herbal product helped my stomach to heal and work properly again. This took me down the path of learning how our food is our medicine, especially the fruits, herbs, legumes, nuts, oils, seeds and vegetables.

Thank you to my amazing family and friends who have walked this path with me and have taught me so much in one way or the other. You all are a huge blessing!

CHAPTER 1

Holistic Healing Techniques

THE ORIGINAL SETTLERS OF ALL THE COUNTRIES AROUND THE WORLD HAD AMAZING forms of healing. They used the medicines and energies of the land and spirit realm for healing the mind, body and soul. Working with Mother Earth and connecting with God/Creator brought many healing techniques that the medicine men and medicine women learned to use. These teachings were passed on to people in the community who had the same soul path. The children who were destined for this path of healing were taught at a very early age. This information that they learned was also shared among the other communities around the world.

A lot of the teachings were lost due to the fact that healing options were taken away from the indigenous peoples and those who were called witches and the right to live with Mother Earth. In the the east in countries like China, India and Japan: many of the healing techniques were retained and are still being used to this day. They shared acupuncture, acupressure and the knowledge of working with the body's meridians along with incorporating herbs and healthier energy practices. In India, there was the use of meditation and Ayurveda medicines, which included food planning. All above healing methods taught one how to heal the body, mind and spirit.

In the early 1970s, some of the eastern healing techniques started to come back to the west in both Canada and the United States. This started with meditations, massage therapy and chiropractic work. At this time, more books were being published on how the plants of the earth could be used as a medicine instead of the chemicals that were being used by the pharmaceutical companies. In 2016, there are so many ways of practising holistic healing that it is hard to keep up with all the new techniques.

This chapter is to share some of the healing techniques that are available to us today. Each will have a brief description, and it is up to you to research more on what you are most intrigued and comfortable with. We don't all enjoy the same teachings or ideas, yet now have many options to choose from. If you are unsure, try something out see how it reacts with you and the changes it brings to you. I have tried a few techniques. My favourite healing techniques are the following: essential oils, herbs, Reiki and reflexology. What are yours?

One should never take ownership of a disease. Refrain from saying things like: "my diabetes, my asthma, my sick cell."

Start the healing process by putting it out into the universe and with your body that this discomfort is only temporarily. That illness does not belong to you. Focus on the positive steps you will make to release any sickness from your body.

Disclaimer: Kimberley Anne Buckler is not a healthcare professional and no part of the book or her writings is to be regarded as medical advice. In the event that you use any of the information that she has provided for her readers, assume full responsibility for your understanding, actions and the results.

Accessing Bars
A neuroscientist, Dr. Fannin, found that there are thirty-two bars in the head that connect your thoughts and attitudes. When the bars are not cleared, we are healed back. When working with the bars, a person is able to release thought patterns that we have been holding onto from other lives, whether it be financial success, health, creativity or more. This healing technique was started in the 1990s, now being taught around the world.

Acutonics
Acutonics is done with tuning forks that are calibrated to the frequencies and harmonic resonances of the celestial bodies. Known as "the Music of the Spheres," the vibrations of the tuning forks resonates with every cell in our body and helps to provide healing to the physical, mental, emotional and spiritual bodies.

Acupuncture
Acupuncture is a treatment involving the use of fine needles. The needles stimulate the meridians of the body. This helps to increase the flow of Qi, essential to the well-being of the spiritual, mental, physical and emotional state. Acupuncture is used to relieve headaches, depression, reduces allergies and works with the emotional well-being.

Akashic Records
The Akashic records hold the information on your past lives and provides the information on how you can release the patterns that have repeated themselves from lifetime to lifetime. These patterns can show emotional abuse - mental - physical, anger, fear, frustration, physical ailments and unhealthy belief systems. When the records are accessed on your behalf, the healing work is interactive, and you can take a conscious part in seeing the events, healing and releasing the patterns and emotions.

Aromatherapy
Essential oils are used for aromatherapy. The oils are infused into the air so that it can be spread over a larger area. The oils can be used for their antibacterial to help clean the air. The oils can bring a pleasant smell to the air and provide a relaxing energy. The use of aromatherapy is a lot safer for the environment than the use of air refreshers and disinfectants that are made with chemicals that cause damage to our neurological system and liver. The oils do not contain the chemicals that cause neurological damage to the body.

Ayurveda
Ayurveda was created by the Vedic civilization of India. The system brings together the use of the earth, water, air, fire and space. The body needs the proper balance to sustain a health life. With the use of energy work for healing, eating the proper foods for the body type and meditation for spiritual balance, a person can have a healthier balance in all areas of their life.

Biofield Medicine
Biofield Medicine is working with the energy fields around the body to help promote healing on all levels. Working with the energies within the body and around the body, one can heal faster after surgeries and release old energies that we may be still holding onto. Craniosacral therapy, Healing Touch, Therapeutic Touch and Reiki are examples of Biofield Medicine.

Blood Analysis
Poor health conditions can be revealed through the analysis of dry or live blood samples. These samples can show parasites, toxins and many more imbalances in the human system from hormone imbalance to chronic fatigue. This provides a basis for where to start with the healing process and what the body needs to work on first.

Body Talk
Body talk is done by taping on the body to access the inner wisdom and memories of the body to balance the system and prevent poor health issues from reoccurring. Body talk is used to heal the energy circuits within the body along with releasing old habits and fears that we hold onto.

Body Work
Body work can be performed by the use of different healing techniques such as massage therapy, acupressure, chiropractic, Rolfing, physical therapy and energy work. The result is the balancing of the physical and emotional state of being, working with the structure of the body and releasing blocks.

Brain Gym
Brain Gym is the use of educational kinesiology. This form of healing helps to redevelop the brains neural pathways through physical movement in order to reprogram and improve our concentration, reading, memory, listening and confidence.

Chakra Balancing
Our bodies have seven major chakras or energy centres: root, sacral, solar plexus, heart, throat, third eye and crown chakra. When these chakras become blocked, our physical, emotional and spiritual well-being can be affected in our daily living. Chakra balancing can be achieved through many remedies and techniques. Some of the methods we can use are aromatherapy, crystals, colour therapy, massage, meditation, prayer, sound and music therapy, reflexology, Reiki, tuning forks, yoga and visualization.

Chiropractor
Chiropractors work mainly with the spine, making adjustments to the skeletal system. These adjustments can release pinched nerves, headaches, unbalanced hips and many more ailments that can affect the health and mobility of the client. Chiropractors are one of the first alternative methods of healing that was accepted in the Western countries.

Clearings for Home and Business
Smudging is done with sage to clear rooms/buildings of negative or old energy. Smudging can also release emotional imprints that have been left behind from unpleasant situations and events. Smudging can be used to help release entities or spirits from areas that they are occupying. Tools for clearing are energy work, sage, smudge wand sweetgrass,

Coaching
Coaching can be provided and applied to many different areas of our lives. A motivational coach helps the client to recognize how one is allowing misguided believes or practices to get in the way of going forward and reaching new goals.

Counselling
Similar to the coach, this is a person who can empathize and mirror another person's experiences in order to help the client to resolve the problem or issue at hand. Counselling helps to provide the support that a person needs to go forward in their life.

Craniosacral Therapy
Craniosacral therapy was developed by John Upledger. He discovered a gentle form of healing, working with the pulse of the cranial system to release blocks that have occurred from physical and emotional stress and trauma. Craniosacral therapy is administered through monitoring the rhythm of the cerebrospinal fluid's flow through the system. The movable skull, sacrum and coccyx are attached to membranes, encompassing the cerebrospinal fluid. Experienced clinicians can detect motion or blocked areas. Light, hands-on touch assists hydraulic forces to improve the body's internal system, thus strengthening the body's ability to heal itself. By freeing tension from the spinal cord, the cerebral spinal flows more freely. Craniosacral therapy optimizes rhythm of the spinal fluid and influences the whole body. It is relaxing, safe and effective; and Craniosacral therapy may heal or alleviate numerous conditions including migraines, chronic fatigue, motor coordination impairments, stress and tension, TMJ and orthopedic problems.

Crystal Healing
Each crystal has different healing properties and different vibrational energy. Crystals provide energy healing for the physical, emotional and spiritual well-being. Crystals are a wonderful asset and healing tool to have in your home and office. Crystals have been used since the beginning of time in many healing practices. They carry the energies of both heaven and earth.

Cupping
Cupping is used with the Chinese medicine techniques. Either a bamboo cup or a glass is vacuumed to the body of the client to increase circulation and extract or drain the body of the cold or damp evils (blocks) from the body.

Curanderismo
This is a Latin American healing system used in the United States. This healing system was brought up from Mexico, and some of the medicines used in Mexico are used. This method of healing uses energy work, medicines and belief practices that may include the supernatural world.

Doula
A doula helps a mother to go through the birthing process with compassionate and the knowledge to provide a safe environment. The birthing process can be long, and the supporting doula can help the mother be more comfortable and at ease with what she is experiencing during the pregnancy and birthing time. The doula goes through years of training for this work.

Dowsing
Dowsing is a form of neutralizing and curing energies in your environment that have a negative impact. Dowsing can be done to find electromagnetic frequencies in your home and is also used to find non-beneficial energies. These energies can make a person sick, physically and emotionally until they are removed. Dowsing rods are used to find water and to help clear energies.

Ear Candling
Use of wax covered cotton to help clear the sinuses, equalizes pressure in the head and boosts the immune system. This can help to decrease candida, enhance the hearing, healing infections, brings relief to the sinus and more. The use of ear candles is illegal in Canada.

Entity and Spirit Clearings
Often different elemental entities, heavy energies or dark spirits attach themselves to property, humans and animals. They are looking for another source of energy. The universe uses light workers to help release spirits and entities that are stuck to the earth. These energies do not like strong sources of light energy. When the entities are attached to someone, the person may feel sick or get the chills. As the entity or dark spirit is exposed to higher vibrational energies such as Reiki energy or crystal energy, their energy changes, and it is easier to release them for safe processing.

Essential Oils
Essential oils can be used everyday in your home, office and clinic. Essential oils have different healing properties, from being a disinfectant and antibacterial to being soothing and relaxing. Essential oils are extracted from the plant world to help heal the human body of all ages, pets and farm animals along with being used as cleaning and for disinfecting the living or work area.

Feng Shui
Using the Chinese art of placement, we can balance and enhance the energy flow in our living and work spaces. An area with a balanced (uncluttered) sense of feeling will increase the Qi energy in our physical and emotional well-being. This may include using water fountains, mirrors, crystals and other methods of increasing the energy in the home or office.

Folk Medicine
This is the use of traditional healing practices that are not recognized by government bodies, like a lot of the other practices listed in this chapter. One may use prayer, meals for healing and other natural methods to enhance the well-being of the patient.

Guided Imagery
Guided imagery is a practice of visualizing better health for the body. This is a method of positive thinking and visualizing a state of healthier well-being to overcome any illness or setbacks that one may be experiencing. An example is if a child had cancer, the child could visualize a Pac-Man character going through his or her body to eat all the cancer cells. This imagery can help the person stay in a positive state, and it can slow down the cancer growth.

Healing Touch
Healing touch is a therapeutic treatment that assists people by restoration of balance in the human energy field. A complimentary medicine, healing touch helps decrease pain, increase effectiveness of conventional medicine, relieves anxiety and helps promote the self-healing processes. This is done by placement of the hands 1 – 6 inches above the body surface.

Health Care Products
We are looking for products that are environmentally safe and beneficial that do not have any harmful chemicals. Many of the products in the market place have ingredients that are toxic externally and internally. From bath soaps to toothpaste, from air fresheners to cleansers, they are brands names that people have used for years, and the toxicity tests are finally being released.

Health Foods
These are organic foods that enhance our health through using more due care with the growth and production for the ingredients that are added to the final product. For many of us, store shelf foods and additives are no longer acceptable in our daily lives. Many people require specific diets and ingredients to ensure good health. For example, many people have reactions physically and mentally

when they consume gluten found in different forms of flour. Young children can have huge emotional swings from the yellow and red food dyes that are used in canned goods and juices. We now have a larger selection of food products that are better for our body types and requirements.

Herbs & Herbal Medicine
Learning how to heal the whole body with the use of herbs: roots, leaves, stems, flowers, seed, bark, and root. Herbs can be used dried, in extracts and in combination with other herbs, tinctures and poultices. Herbs have been used for thousands of years with a lot of success. The compounds of the herbs works together as a whole, while promoting the healing of the body and or organs. Herbology students learn the anatomy of the body and how the body works in unison. The herbalist has learned all the healing components of the herbs, where they are grown and how they can most effectively be used for different ailments.

Homeopathy
Homeopathy is carried out using natural resources from plants, minerals and animals. These essences have the healing and energy pattern of the substance is used to treat several different ailments. The essences are placed into tablets and are dissolved under the tongue.

Hot Stone Therapy
The use of water treated stones that have been heated up. The stones are placed on the back to help open the meridians and will also help to relax the muscles of the body.

Hypnotherapy
The use of hypnotherapy can provide changes in the thought pattern to enhance a person's physical and emotional state of being. Hypnotherapy can be used to help a person to quit smoking, lose weight, release negative images or traumas and work with releasing physical pain. This process is done in a trance like state. Hypnotherapy reaches all five states of consciousness.

Ion Cleanses (Foot Bath):
Detoxify the body through the bottom of the feet. This draws out the harmful build-up of toxins, heavy metals, candida and more. This process has been used for several diseases such as multiple sclerosis (MS), liver diseases and yeast infections

Iridology
This technique uses the study of the iris to find the strengths and weakness of the body, along with detection of weakened organs and toxins in the body. This can reveal the levels of health and indicates where additional healing is required.

Kinesiology
Kinesiology is the science of energy balancing and is grounded in both the study of anatomy and physiology. With this healing system, you will learn how your muscles become monitors of stress and imbalances within your body. Kinesiology

is done with muscle testing, and can correct many imbalances that may relate to stress, nutrition, learning problems, minor injuries and other issues in our lives. It can also help to strengthen self-esteem, self-confidence, lessen fears and more.

Light Worker
"A light worker is determined by his or her mission. Light workers share light and love around the globe with others. By sharing their light, light workers empower others towards their own pattern shifts and spiritual enlightenment. Light workers, ultimately, seek to teach others who they each have their own, special, spiritual energy. Light workers also show others who they are free to search and interconnect with the cosmological life force energy inherent to us all. The focus of a light worker is to create heaven on earth through manifesting Christ consciousness on earth's plane."

Massage Therapy
Relaxation massage can decrease stress, improve the immune system and circulation along with enhancing a person's health and well-being.

Therapeutic massage is used to relax the client with a gentle massage. This method is a wonderful self- pampering healing method.

Deep Tissue Massage is a massage that is helpful for stress, bad posture, excessive fitness training, prolonged computer work, and any other overuse of muscles that can cause muscle stiffness, back and neck pain and headaches. Deep tissue massage is a stretching treatment which releases stiffness and soreness. Deep tissue massage penetrates deeper layers of muscles by squeezing and stretching muscles through skillful hand movements and pressure while stimulating blood circulation. With regular deep tissue massage treatment, constrained muscles become loose and flexible, reducing pain and increasing range of motion. Intensity of deep tissue massage is directed by the client to reach a comfortable level of treatment.

Meditation
Meditation can enhance your spiritual growth by learning to clear the mind, heal the body and listen from within. It is used in cancer clinics worldwide and at home, outside and even while being immersed in a project or exercise program. Meditation is used to be in the moment and calm the mind. Some of the ways of meditating can be done by using music, being in silence, watching a candle flame, walking and gardening.

Natural Healing
Uses methods of healing that are derived from natural sources such as herbs, organic products and energy while working with holistic/alternative practitioners to learn how to heal the whole body physically, emotionally, mentally and spiritually. As each state of well-being is enhanced, we can live a more balanced and happier life.

Naturopathy / Naturopathic Physician
A physician who will provide better health for their client's by using nutrition, homeopathy, herbal medicine and other natural methods without using

pharmaceutical treatments. The naturopathic physician looks for the root cause and goes forward to heal the body using techniques that best suits the client at that time.

Neuro Acoustic Therapy
This method provides healing for the body by using different sound vibrations at various frequencies.

Neuro Linguistic Programming
A form of healing by retraining a new thought process to learn how to create new positive ways in order to approach personal problems, fears, self-esteem and more.

Nutritional Therapy
To implement a nutritional diet that will improve the health of the organs, blood and body. This could be from the use of vitamins and minerals to specific food products. Each body has its own requirements due to lifestyles and needs to be nourished to replace what the body uses on a daily basis.

Organic Gardening, Produce and Products
Organic garden is the process of learning how to enhance the soil for our gardens to grow vegetables, herbs and other plants without the use of chemicals. This method of gardening will be without the use of herbicides or pesticides.

Orthomolecular Medicine
Orthomolecular Medicine helps to restore the body by adjusting any imbalances that are in the person's biochemistry. This can be obtained by using amino acids, fatty acids, minerals, trace elements and vitamins.

Past Life Regression
Past life regression is the use of hypnosis to provide a deep state of relaxation to reach beyond the veil of your conscious mind, accessing your soul's memory. This is a method to help us release patterns from other lives or even this present life that we seem to keep repeating in this lifetime.

Psych-K
This is a rebalancing of the belief system to release old thinking patterns in order to go forward in better health and happiness.

Psychic Readings
Psychic readings are provided by working with our intuition, listening to our spirit guides, angels and other spirits connecting with those who have passed over to share other messages. Readings can access information that will help to guide you now and in the future. Some of the methods used are reading a person's aura, use of cards, empathic information and the use of object such as pictures or crystals.

Pranic Healing
Pranic Healing was founded by Grand Master Choa Kok Sui. Pranic Healing works with the physical body and the non-physical energy body. This method provides cleaning of the energy body to heal and free the physical body from thought restraints, chord attachments and more.

Qi Gong (Chi-Kung)
This is the use of meditation, breathing patterns and movement to increase the energy flow through the body. It is used to cure diseases and for promoting good health and well-being.

Raindrop Therapy
Balancing and detoxifying treatment using essential oils.

Rayid
The iris in your eyes can reveal personal characteristics, alone with strengths and behaviour patterns. Using the Rayid method helps to provide a balance with the physical, emotional, mental and spiritual well-being. This method shows what is out of balance in the body.

Reconnective Healing
"Connecting us to the universe and to our very essence, not just through a new set of healing frequencies but through a new bandwidth." Reconnective Healing is a form of healing that is here on the planet for the very first time. It reconnects us to the fullness of the universe as it reconnects us to the fullness of our beings and of who we are. The reality of its existence has demonstrated itself clearly in practice as well as in science laboratories.

The reconnection is the umbrella process of reconnecting to the universe, which allows Reconnective Healing to take place. These healings and evolutionary frequencies are of a new bandwidth brought in via a spectrum of light and information. It is through the reconnection that we are able to interact with these new levels of light and information.

Reflexology
Reflexology is a gentle stimulation of different areas of the feet, hands and ears to promote healing through the meridians that connect to the organs in the body. Reflexology promotes relaxation and healing along with the elimination of toxins.

Foot reflexology is an ancient art practised by early Egyptians. Foot reflexology is a science founded on the basis that areas of the feet are comprised of zones and reflex areas that correspond to all glands, organs and bodily systems. Foot reflexology is a technique whereby pressure is applied to these areas resulting in stress reduction by using thumb, finger and hand methods. Using foot reflexology promotes physiological improvements in the body. This method restores natural balance and revitalization from within.

Reiki
Dr. Usui from Japan created the Reiki system of spiritual healing. This is the use of the universal life force energy, releasing of blocks and toxins to promote healing of your spiritual, physical and emotional well-being. Reiki is practised on a spiritual basis; the energy is God's energy or universal energy. Reiki is used to release stress, provide healing after surgeries, and even enhance healing to help avoid future health problems. Reiki is being used in hospitals and clinics around the world.

Sacred Healing Tools
Some examples of sacred healing tools are energy charged pendulums, charged and programmed chakra crystals for use in healing, to add to the altar or to wear in a beaded leather bag. Beaded bags and sacred rawhide rattles are sewn in ceremony with a prayer in every stitch. Meditation bowls can be created when in a meditative state.

Shamanic Healing
Shamanic healing is going back to the ancient healing of our ancestors. Whether one uses herbs, crystals, spirit guides or other ancient methods, the shamanic healer works with creator and source to provide healing for the client. This can also include soul retrieval, dream interpretation, vision quests, negative energy release and journeying.

Shen
The Shen Physio-Emotional Release Therapy was developed by Richard Pavek in 1977. This method is taught by learning how the emotions have an unhealthy effect on the body when the emotions are held onto. The Shen practitioner can assist to release the painful emotions from the body in a safe manner.

Spa Therapy
Spa therapy can include different forms of therapy to provide a relaxed state of mind and body while promoting self-healing and personal pampering. Using fragrances through spa and aromatherapy provides for a revitalizing experience and may encourage natural self-healing mechanisms. Spa and aromatherapy work so well together with the simple use of extracts, essences and other fragrances that have been proven to help individuals with colds, flu, burns, insomnia, mental depression, headaches, neuromuscular pain and even stress.

T'ai Chi
T'ai Chi is an energy flowing exercise that works on many levels, physical conditioning, strength, flexibility and resilience. This method works with mental focus, clarity along with creating proper flow and balance of the Chi throughout the body.

T'ai Chi Massage
A client is fully clothed and lies on a mat on the floor so that practitioner can apply stretches on the client to open the joints and stimulate the blood flow.

Theta Healing
Theta Healing is a powerful healing technique that addresses the limiting subconscious beliefs that hold us back from reaching our fullest potential, optimal health and joy. Using Theta Healing our limiting subconscious beliefs are instantly and permanently shifted into beliefs that are self-empowering and aligned with what we desire.

Therapeutic Touch
Gentle healing done in a comfortable setting to smooth out, balance and energize the client's energy field. Therapeutic Touch was developed by nurses, Delores Krieger and Dora Kunz.

Touch for Health
The use of muscle testing is done in order to find imbalances within the body. Using muscle manipulation, acupressure like treatments, some cranial sacral therapy moves and some may use nutritional or herbal practices.

Traditional Chinese Medicine
Traditional Chinese medicine has been used for over thousands of years in China. This is the use of herbal medicines, acupuncture, Tai Chi and other body and mind healing practices to bring balance to the body. These practices also help to prevent future health problems.

Transcendental Meditation
Transcendental Meditation became popular in the American countries in the 1970s. This is a form of meditation using mantras to help calm the mind and body in order to promote inner peace.

Transpersonal Development Therapy
Transpersonal Development Therapy recognizes the importance of the intuitive nature along with transpersonal transcendental experiences which can be used as a valuable growth opportunity. In other words, transpersonal development therapy recognizes the psychic and spiritual levels of consciousness and incorporates them into traditional practices such as symptom relief and behaviour changes:

Vibro Acoustic Sound Therapy
A client receives the therapy by lying on a table which supplies a special sound frequency which vibrates throughout the table and the client's body. The vibration helps to release blocks and also helps to increase the vibrational level of the body.

Visceral Manipulation
This is a manual therapy usually done with massage or Craniosacral therapy to encourage the normal mobility, motion and tone of the viscera and connective tissues.

Whole Brain Integration
This is a method that works with the left and right side of the brain using cross body exercises. This aids in more effective cognition, physical and mental abilities, along with releasing stress, depression and learning difficulties.

Yoga
Using slow movements and breathing techniques to increase concentration, strength and health and well-being. Yoga can be used as a calming of the mind and nervous system.

> ~~~ The above treatments could have much longer explanations, and there may be many that are missing. This is to give you an idea of what is out there and hopefully you can find the process that best suits you.. ~~~

CHAPTER 2

Energy Healing

THE REASON FOR ENERGY HEALING TO HAVE A CHAPTER ON ITS OWN IS THAT THIS TYPE of work is mentioned several times in Chapter 1. Energy healing is very powerful as it can create the opportunity to assist in making changes to the body. Energy work is a natural alchemy of creating a new and heathier lifestyle. Energy healing is a safe and ancient method of healing that provides lasting changes to the body physically, emotionally, mentally and spiritually. This method of healing has been provided since the beginning of history, but some of the cultures discontinued this technique as people were taught to fear this type of healing.

Over the last several years the Western world has been reintroduced to alternative healing, starting with the hippie days of the later 1960s. This is when the practice of meditation and the messages for love and peace started to show up in society and become more than a trend. There were rallies to promote peace that were associated with the demand to stop the wars in the east and the desire to live a more peaceful life. The young adults were practising meditation, eating raw foods and living with Mother Earth's resources.

During this time and even today many people are still living in fear and unaccepting of natural ways of healing due to upbringing and beliefs passed on from parents, grandparents and guardians.

The practice of energy healing has helped many people release these old beliefs and thought patterns that have been affecting their bodies and creating diseases. Energy healing can release the fears and other emotional imprints that stay with us from the time we are born, and in some cases from previous lives. When a person holds on to a false belief from a time of distress or something someone judgementally said to them, this can create an emotional imprint that will harm the body in many ways.

If I was told that I was dumb and could not do anything right, this statement may cause me to give up trying again and create a sense of uselessness, and myself confidence would be destroyed. This action will then lead to severe anxiety in school during tests and around classmates. Later on I might not pursue the work of my dreams, as I am scared that I will fail. This verbal abuse I have heard can also create other physical ailments such as ulcers, bowl diseases, addictions to alcohol and drugs or poor eating habits. Sometimes we can ignore the words, but many times it sticks to us till we find a way to release and heal the mental harm it caused.

After something like this happens to a child or an adult, the body can create energetic imprints or emotions that harm the person and hold their spirit and soul from going forward to achieve amazing feats or providing the services to mankind that they were brought here for. This is where the energetic healing comes in. When someone takes a prescription from the doctor for the depression, the chemicals would only be masking the cause and will not heal the original source from where depression started. Energy work would help to release the belief patterns, hurt and sorrow that the person's mind and body is holding onto. The general rule is if a person wants to make a lasting change in their life, they will take that extra step to make it happen, and that is where they will search out a practitioner or coach that can see the blocks or beliefs and help you to release them.

Energetic blocks can be released through several methods. The ones that I am more familiar with and work with are through meditation and done with Reiki. After several years of practising both methods, I found we could connect to the soul or our higher self and that of the clients. We can get past the ego state of the client and allow the changes to come in. With Reiki I ask the higher self of the person that is being worked on if we can go to deeper levels of the belief system and release that imprint of the thought pattern or emotion. As soon as the connection and agreement with the soul is made, I can feel the shift in the person that I am working on.

That is where sometimes the fear of doubt will come in for people. Many are still sceptical of how energy can change something for the good or heal our bodies. We can stop and take the time to think of the effect of sharing a hug with a friend when they are sad. Why do you want to give them a hug? Was it to help them feel better? How do you feel after you have received a hug when you are sad? Did you feel better? You feel that someone really cares. You feel like someone has taken a load off your shoulders, and you know that you can continue on with a stronger sense of purpose. Energy healing is pretty much the same, but we are going deeper to find and release the cause of the energetic imprint. After practising and being able to learn how to connect with the client, one can see or know when all of the trauma started.

Our bodies are sources of energy, as we consist of water and matter. When water is processed farther, it creates energy. When the currents of energy flow freely and productively, we have clouds and wind that creates the accumulation of water that brings us rain. Rain goes to the earth providing the moisture for the plants to grow. These plants can provide shelter and food to look after the human body along with providing the same for the animal kingdom. When the sources of energy are pure and clean, then the outcome is much healthier.

ENERGY IS TRANSFERRED FROM SOURCE: GOD / CREATOR / MOTHER EARTH

When we connect to God, we are provided with the energy to transfer to the person that is seeking the healing. This energy is pure unconditional love. Just like energy going through the phone line or electrical wire. When the energy reaches its destination, it clears out imprints from physical, mentally, emotional and spiritual abuse. This is like when the energy from the wire is turned on, the light goes on or something will start to work. When we bring new clean energy into our bodies, it clears the way for better health.

When the source of energy is toxic, then the growth becomes distorted and stunted. When water is polluted, the other living entities around it also become sick and unable to reproduce healthy offspring or create a cancerous-like environment. This all can be seen in the human body through the chakras, the seven main energy centres of the human body. When the human body holds onto negative thought patterns or consumes outside toxins, the chakra centres become blocked and the body then manifests illnesses and is stuck in its growth.

We have seven major chakras in our body/energy field. These chakras flow with ease when the body, mind and spirit are synchronized and the person is living a healthy and vibrant lifestyle. Each charka has its own area of the body. They start from the pelvic area and go to the crown of the body. The chakras are energetically connected to the organs in the body. An example is if I become really worried about my finances. My root chakra can become clogged as the heavy energy and worry builds an unhealthy effect on the chakra in my body. My lower back might feel sore, or I might become lethargic. Until the chakra becomes clear again, I will get the same feelings day after day.

Seven Major Chakras

From the pelvic area on our body up to above our head we have seven major chakras, and they are as follows:

CHAKRA 1: ROOT

Location: pelvic area.

Areas of the body that are affected: adrenals, feet, legs, pelvis, reproductive system, tail bone, testes, vagina.

Requirement: Survival and stability. The needs to be able to survive are clothing, food, medical care, shelter.

Discomfort when needs not met: anorexia, bone disorders, constipation, fears, hemorrhoids, knee troubles or sciatica. Being unable to focus or be still.

CHAKRA 2: SACRAL

Location: by our belly button.

Areas of the body that are affected: abdomen, gonads, kidneys, ovaries, spleen, urinary tract, uterus.

Requirement: Sexuality and Emotions. We need to have pleasure and relaxation in life. We need to be able to feel our own emotions with ease.

Discomfort when needs not met: emotional instability, isolation, numbness sexual problems and stiffness.

** Empaths can also sense the emotions of others around them. When they pick up one or more emotions above their own, it can be hard to handle the intensity of what they are feeling. When there is no filter for the incoming emotions, a person will have the three times the feeling of sadness, happiness and anxiety than a normal person would feel.

CHAKRA 3: SOLAR PLEXUS

Location: by the junction at the bottom of our rib cage.

Areas of the body that are affected: digestive system, bile, gall bladder, liver, pancreas, small intestine, stomach.

Requirement: To stand in our power, to follow our intuition. The feeling of purpose and strength.

Discomfort when needs not met: digestion troubles, domination, fatigue, timidity, ulcers. Our intuition also is a warning system for us to follow. Intuition will let us know if something feels right or wrong. If something feels wrong, you might feel sick or nervous.

CHAKRA 4: HEART

Location: Heart area.

Areas of the body that are affected: allergies, blood pressure, circulation, heart, immune system, lung, lymph, thymus.

Requirement: Self love, love for others. This will provide balance, compassion.

Discomfort when needs not met: co-dependence, depression, loneliness.

CHAKRA 5: THROAT

Location: throat.

Areas of the body that are affected: ears, neck, parathyroid, respiratory system, sinus, throat, thyroid.

Requirement: Clear communication to speak the truth with ease. We can speak our truth in a gentle way so that we can be heard. Sometimes we are scared to say something in fear that we may be rejected as a friend or may make someone mad in a relationship. When we speak from our hearts, the words are kinder and the message is stronger.

Discomfort when needs not met: communication skills are poor, sore throat, stiff neck, scared of other person's reactions to what we say, unable to speak up.

CHARKA 6: OUR THIRD EYE

Location: the forehead.

Areas of the body that are affected: autonomic system, brow, eyes, hypothalamus, nervous system, pituitary gland.

Requirement: imagination, intuition, perception, premonitions and psychic abilities to see the spirit realm, to have the sixth sense of knowing things that others might not know or see.

Discomfort when needs not met: hallucinations, headaches, nightmares, unable to filter incoming information from other sources.

** These people who are diagnosed as being ADD, schizophrenic and border line multi personality and have a hard time. I truly believe that these amazing people see, feel, and communicate information or thoughts from other people around them or from the spirit realm and or other dimensions. They have not learned how to filter the incoming information.

CHAKRA 7: CROWN:

Location: above the head.

Areas of the body that are affected: central nervous system, cerebral cortex, crown, hair, head, pineal gland, upper spine.

Requirement: The right to know, knowledge, understanding, spiritual connection, wisdom.

Discomfort when needs not met: apathy, confusion, overly intellectual, will only believe things that are proven true.

It is important for our first seven chakras to be unblocked and healthy. This is a requirement to live a healthy life on Mother Earth and be connected to both God and our soul. We also have an advanced chakra system, which are above the first seven chakras, extending above our head towards the heavens.

CHAKRA 8

Energy centre of divine love, of spiritual compassion and spiritual selflessness. Your karmic residue that activates spiritual skills contained in the seventh chakra.

CHAKRA 9
Soul blueprint (the individual's total skills and abilities learned in all the lifetimes)

CHAKRA 10
Divine creativity, synchronicity of life; the merging of the masculine and feminine within, unlocking of skills contained in the ninth chakra

CHAKRA 11
Path work to the soul, the individual's ability to acquire advanced spiritual skills (travel beyond the limits of time and space, teleportation, bi-location, instantaneous precipitation of thoughts, telekinesis in some cases)

CHAKRA 12
Connection to the monadic level of divinity, advanced spiritual skills, ascension, connection to the cosmos and beyond

Over the last several years, while watching people, listening to them speak, seeing how they react, one can see why their bodies are acting out and why they are in physical or mental pain. I will use myself as an example again. A few years ago, I was working in my veggie garden, mad as a hatter because I was going to have to physically dig up the garden with a shovel and not have some help. My hip got sore and almost seized up. Right away the realization kicked in that I was holding onto anger, control and resentment. These emotions were affecting both my stomach and my hip. When I looked at the situation differently and saw the blessings of having an amazing space for the veggie garden, having the strength and body to be able to dig the garden and having the seeds to grow in the garden, the discomfort went away within half an hour. About a week after this happened while weeding at a friend's farm, the same discomfort happened again. I was mad because I wanted to work in a different part of the garden, and I was resenting a couple of people there. As soon as the discomfort started to happen, within I asked what was needed to be able see the situation on a different level and recognize the pattern. Again, the resentment and anger showed itself and the realization of how I was viewing situations and building a mountain of emotional turmoil into pain. Right away all the answers came. I needed to recognize the fact that I was there to help my friends out, and that help may not always be the way we imagine it, and to do the best we can.

Next is another example of how the throat chakra can be blocked and lead to discomfort within the body. For the most part of my 20s and early 30s, I was able to express, speak up about how things affected me, or seeing the ripple effect of other people's actions and the accountability. The last part of the 30s and 40s my communication skills went downhill. I was not expressing how I felt and not relaying the ripple effect of what others were doing around me took its toll. After many years of being able to share from the heart, I noticed that my communication skills were gone. Was I scared of losing family members? Was I scared of making someone mad? After a couple of bouts of a sore throat to finally getting a case of laryngitis right before a major event to promote my work, I got the message. There were many people around me that were taking advantage of my generosity, or thought they could continue to be abusive, and maybe they thought that being the kind soul I was, I would let it go. After approaching three different people to share from my heart what was wrong and setting boundaries, I have not since had the same problem. We need to learn to communicate from the heart and share how one is being affected by another's negative patterns. Sometimes we need to walk away from the relationship and let that person go. When the energy that is being shared is not mutual, it can have a negative effect.

When all seven of the chakras in the body are cleared, open and the energy is flowing freely, a person can live a life of peacefulness and good health. As this becomes more the norm and reality becomes more about happiness and being able to enjoy life. We can learn to enjoy being in this new state of well-being. We will then also find that we are not using stimulants for happiness such as alcohol, food and drugs. Happiness is internal and one can now see all the beauty in the world around them.

When we reach the state of heightened personal well-being, one can recognize when something does not feel right. As this state of personal bliss is reached, we can see others in a different light and know that they too may be having a tough time and have their own journey to travel. It is up to them as individuals to learn how they can personally heal themselves within and to experience the life that they are meant to live. When they are ready to make the energetic shifts, they will, but not until they are truly ready.

There are times when a person will make changes for the better then go backwards as they are uncomfortable with this new feeling. Sometimes they have the sense that they will have more responsibilities, and that can scare them too. When we make that commitment and allow the growth to settle in, we come to the point where we do not regress, as the old anger, unhappiness or resentment no longer feels comfortable. Then we will do anything we can to obtain the peace and harmony that we desire.

In the meantime, we can take the time to think twice about what we say to others and provide each and every person a kind word and support to pursue what they are capable of doing. It is not our decision what someone else does or how they lead their life. It is not energetically good to hold someone back either. It is not healthy to be jealous because someone is good at something and you are not. Maybe your strengths or gifts could be somewhere else that you have yet to explore or allowed yourself to see or try.

Sometimes we are raised and taught ego state habits. These are old thinking habits and actions that are very low energy. I am so grateful to have had both my parents. My mom was here till I was eight years old, and she taught me the love of a mother and to live in harmony and with strength. My father taught me how to be here first for my children, as he changed what he had witnessed as a child. Many people did not have these blessings, and life has not been easy for them. They are taught as a child to fear the unknown, to be scared of God, that there is a real hell, and to judge other people because they do not look the same or do things the same way. All of this can create the same energetic imprints within our spirit and on our body. This can close doors to success.

We need to stop and think how we look at life, and see what we can do energetically to see our lives with a different view and know we are the creator of our daily lives, and we can make significant changes. There are many ways of providing energy work: Reiki, reflexology, Craniosacral therapy and Healing Touch. Many of these ways are listed in Chapter 1.

When we apply energy work to our healing process, the releases that occur can be much more powerful than going to counselling for years. The energy practitioner can also provide some amazing insights into how or when the discomfort started in the first place.

When we are seeking a practitioner in this field, we seem to be drawn to the right person at the right time. If at any time I had an uncomfortable experience with the practitioner, that was something for me to learn from. Then I would seek someone that would empower me to grow.

CHAPTER 3

Healing Property Terms

THIS CHAPTER IS ON SOME OF THE TERMINOLOGY FOR HEALING PROPERTIES THAT Mother Earth provides with the food that we consume or products that we use such as herbs and oils. Whether it be dairy, fruit, grains, herbs, legumes, meat, nuts or vegetables, the food we consume contributes to our health.

Chapters 6 to 14 cover a lot of the options that we have that provide the nutrients for our bodies. These nutrients have a larger effect than what we realize. When our food can provide the puzzle pieces to keep our organs healthy, the food can also provide healing abilities that you cannot find in manufactured medicine. In Chapter 15 we will have a cross reference for all the food groups, including the essential oils and herbs. You will see a quick reference for what you can use for as an alterative and also what can be used for asthma or diabetes prevention.

Alterative: A substance that cleanses the blood. It can alter the process of the nutrition we consume, work with the excrement and restore the organs of the system to a healthy action. It can stimulate the lymphatic glands and the endocrine glands.

Analgesic: A substance used to reduce pain.

Anodyne: Pain relieving compound that is used to help with pain that is experienced through the brain and nervous system.

Anthelmintic: Substance that kills intestinal worms.

Anti-aging: Slows down the aging process of the organs, especially the skin and hair.

Antibacterial: Wards off and fights bacterial infections.

Antibiotic: A natural antibiotic that can fight off or destroy unhealthy living organisms that are living in the body. It will also assist with healing the body at the same time. A natural antibiotic will not kill the good bacteria in our body.

Anti-cancer: Helps to destroy cancerous cells in the body. When you use a product that has anti-cancer properties, it will help to clean the blood and strengthen the liver.

Anti-catarrhal: This helps the body to remove excess mucous.

Anti-coagulant: Used to stop the blood from coagulating or clotting. Helps to thin the blood.

Anti-convulsion: Helps to lessen or prevents convulsive attacks that can happen with epilepsy. An anti-convulsion would help the body to relax more and allow the brain to create less electrical charges.

Antidepressant: Used to lessen or treat depression. A natural antidepressant will help to restore the body while helping the mind to feel calmer without the harsh side effects that pharmaceuticals can cause. The idea is to heal the mind and body so that a person does not become dependent on the antidepressants.

Anti-diabetic: Used to treat diabetes or aid in lessening diabetic attacks. An action that can help to regulate the blood sugar levels.

Antidote: Used to counteract the effect of a toxic substance or poison.

Anti-emetic: Helps to lessen or prevent vomiting that can occur from situations such as motion sickness.

Anti-flatulent: Used to reduce intestinal gas.

Antifungal: Helps to prevent or destroy the growth of fungi on or in the body.

Antihistamine: When the body reacts to allergens, it creates a histamine. This can cause breathing troubles and create a rash on the skin. The antihistamine helps to counteract this reaction.

Anti-infectious: A substance that provides the body with protection from airborne viruses.

Anti-inflammatory: Reduces the inflammation of the body organs such as in the bowels, muscles, organs and skin.

Anti-malarial: Malaria Is a disease that is caught by infected mosquitoes generally found in tropical and subtropical climates. This can also be transmitted from person to person and by using dirty needles.

Antimicrobial: Kills or stops the growth of microscopic organisms such as bacteria and fungus.

Antioxidant: Antioxidants protect our cells against free radicals that cause diseases like cancer. Free radicals are the chemicals that our bodies absorb from different elements in the environment. Some of these free radicals are in the chemicals from different cleaning or manufactured products that are used in households and businesses.

Anti-parasitic: An agent that will kill the parasites in the blood, bowels and intestines.

Anti-perspirant: A substance that helps to control body odour and sweat effectively.

Anti-pyretic: Used to prevent or to reduce a fever.

Antiscorbutic: A substance that is a blood cleanser and can prevent illnesses like scurvy. The antiscorbutic has a medium to a large amount of vitamin C.

Antiseptic: Stops or slows the growth of microorganisms

Antispasmodic: Stops or relieves spasms, such as muscle or stomach spasms.

Anti-suppressant: To curb the appetite, cravings or the need to use something that is causing ill health.

Antitoxin: antidote to stop the poisoning from a microorganism, like a snake or spider bite.

Anti-tumour: To reduce the size of a tumour and help the body to heal on a cellular level.

Antiviral: Helps to treat and stop viruses that are passed from person to person.

Anxiety: To help reduce the effects anxiety has on the mind and body.

Aperient: To gently move the bowels to bring relief from constipation.

Astringent: Helps the skin tighten, especially for minor cuts to help stop the bleeding.

Carminative: Helps to prevents formation of stomach gas.

Cathartic: Promotes evacuation of the bowel. It can also assist in the purging of the liver and gall bladder to help clean the organs.

Decongestive: A substance that is used to relieve lung congestion, expectorant causing person to expel excess phlegm from the lungs.

Demulcent: A salve, oil or other agent that soothes and relieves skin discomfort.

Diaphoretic: Opens the pores of the skin to stimulate sweating and raise body temperature.

Diuretic: A compound that promotes production and excretion of urine. A diuretic will collect and eliminate excess fluids through the urinary tract.

Emetic: A substance that induces vomiting. Used for some cases of drug overdoses or types of poisoning.

Emmenagogue: Used to induce menstruation.

Emollient: An agent that soothes and softens the skin.

Expectorant: To help promote the secretion of sputum that has built up in the air passages.

Fungicide: A substance that helps to kill the fungus that has built up in the body.

Hepatic: Works to cleanse the liver and strengthen the function of the organ.

Laxative: To help the bowels loosen for better elimination of the waste.

Nervine: Used to settle the nervous system.

Parturient: A tonic that is used to assist in giving birth.

Pectoral: A substance that would help with the development of the chest muscles.

Pulmonary: The lungs and the respiratory system.

Purgative: A substance used to purge or cleanse, especially by causing evacuation of the bowels.

Relaxant: To help the body and mind relax.

Restorative: To be able stimulate the nervous system to function in a healthier manner.

Rubefacient: This is a substance that is used as an external application to the skin. It reduces the redness of the skin by causing the dilation of the capillaries and provides an increase in blood circulation.

Soothing: To have a calming effect.

Stimulant: A stimulant is used to increase the action and strengthening of a body organ.

Stomachic: Aids in the digestion and can improve your appetite.

Tonic: A tonic is a liquid composition using Mother Earth's medicines that can be ingested to help heal the body.

Vermicide: An agent that kills worms in the intestines.

CHAPTER 4

Proper Nutrition Essentials: Minerals, Vitamins, Oils, Enzymes, Proteins and Antioxidants

HEALING THE BODY PHYSICALLY, EMOTIONAL AND SPIRITUALLY CAN BE DONE IN SEVERAL ways: lifestyle, thinking patterns, releasing blocks and nurturing the human body organs properly. We can start by cleansing the body of toxins, using things like roots, plants and oils. Many herbs and plants have very powerful healing properties, but one must make sure that what they are using is compatible with their body.

Herbs, plants and supplements help our bodies stay in a higher state of vibration, bringing us to a point where it is harder for the body to create a sickness. Know that there are many options out there. We just need to be open to them.

During the 1960s, when the promotion of fast foods and prepared foods began, a lot of food: fruit, grains, herbs, vegetables and meat were grown and produced in a person's own yard, if they had the property. The food was eaten during the season then stored for use over the sparse months. During the 1960s if you were to buy your food in the grocery store, it was a sign that you were rich. This is where the quality of our food started to go downhill. The stores could not keep up, chemicals were being created to produce bigger crops and the herbicide and pesticide use got out of hand. People stopped growing their own food in their yards to preserve for the winter months. More was expected to be on the shelves. People wanted selection instead of learning how to make the food on their own. People started to get sick. If you were blessed with being raised on a farm, you learned how to grow, harvest and preserve for the leaner months. You stayed healthy.

Our bodies need the proper balance of nutrients: minerals, vitamins, oils and proteins. When the body is deprived of these, our organs do not function very well and start to fail. For example, our brain is one of the organs that enables us to think and function on a daily basis. When the body is lacking in the minerals and vitamins, we become lethargic, unable to think, focus and complete simple tasks. The oils and proteins also provide the nutrients for our brains to function while producing the proper enzymes and hormones to regulate other parts of the body.

Minerals / Elements

The minerals that are found in our food sources help the body to function in so many ways. Minerals in our food help the body to derive energy from the foods that we consume and encourage the minerals to work on a cellular level.

Minerals work together with each other and with the aid of the vitamins from our foods. Many ailments of the body are due to the body not producing enough of the chemicals that are needed to operate, and this happens by not consuming the proper foods. If one were to have a straight diet of meat and bread or just pastas with little or no vegetables, one would be starving oneself of what their body really needs.

When you sit down to a meal, whether it is breakfast, lunch, dinner or a snack, what are you putting into your temple? I have heard this saying many times: Our body is a temple, how are we going to treat it? Treat it with fatty foods, preservatives and sugars and you will create a temple of sickness, physically, mentally, emotionally and spiritually. Treat your body with herbs, vegetables, fruits, proteins (legumes and plant protein) and grains and your body will resonate with a much higher frequency and the organs operate a lot better.

BORON

Boron is for the bones, muscles, brain function and alertness, and it aids in preventing postmenopausal osteoporosis. Boron also helps the body to derive energy from the fats and sugar, and in essential in maintaining the vitamin D level. Boron helps the body to metabolize calcium, phosphorus and magnesium.

Food Sources:
Fruits: apple, grape, pear, Saskatoon berry, strawberry.

Grains: barley, buckwheat, cereal grain, corn, oats, quinoa, rice (brown and white), rye, spelt, wheat.

Legumes: carob, garbanzo, navy, peanut

Nuts, Oils & Seeds:

Nuts: almond, Brazil nut, cashew, coconut, hazelnut, macadamia, pecan, pistachio, walnut

Seeds: chia seed, flaxseed, sesame seed, sunflower seed

Vegetables: carrots, Swiss chard.

CALCIUM

Calcium is essential for the development of bones and teeth. Calcium helps to maintain the gums, regular heartbeat, nerve pulse transmission, prevents cardiovascular disease, lowers cholesterol, helps with blood clotting, prevents cancer, stops the absorption of lead and is essential for proper muscle growth. Calcium promotes energy, aids in the structure of our RNA and DNA, aids in the activation of enzymes. During pregnancy, calcium is essential in avoiding the development of pre-eclampsia (greatest cause of maternal death) and can help to lower high blood pressure of the mother. A deficiency of calcium can cause depression, convulsions, rickets, delusions, muscle spasms, loss of hearing and osteoporosis.

Food Sources:

Dairy: butter, buttermilk, cheese, goat milk, milk, whey.

Fruits: apple, apricot, avocado, blackberry, blueberry, cherry, choke cherry, cranberry, currant, date, fig, goji berry, gooseberry, grape, grapefruit, guava, kiwi, lemon, lime, mango, orange, papaya, passion fruit, peach, pear, pineapple, plum, raspberry, rhubarb, Saskatoon berry, strawberries, tangerine, watermelon.

Grains: oats, quinoa, spelt, wheat, wheat (bran and germ).

Herbs: alfalfa, aloe vera, amaranth, angelica, anise seed, antler, astragalus, barberry, basil, bayberry, bearberry, bilberry, birch, black cohosh, black walnut, blessed thistle, blue cohosh, borage, burdock, butcher's broom, calendula, caraway seed, cascara sagrada, catnip, cayenne, chamomile, chaparral, chickweed, chlorella, cilantro, cinnamon, clove, comfrey, dandelion, echinacea, eyebright, fennel, garlic, gentian, ginger, ginseng, goldenseal, green tea, hawthorn, hops, horseradish, horsetail, Irish moss, juniper, lemongrass, liquorice root, marjoram, marshmallow, milk thistle, nettle, oatstraw, olive leaf, oregano, parsley, peppermint, plantain, pokeweed, primrose, raspberry leaves, red clover, rose hips, rosemary, sage, skullcap, slippery elm, spearmint, turkey rhubarb, turmeric, white oak bark, wormwood, yellow dock.

Legumes: bean (black, red and white), black-eyed peas, carob, garbanzo, kidney bean, lentil, lima, navy, peanut, pinto, soybean.

Meat:

Beef: calf liver, beef liver,

Lake, ocean, river, sea: salmon and sardines

Poultry: eggs, turkey

Nuts, Oils & Seeds:

Nuts: almond, Brazil nut, cashew, coconut, hazelnut, macadamia, pecan, pine nut, pistachio, walnut

Oils: sesame seed oil

Seeds: chia seed, cacao, flaxseed, mustard seed, pumpkin seed, sesame seed, sunflower seed

Vegetables: artichoke, asparagus, bean, beet greens, broccoli, Brussel sprouts, cabbage, carrot, celery, collard, corn, cucumber, dulse, kale, kelp, kohlrabi, lettuce (romaine), mustard green, onion (green and red), parsnip, pepper (bell), potato, pumpkin, radish, rutabaga, spinach, squash, sweet potato, Swiss chard, turnip and turnip greens.

CHROMIUM

Chromium is used for helping to regulate the sugar levels and is helpful for those with diabetes and hypoglycemia, along with reducing body fat. Chromium helps the body to synthesize cholesterol, fats and proteins. Excellent during pregnancy to help the fetus develop properly and to keep the mother's blood sugar level low. Sugars deplete our chromium levels from alcohol consumption to too much sugary foods and flour in our diets. When our bodies do not get enough chromium, we become lethargic, diabetic, have kidney problems and poor liver function. The best form of chromium to take is chromium picolinate.

Food Sources:
Dairy: cheese, buttermilk, goat milk, milk.

Grains: corn, couscous, quinoa, rice (brown and white), rye, wheat.

Herbs: black cohosh, burdock, butcher's broom, catnip, cinnamon, eyebright, gentian, hawthorn, hops, horsetail, juniper, licorice, nettle, oat straw, red clover, sarsaparilla, yarrow.

Legumes: bean (black, red and white), carob, garbanzo, kidney bean, lentil, lima, navy, pinto, soybean.

Meats:

Beef: beef: calf liver, beef liver

Poultry: eggs

Vegetables: broccoli, Brussel sprout, corn, dulse, lettuce(romaine), mushroom, potato, sweet potato.

Caution: Those with diabetes must be careful, especially those who are insulin dependent.

COPPER

Copper aids in the proper formation of the blood cells. It works with the help of vitamin C and Zinc. Copper helps with healthy nerves, joints, energy production, the healing process of the body, hair colouring, skin colouring and with our taste buds. The lack of copper can cause osteoporosis, anemia, diarrhea, baldness, poor respiratory health, increased blood fat level and skin sores. The body can also have too much copper, which can cause depression, vomiting, nervousness and muscle and joint pains (flu like symptoms). Too much copper can also be destructive for the eyes.

Food Sources:
Fruits: avocado, banana, blackberry, blueberry, cantaloupe, cherry, cranberry, currant, date, fig, goji berry, grape, grapefruit, kiwi, lemon, lime, mango, orange, papaya, passion fruit, peach, pear, pineapple, plum, raspberry, strawberry, tangerine, watermelon.

Grains: barley, corn, oats, spelt, wheat bran.

Herbs: alfalfa, birch, burdock, caraway seed, chlorella, cinnamon, comfrey, eyebright, fenugreek, garlic, goldenseal, kelp, lobelia, nettle, oregano, slippery elm, valerian, witch hazel, yarrow

Legumes: bean (black, red and white), black-eyed peas, carob, garbanzo, kidney bean, lentil, lima, navy, pinto, soybean

Legume: peanut

Meat: Lake, ocean, river, sea: salmon

Nuts, Oils & Seeds:

Nuts: almond, Brazil nut, cashew, coconut, hazelnut, pecan, pine nut, pistachio, walnut

Seeds: chia seed, flaxseed, mustard seed, pumpkin seed, sesame seed, sunflower seed.

Vegetables: asparagus, bean; lima, bean(snap), beet, beet green, broccoli, Brussel sprouts, cabbage, carrot, celery, collard, corn, cucumber, kale, kelp, kohlrabi, lettuce (romaine), mushroom, mustard green, onion (green and red), parsnip, pea, pepper (bell), pumpkin, radish, rutabaga, spinach, squash, sweet potato, Swiss chard, turnip and turnip greens.

Caution: We need very little. Taking up to10 milligrams can cause problems.

GERMANIUM

This mineral is best used in the organic form. it helps to improve the cellular oxygenation. Germanium helps the body to detoxify, supports the immune system and helps fight pain. A study in Japan showed that the intake of 100 – 300 mg brought about a significant decrease in arthritis, allergies, candida, cancer, viral infections and AIDS.

Food Sources:
Fruits: rhubarb

Herbs: aloe vera, comfrey, garlic, ginseng

Vegetables: broccoli, celery, garlic, onion (green and red)

IODINE

Iodine is a requirement for the proper functioning of the thyroid gland and is used for the goitre. It also helps with our metabolism for excess fat and aids in our physical and mental growth. Tests have shown that the children who do not receive enough iodine are linked to mental disabilities. Our bodies only require a little amount of iodine. The lack of iodine can cause mouth sores, diarrhea, weight gain, and fatigue. Note: If you have an underactive thyroid, you must be careful not to over consuming some of the foods.

Food Sources:
Herbs: cinnamon, eyebright, Irish moss, kelp, liquorice root, kelp, lemongrass, liquorice root, lobelia, spearmint, yarrow

Legumes: lima beans

Meats: lake, ocean, river, sea: fish: saltwater halibut, herring, mackerel, sardines, tuna

Nuts, Oils & Seeds: Seeds: sesame seeds

Vegetables: artichoke, asparagus, dulse, garlic, kelp, mushroom, spinach, squash, Swiss chard, turnip greens

IRON

Iron is very important for our red blood cells and for a good immune system and energy. The lack of the intake of iron is related to many things: too much phosphorus in diet, too many antacids, too much tea or coffee intake, intestinal bleeding and heavy and/or continuous menstrual cycles. Too little and too much iron can have so many effects. The lack of iron can cause tiredness, anemia, dizziness, hair loss, effects on the mouth and nail and obesity. Too much iron can cause heart disease, liver problems, diabetes and other discomforts. Be careful of your supplements – do you need the iron supplements, or can you get enough of it in your foods? Some of the iron supplements can cause constipation, so you may want to try a liquid supplement.

Food Sources:
Dairy: whey, yogurt

Fruits: apricot, avocado, banana, blackberry, blueberry, cantaloupe, cherry, chokecherry, cranberry, currant, date, fig, goji berry, gooseberry, grape, grapefruit, guava, kiwi, lemon, lime, mango, orange, papaya, passion fruit, peach, pear, pineapple, plum, raspberry, rhubarb, Saskatoon, strawberry, tangerine, watermelon

Grains: corn, millet, oats, quinoa, rice (brown and white), rye, spelt, wheat, wheat (bran and germ).

Herbs: agrimony, alfalfa, aloe vera, amaranth, anise seed, antler, astragalus, barberry, basil, bayberry, bearberry, bilberry, birch, black cohosh, black walnut, blessed thistle, blue cohosh, borage, burdock, butcher's broom, caraway seed, cascara sagrada, catnip, cayenne, chamomile, chickweed, chlorella, cilantro, cinnamon, clove, comfrey, dandelion, echinacea, eyebright, fennel seed, fenugreek, garlic, gentian, ginger, ginseng, goldenseal, green tea, hawthorn, horseradish, horsetail, Irish moss, juniper, kelp, lemongrass, licorice, marjoram, marshmallow, milk thistle, nettle, oatstraw, oregano, parsley, Pau d'arco, peppermint, plantain, pokeweed, raspberry leaves, red clover, rose hips, rosemary, sage, skullcap, slippery elm, spearmint, thyme, turmeric, white oak bark, yarrow, yellow dock

Legumes: bean (black, red and white), black-eyed peas, carob, garbanzo, kidney bean, lentil, lima, navy, peanut, pinto, soybean

Meats:

Beef: beef, beef: calf liver, beef kidney, beef liver

Pork

Lake, ocean, river, sea: clams

Poultry: chicken, egg, turkey

Nuts, Oils & Seeds:

Nuts: almond, Brazil nut, cashew, coconut, hazelnut, macadamia, pecan, pine nut, pistachio, walnut

Oils: coconut oil, olive oil, sesame seed oil

Seeds: chia seed, cacao, flaxseed, hemp seed, mustard seed, pumpkin seed, sesame seed, sunflower seed

Vegetables: asparagus, bean (lima and snap), beet - beet green, broccoli, Brussel sprout, cabbage, carrot, cauliflower, celery, collard, corn, cucumber, dulse, garlic, kale, kelp, kohlrabi, lettuce (iceberg and romaine), mustard green, onion (green and red), parsnips, pea, peppers (bell), potato, pumpkin, radish, rutabaga, spinach, squash, sweet potato, Swiss chard, turnip.

Caution: It is recommended not to take iron supplements unless you have been diagnosed as having a low iron intake. Iron should not be taken at the same time as vitamin E.

MAGNESIUM

Magnesium is essential in enzyme activity that helps with your energy production. Magnesium works well with calcium and potassium. Magnesium is important for our nerve and muscle impulses. It helps us to feel a lot more peaceful and lessens our nervousness and states of irritability. The lack of magnesium can also effect a female's menstrual cycle, cause kidney stones, insomnia and more. Magnesium helps to protect our arterial linings. It is important that pregnant females take a magnesium supplement during the pregnancy to avoid cerebral palsy in the baby. Other problems that occur with the lack of magnesium are seizures, tantrums, diabetes, hypertension, fatal cardiac arrhythmia and irritable bowel syndrome.

Food Sources:
Dairy: cheese, buttermilk, goat's milk, milk, whey, yogurt.

Fruits: apple, apricot, avocado, banana, blackberry, blueberry, cantaloupe, cherry, chokecherry, cranberry, currant, date, fig, gooseberry, grape, grapefruit, guava, kiwi, lemon, lime, mango, orange, papaya, passion fruit, peach, pear, pineapple, plum, raspberry, rhubarb, Saskatoon, strawberry, tangerine, watermelon.

Grains: barley, buckwheat, corn, millet, oats, quinoa, rice (brown and white), rye, spelt, wheat, wheat (bran and germ).

Herbs: alfalfa, aloe vera, amaranth, anise seed, astragalus, barberry, basil, bayberry, bearberry, bilberry, birch, black cohosh, black walnut, blue cohosh, borage, buchu, burdock, butcher's broom, caraway seed, cascara sagrada, catnip, cayenne, chaparral, chickweed, chlorella, cilantro, clove, comfrey, dandelion, echinacea, eyebright, fennel seed, fenugreek, garlic, gentian, ginger, ginseng, goldenseal, green tea, hawthorn, hops, horseradish, horsetail, Irish moss, juniper, kelp, lemongrass, licorice, marjoram, marshmallow, milk thistle, nettle, oatstraw, oregano, parsley, peppermint, plantain, primrose, raspberry leaves, red clover, rose hips, rosemary, sage, skullcap, slippery elm, spearmint, valerian, white oak bark.

Legumes: bean (black, red and white), black-eyed peas, carob, garbanzo, kidney bean, lentil, lima, navy, peanut, pinto, soybean.

Meats:

Lake, ocean, river, sea: clams and salmon

Poultry: chicken, egg, turkey

Nuts, Oils & Seeds:

Nuts: almond, Brazil nut, cashew, coconut, hazelnut, macadamia, pecan, pine nut, pistachio, walnut

Oils: cotton seed oil, sesame seed oil, walnut oil

Seeds: chia seed, cacao, flaxseed, hemp seed, mustard seed, pumpkin seed, sesame seed, sunflower seed

Vegetables: artichoke, asparagus, bean (lima and snap), beet - beet green, broccoli, Brussel sprout, cabbage, carrot, cauliflower, celery, collard, corn, cucumber, dulse, garlic, kale, kelp, kohlrabi, lettuce (iceberg), mushroom, mustard green, onion (green and red), parsnips, pea, peppers (bell), potato, pumpkin, radish, rutabaga, spinach, squash, sweet potato, Swiss chard, turnip.

Caution: Recent studies have shown that magnesium should be taken with calcium and on a 1:1 proportion. The magnesium helps the body to properly absorb the calcium.

MANGANESE

Manganese is essential for blood sugar regulation, healthy nerves and the immune system. Manganese helps with our protein and fat metabolism, bone growth, joint lubrication, our cartilage and reproduction. It is also essential for those with anemia and mothers who are nursing to use with B1 for a sense of well-being. The lack of manganese can cause confusion, hypertension, heavy perspiration, convulsions, affect the eyes and hearing, heart problems, memory loss, tremors and teeth grinding.

Food Sources:

Fruits: apricot, avocado, banana, blackberry, blueberry, cherry, chokecherry, cranberry, currant, date, fig, grape, grapefruit, guava, kiwi, orange, peach, pear, pineapple, raspberry, rhubarb, Saskatoon, strawberry, tangerine, watermelon.

Grains: buckwheat, cereal grain, corn, oats, quinoa, rice (white), spelt, wheat, wheat (bran and germ).

Herbs: amaranth, anise seed, astragalus, barberry, basil, bayberry, bearberry, bilberry, black cohosh, black walnut, blessed thistle, blue cohosh, buchu, burdock, butcher's broom, cascara sagrada, catnip, chickweed, cilantro, cinnamon, clove, comfrey, dandelion, echinacea, eyebright, fennel seed, fenugreek, garlic, gentian, ginger, ginseng, goldenseal, green tea, hawthorn, Irish moss, juniper, kelp, lemongrass, licorice, marshmallow, milk thistle, nettle, oatstraw, oregano, parsley, peppermint, primrose, raspberry leaves, red clover, rose hips, rosemary, sage, skullcap, slippery elm, turmeric, white oak bark, witch hazel, wormwood, yarrow, yellow dock.

Legumes: bean (black, red and white), black-eyed peas, carob, garbanzo, kidney bean, lentil, navy, peanut, pinto, soybean.

Meats: Poultry: egg yolk.

Nuts, Oils & Seeds:

Nuts: Brazil nut, cashew, coconut, hazelnut, macadamia, pecan, pine nut, pistachio, walnut

Seeds: sesame seed

Vegetables: asparagus, broccoli, Brussel sprout, carrot, cauliflower, celery, collard, corn, cucumber, garlic, kale, kelp, kohlrabi, lettuce (iceberg and romaine), mushroom, mustard green, onion (red), parsnips, pea, peppers (bell), pumpkin, radish, rutabaga, spinach, squash, sweet potato, Swiss chard, turnip.

MOLYBDENUM

Molybdenum is for the metabolism of our nitrogen that is required for normal cell function. Molybdenum will also help to activate some of the enzymes, and we only need a little bit of it. Our liver, kidneys and bones hold the mineral along with it helping with our teeth. It helps to prevent gum disease, mouth disorders and cancer. Impotency for older men can be linked to the lack of molybdenum. Those who eat a lot of processed foods are susceptible to a deficiency.

Food Sources:
Grains: cereal grain.

Legumes: black, kidney bean, lentil, lima.

Meats: Beef: beef liver.

Nuts, Oils & Seeds:

Nuts: walnut

Seeds: sesame seed

Vegetables: asparagus, beans (lima and snap), carrots, celery, lettuce (romaine), parsnips, peas, spinach, Swiss chard.

Caution: Too much of this mineral can slow down copper metabolism.

PHOSPHORUS

Phosphorus is necessary for our kidney function, heart rhythm, to help clot the blood, along with bone and teeth formation. Phosphorus will help our body change the food to energy and aids in the utilization of vitamins. Effects of too little phosphorus are trembling, weight changes, weakness, tiredness, anxiety and troubles with breathing. We can consume too much of this mineral by eating too much processed foods. Vitamin D works well with phosphorus and can increase the strength of the mineral.

Food Sources:

Dairy: butter, cheese, buttermilk, goat's milk, milk, whey, yogurt.

Fruits: apple, avocado, banana, blackberry, blueberry, cherry, cranberry, currant, grape, grapefruit, guava, lemon, lime, mango, orange, papaya, passion fruit, peach, pear, plum, raspberry, rhubarb, strawberry, tangerine, watermelon.

Grains: barley, buckwheat, cereal grain, corn, millet, oats, quinoa, rice (brown and white), rye, spelt, wheat, wheat (bran and germ).

Herbs: alfalfa, aloe vera, amaranth, anise seed, barberry, basil, bayberry, bearberry, bilberry, birch, black cohosh, black walnut, blessed thistle, blue cohosh, borage, buchu, burdock, butcher's broom, calendula, caraway seed, cascara sagrada, catnip, cayenne, chickweed, cilantro, cinnamon, clove, comfrey, dandelion, echinacea, eyebright, fennel seed, garlic, gentian, ginger, ginseng, goldenseal, green tea, hawthorn, horseradish, horsetail, Irish moss, juniper, kelp, lemongrass, licorice, marjoram, marshmallow, milk thistle, nettle, oatstraw, parsley, peppermint, pokeweed, primrose, raspberry leaves, red clover, rose hips, rosemary, sage, skullcap, slippery elm, turmeric, white oak bark, yellow dock.

Legumes: bean (black and white), black-eyed peas, black-eyed peas, carob, garbanzo, kidney bean, lentil, lima, navy, peanut, pinto, soybean.

Meats:

Beef: beef, beef liver

Lake, ocean, river, sea: salmon

Lamb

Pork

Poultry: egg, turkey

Nuts, Oils & Seeds:

Nuts: almond, Brazil nut, cashew, coconut, hazelnut, pecan, pine nut, pistachio, walnut

Oils: walnut oil

Seeds: chia seed, flaxseed, hemp seed, mustard seed, pumpkin seed, sesame seed, sunflower seed

Vegetables: artichoke, asparagus, bean (lima and snap), beet - beet green, broccoli, Brussel sprout, cabbage, carrot, cauliflower, celery, collard, corn, cucumber, garlic, kale, kelp, kohlrabi, lettuce (iceberg and romaine), mushroom, mustard green, onion (green and red), parsnips, pea, peppers (bell), potato, pumpkin, radish, rutabaga, spinach, squash, sweet potato, Swiss chard, turnip and turnip greens.

POTASSIUM

Potassium works with the contractions of our muscles, nervous system and our heart rhythm. Potassium and sodium work together with the balance of water in our systems. Our cell membranes require the proper chemical reactions to transmit electrical pulses and potassium helps to regulate it, which is essential for proper blood pressure. This aids in the transfer of the required nutrients that our cells need. Potassium works together with magnesium, and as we age, we may require more to obtain the right balance. When our body is lacking in potassium, we may experience chills, constipation, diarrhea, edema, thirst, irregular heartbeat, dry skin, high cholesterol, insomnia, sore muscles, headaches and more.

Food Sources:
Dairy: whey, yogurt.

Fruits: apple, apricot, avocado, banana, blackberry, blueberry, cantaloupe, cherry, chokecherry, cranberry, currant, date, fig, goji berry, gooseberry, grape, grapefruit, guava, kiwi, lemon, lime, mango, orange, papaya, passion fruit, peach, pear, pineapple, plum, raspberry, rhubarb, Saskatoon, strawberry, tangerine, watermelon.

Grains: barley, buckwheat, corn, millet, oats, quinoa, rice: brown, rice (white), rye, spelt, wheat, wheat: bran, wheat (germ).

Herbs: alfalfa, aloe vera, amaranth, anise seed, astragalus, barberry, bayberry, bearberry, bilberry, birch, black cohosh, black walnut, blessed thistle, blue cohosh, borage, buchu, burdock, butcher's broom, caraway seed, cascara sagrada, catnip, cayenne, chamomile, chickweed, cilantro, cinnamon, clove, comfrey, dandelion, echinacea, eyebright, fennel seed, garlic, gentian, ginger, ginseng, goldenseal, green tea, hawthorn, hops, horseradish, Irish moss, juniper, kelp, lemongrass, licorice, marjoram, marshmallow, milk thistle, myrrh, nettle, oatstraw, oregano, parsley, peppermint, plantain, primrose, raspberry leaves, red clover, rose hips, rosemary, sage, skullcap, slippery elm, spearmint, turmeric, valerian, white oak bark, wormwood, yarrow.

Legumes: bean (black, red and white), black-eyed peas, carob, garbanzo, kidney bean, lentil, lima, navy, peanut, pinto, soybean.

Meats:

Lake, ocean, river, sea: saltwater, halibut, herring, mackerel, tuna

Poultry: chicken, turkey

Nuts, Oils & Seeds:

Nuts: almond, Brazil nut, cashew, coconut, hazelnut, macadamia, pecan, pine nut, pistachio, walnut

Oils: sesame seed oil

Seeds: chia seed, cacao, flaxseed, mustard seed, pumpkin seed, sunflower seed

Vegetables: artichoke, asparagus, bean (lima and snap), beet - beet green, broccoli, Brussel sprout, cabbage, carrot, cauliflower, celery, collard, corn, dulse, garlic, kale, kelp, kohlrabi, lettuce (iceberg, and romaine), mushroom, mustard green, onion (green and red), parsnips, pea, peppers (bell), potato, pumpkin, radish, rutabaga, spinach, squash, sweet potato, Swiss chard, turnip and turnip greens.

SELENIUM

Antioxidant, cancer prevention, immunity booster, improves thyroid function, aids in the development of the fetus during pregnancy. Selenium is found in liver, sea food, grains and veggies. Selenium deficiency can cause warts to grow.

When our bodies start to oxidize, it is the same as getting rusty on the inside. Selenium helps as an antioxidant for the lipids. It works well with vitamin E. Our thyroid controls our fat metabolism, and the selenium helps to regulate the thyroid hormone along with preventing certain tumours. For men, selenium can help to prevent prostate and lung cancer. Selenium has been helpful in creating antibodies with vitamin E, which aids in treating AIDS, liver cirrhosis, enlarged prostates, tissue elasticity and high blood pressure. The lack of selenium will contribute to heart disease, cancer, infections, poor liver function, exhaustion and sterility. Too much selenium can also cause health problems.

Food Sources:
Fruits: blackberry, currant, goji berry, guava, mango, orange, papaya, rhubarb, strawberry, watermelon.

Grains: buckwheat, quinoa, rice (brown and white), spelt, wheat, wheat (bran and germ).

Herbs: barberry, bayberry, bearberry, bilberry, black cohosh, black walnut, blessed thistle, blue cohosh, buchu, burdock, butcher's broom, cascara sagrada, catnip, cayenne, chamomile, chaparral, chickweed, cilantro, comfrey, dandelion, echinacea, eyebright, fennel seed, fenugreek, garlic, gentian, ginger, ginseng, goldenseal, hawthorn, hops, horsetail, juniper, lemongrass, liquorice root, lobelia, marshmallow, milk thistle, nettle, oat straw, parsley, peppermint, raspberry leaf, red clover, rose hips, sarsaparilla, slippery elm, white oak bark, yarrow, yellow dock.

Legumes: bean (red), black-eyed peas, carob, garbanzo, lentil, peanut

Meats:

Beef: beef, beef kidney,

Lake, ocean, river, sea: clams, salmon, tuna

Lamb: lamb

Pork: pork

Poultry: chicken, turkey

Nuts, Oils & Seeds:

Nuts: Brazil nut, cashew, coconut, hazelnut, pecan, pine nut, pistachio, walnut

Oils: walnut oil

Seeds: flaxseed, mustard seed, sesame seed, sunflower seed

Vegetables: asparagus, broccoli, cabbage, corn, dulse, garlic, kelp, mushroom, onion (green and red), parsnips, pea, potato, pumpkin, radish, spinach, squash, sweet potato, Swiss chard.

SILICON

Silicon provides the collagen development that we need for our bones. Our hair, nails and skin need the silicon in the connective tissues. Silicon helps to absorb the calcium for the formation of our bones. It also helps to keep our arteries flexible and for the prevention of cardiovascular disease. Silicon aids in decreasing aging, is good the immune system and helps to heal the effects that our bodies have from absorbing aluminum.

Food Sources:
Grains: rice (brown and white).

Herbs: alfalfa, barberry, bayberry, bilberry, birch, black cohosh, black walnut, blessed thistle, blue cohosh, buchu, burdock, butcher's broom, caraway seed, cascara sagrada, catnip, chickweed, ginseng, hawthorn, hops, horsetail, kelp, liquorice root, marjoram, nettle, oat straw, raspberry, thyme.

Legumes: soy beans.

Nuts, Oils & Seeds: Seed: sunflower seed

Veggies: beet, peppers (bell).

SODIUM

One may be low on sodium in excessive heat and without proper intake of water or if on diuretics for low blood pressure. Sodium balances our water along with the PH levels. There can be too much intake of sodium, causing water retention and swollen legs and ankles, high blood pressure, potassium deficiency, liver and kidney distress. There are cases when sea salt has been recommended for those with fibromyalgia. The sodium helps with nerve transmission and muscle contraction. When one is low on sodium, one can experience confusion, dizziness, stomach cramps, nausea, dehydration, hallucination, memory loss, lack of coordination, headaches, infections, weight loss and seizures.

Food Sources:
(almost all foods contain sodium)

Dairy: buttermilk, whey, yogurt.

Fruits: passion fruit, Saskatoon berry.

Grains: quinoa, spelt, wheat, wheat germ.

Herbs: alfalfa, aloe vera, birch, caraway seed, cilantro, clove, comfrey, dandelion, garlic, hawthorn, Irish moss, lobelia, marjoram, nettle, parsley, red clover, rosemary, sage.

Legumes: bean (red and white), carob, garbanzo, kidney bean, peanut

Meats: Poultry: turkey.

Nuts, Oils & Seeds:

Nut: coconut

Seeds: cacao, flaxseed

Vegetables: artichoke, bean (lima and snap), beet, broccoli, cabbage, cauliflower, celery, corn, dulse, kelp, kohlrabi, onion (green), parsnips, pumpkin, rutabaga, spinach, squash, sweet potato, Swiss chard.

SULFUR

For the amino acids in our bodies, sulfur is the acid forming chemical. Sulfur helps to disinfect our blood. It is bacteria resistant, helps to resist the oxidation of the body for proper bile secretion and aids in protecting us from pollution.

(Some are sensitive to too much sulfur. Drugs with sulfur has been known to cause yeast infections).

Food Sources:
Grains: wheat: germ.

Herbs: alfalfa, aloe vera, bilberry, burdock, catnip, cayenne, chaparral, chickweed, eyebright, fennel, garlic, hawthorn, horseradish, horsetail, Irish moss, kelp, lobelia, myrrh, nettle, parsley, plantain, raspberry leaf, sage, spearmint, thyme, yarrow.

Legumes: bean (black, red and white), carob, garbanzo, kidney bean, lentil, lima, navy, pinto, soybean.

Meats:

Lake, ocean, river, sea: fish: fresh water fish: salt water, halibut, herring, mackerel, salmon, sardines, tuna.

Poultry: eggs

Nuts, Oils & Seeds: Seed: cacao

Vegetables: Brussel sprouts, cabbage, garlic, kale, onion (green and red), turnip.

VANADIUM

Vanadium is known as a trace mineral. For the formation of our teeth and bones, we need vanadium. Our cellular metabolism and growth production need the vanadium. This mineral can aid in improving our insulin levels, and if one is taking chromium, they must make sure that they take these two minerals at a different time. When we lack in vanadium, we can experience kidney problems and cardio-vascular distress. This mineral is important for infant survival and reproductive ability. Use of tobacco can impair our levels of vanadium.

Food Sources:
Grains: barley, buckwheat, cereal grain, corn, millet, rice (brown and white), rye.

Vegetables: bean (snap), radish.

ZINC

Growth of the reproductive organs and the function of the prostate glands. Zinc is used for oily skin, healing of diaper rashes, collagen formation and our immune system. It aids in our sense of smell and taste, protects our liver, for bone formation, fighting of free radicals and sore throat due to colds. Zinc works well with both vitamin E and A. The lack of zinc can cause fingernails to thin and get white spots, affect our taste and smell, acne, hair loss, fatigue, impaired night vision, skin lesions, infections, impotency and problems with the prostate.

Food Sources:
Dairy: buttermilk, whey.

Fruit: avocado, blackberry, blueberry, cranberry, currant, goji berry, grapefruit, grape, guava, kiwi, lemon, orange, papaya, passion fruit, peach, plum, raspberry, rhubarb, Saskatoon, tangerine, watermelon.

Grains: barley, buckwheat, cereal grain, corn, millet, oats, quinoa, rice (brown and white), rye, spelt, wheat, wheat bran and germ).

Herbs: alfalfa, aloe vera, amaranth, anise seed, astragalus, barberry, bayberry, bearberry, bilberry, black cohosh, blessed thistle, blue cohosh, borage, buchu, burdock, butcher's broom, caraway seed, cascara sagrada, catnip, cayenne, camomile, chaparral, chickweed, chlorella, cilantro, cinnamon, clove, comfrey, dandelion, echinacea, eyebright, garlic, ginger, ginseng, goldenseal, green tea, hawthorn, hops, horsetail, Irish moss, juniper, kelp, lemongrass, licorice, marjoram, marshmallow, milk thistle, nettle, oatstraw, oregano, peppermint, plantain, primrose, raspberry leaves, rose hips, rosemary, sage, sarsaparilla, skullcap, slippery elm, turmeric, valerian, white oak bark, witch hazel.

Legumes: bean (black, red and white), black-eyed peas, carob, garbanzo, kidney bean, lentil, lima, navy, peanut, pinto, soybean.

Meats:

Beef: beef, calf liver, beef liver

Lake, ocean, river, sea: fish: fresh water, fish: oil, fish: saltwater, halibut, herring, mackerel, salmon, sardines, tuna

Lamb: lamb

Pork: pork

Poultry: egg yolk, turkey, clams

Nuts, Oils & Seeds:

Nuts: almond, Brazil nut, cashew, coconut, hazelnut, pecan, pine nut, pistachio, walnut

Oils: walnut oil

Seeds: chia seed, flaxseed, hemp seed, mustard seed, pumpkin seed, sesame seed, sunflower seed

Vegetables: artichoke, asparagus, bean (lima and snap), beet, beet green, broccoli, Brussel sprout, cabbage, corn, dulse, kelp, kohlrabi, mushroom, onion (green and red), parsnips, pea, peppers (bell), potatoes, pumpkin, radish, rutabaga, spinach, squash, sweet potato, Swiss chard, tomatoes, turnip.

VITAMINS

VITAMIN A

Vitamin A helps the eyes adjust to darkness, fight infections, skin problems and cancer. Helps with abnormally heavy menstrual bleeding. Assists with growth in the bones and teeth, structure and function of biologic membranes between cells and adrenal glands (stress). If you are losing your night vision or have an onset of anemia, you may lack in vitamin A. Blindness has occurred in severe cases.

Food Sources:
Dairy: cheese, buttermilk, goat's milk, milk, whey, yogurt.

Fruits: apple, apricot, avocado, banana, blackberry, blueberry, cantaloupe, cherry, chokecherry, cranberry, currant, date, fig, goji berry, gooseberry, grape, guava, kiwi, lemon, lime, mango, orange, papaya, passion fruit, peach, pear, pineapple, plum, raspberry, rhubarb, Saskatoon, strawberry, tangerine, watermelon.

Herbs: agrimony, alfalfa, aloe vera, anise seed, basil, birch, bistort, black cohosh, blessed thistle, borage, burdock root, calendula, caraway seed, catnip, chickweed, chlorella, cilantro, cinnamon, clove, comfrey, dandelion, eyebright, fennel, garlic, ginger, ginseng, hops, horseradish, horsetail, Irish moss, kelp, lemongrass, marjoram, marshmallow, oat straw, oregano, parsley, peppermint, plantain, pokeweed, raspberry leaf, red clover, rosemary, rose hips, rosemary, sage, spearmint, yarrow, yellow dock.

Legumes: black-eyed peas, carob, garbanzo, lima.

Meats:

Beef: beef: calf liver, beef liver

Lake, ocean, river, sea: fish: fresh water, fish oil, salmon, tuna.

Poultry: egg

Nuts, Oils & Seeds:

Nuts: pecan, pistachio

Oils: Siberian pine nut oil

Seeds: hemp seed, pumpkin seed, sunflower seed

Vegetables: asparagus, bean (lima and snap), beet - beet green, broccoli, Brussel sprout, cabbage, carrot, celery, collard, corn, cucumber, dulse, garlic, kale, kelp, kohlrabi, lettuce (iceberg and romaine), mushroom, mustard green, onion (green), parsnips, pea, peppers (bell), potato, pumpkin, radish, rutabaga, spinach, squash, sweet potato, Swiss chard, turnip and turnip greens.

VITAMIN B1 (THIAMIN)

B1 (thiamin) is one of the coenzymes in the energy producing process. Deficiency of thiamin impairs nerve impulses, lack of appetite, production of cellular antibodies is severely diminished, which causes fatigue and depression, pains in chest and abdomen and sometimes eye problems. The lack of B1 leads to pins and needles in feet and sore leg muscles then it will eventually affect the heart muscles. It has helped to slow stuttering in children and improve learning capabilities. Too much coffee and tea, alcohol and oral contraceptives destroy the thiamin our bodies need.

Food Sources:
Dairy: whey, yogurt

Fruits: apple, apricot, avocado, blueberry, cantaloupe, cherry, date, gooseberry, grape, grapefruit, guava, lemon, mango, orange, passion fruit, peach, pineapple, plum, watermelon.

Grains: barley, buckwheat, cereal grain, corn, oats, quinoa, rice: brown, rice: white, rye, spelt, wheat, wheat: bran and germ.

Herbs: agrimony, alfalfa, aloe vera, amaranth, anise seed, barberry, bayberry, bearberry, bilberry, birch, bistort, black cohosh, black walnut, blessed thistle, black cohosh, borage, Buchu, burdock root, butcher's broom, caraway seed, cascara sagrada, catnip, cayenne, chamomile, chaparral, chickweed, chlorella, cilantro, cinnamon, clove, comfrey, dandelion, echinacea, eyebright, fenugreek, garlic, gentian, ginger, ginseng, goldenseal, green tea, hawthorn, hops, horseradish, horsetail, Irish moss, juniper, kelp, lemongrass, liquorice, marjoram, marshmallow, nettle, oat straw, oregano, parsley, peppermint, raspberry leaf, red clover, rose hips, rosemary, sage, skullcap, slippery elm. spearmint, thyme, turmeric, valerian, white oak bark, wormwood, yellow dock.

Legumes: bean (black, red and white), black-eyed peas, carob, garbanzo, kidney bean, lentil, lima, peanut, pinto

Meats:

Beef: beef kidney, beef liver

Lake, ocean, river, sea: fish: fresh water, fish: salt water, halibut, herring, mackerel, salmon, sardines, tuna

Pork: pork

Poultry: chicken, eggs, egg yolk, turkey

Nuts, Oils & Seeds:

Nuts: almond, Brazil nut, cashew, coconut, hazelnut, macadamia, pecan, pine nut, pistachio, walnut

Oils: walnut oil

Seeds: chia seed, cacao, flaxseed, hemp seed, mustard seed, sesame seed, sunflower seed

Vegetables: artichoke, asparagus, bean (lima and snap), beet - beet green, broccoli, Brussel sprout, cabbage, carrot, cauliflower, collard, corn, cucumber, dulse, garlic, kale, kelp, kohlrabi, lettuce (iceberg and romaine), mushroom, mustard green, onion (green and red), parsnips, pea, peppers (bell), potato, pumpkin, radish, rutabaga, spinach, squash, sweet potato, Swiss chard, turnip and turnip greens.

Suggested requirements: Less than 500 mg per day is sufficient. Thiamin is non-toxic.

VITAMIN B2 (RIBOFLAVIN)

B2 in important for our cellular respiration and in the metabolism of the vitamin C from our food. The lack of B2 (Thiamin) shows growth failure. It aids in weight loss, function of eyes, adrenal glands, nerves, skin and mucous membranes, thyroid problems, birth defects and learning disabilities. Signs of a lack of vitamin B2 are exhaustion, inflamed tongue, lips and mouth and sore and teary eyes. Eventually the lack of vitamin B2 affects the red blood cells. Another sign is a greasy scaling by the lips, nose, eyes, ears and scrotum. B2 helps with extroversion, concentration and personal contentment. B2 helps to detoxify harmful chemicals entering your system.

Food Sources:

Dairy: cheese, buttermilk, goat's milk, milk, whey, yogurt.

Fruits: apple, apricot, avocado, blueberry, currant, date, goji berry, grape, grapefruit, guava, lemon, mango, orange, passion fruit, peach, Saskatoon, tangerine.

Grains: barley, buckwheat, cereal grain, corn, millet, oats, quinoa, rye, spelt, wheat, wheat (bran and germ).

Herbs: alfalfa, aloe vera, amaranth, anise seed, barberry, basil, bayberry, bearberry, bilberry, birch, black cohosh, black walnut, blessed thistle, black cohosh, borage, buchu, burdock root, butcher's broom, caraway seed, cascara sagrada, catnip, cayenne, chaparral, chickweed, chlorella, cilantro, cinnamon, clove, comfrey, dandelion, echinacea, eyebright, fenugreek, garlic, gentian, ginger, ginseng, goldenseal, green tea, hawthorn, horseradish, horsetail, Irish moss, juniper, kelp, liquorice, marjoram, marshmallow, nettle, oat straw, oregano, parsley, peppermint, raspberry leaf, red clover, rose hips, sage, skullcap, slippery elm. spearmint, thyme, turmeric, valerian, white oak bark, wormwood, yellow dock

Legumes: bean (black, red and white), black-eyed peas, carob, garbanzo, kidney bean, lentil, navy, peanut, soybean

Meats:

Lake, ocean, river, sea: fish: fresh water, fish: oils, fish: salt water, halibut, herring, mackerel, salmon, sardine, tuna

Poultry: eggs, egg yolk, chicken, turkey

Nuts, Oils & Seeds:

Nuts: almond, Brazil nut, cashew, coconut, hazelnut, pecan, pine nut, pistachio, walnut

Oils: walnut oil

Seeds: chia seed, cacao, hemp seed, sunflower seed

Vegetables: artichoke, asparagus, bean (lima and snap), beet green, broccoli, Brussel sprout, cabbage, carrot, cauliflower, celery, collard, corn, dulse, kale, kelp, kohlrabi, lettuce (iceberg and romaine), mushroom, mustard green, onion (green), parsnips, pea, peppers: bell, potato, pumpkin, rutabaga, spinach, sweet potato, Swiss chard, turnip and turnip greens

Caution: Exercise, weight loss diets and the use of oral contraceptives, tranquilizers and antibiotics uses more Riboflavin and your daily requirements should be increased.

VITAMIN B3 (NIACIN, NICOTINIC ACID, NIACINAMIDE)

B3 is used to treat heart disease, mental illness and arthritis. Assists cellular respiration, and utilization of all major nutrients, widens blood vessels and increases blood flow (which helps to lower high blood cholesterol) and aids in the function of the liver. Lack of B3 affects the skin, gastrointestinal tract and nervous system. This causes the skin to redden, blister, become infected, scaly or harden and this usually occurs when skin is exposed to sunlight or trauma. Causes sores in the mouth, gastric discomfort, vomiting and leads to severe diarrhea. The nervous system is affected by signs of anxiety, fatigue, loss of appetite, headaches, insomnia, depression, hyperactivity, hallucinations, and also smells and tastes are dulled.

Food Sources:

Dairy: cheese, buttermilk, goat's milk, milk, whey, yogurt.

Fruits: apple, apricot, avocado, blackberry, blueberry, cantaloupe, cherry, chokecherry, currant, date, grape, guava, lemon, lime, mango, orange, papaya, peach, pear, raspberry, rhubarb, strawberry, tangerine, watermelon.

Grains: millet, oats, quinoa, rye, spelt, wheat, wheat (bran and germ).

Herbs: agrimony, alfalfa, aloe vera, amaranth, anise seed, barberry, bayberry, bearberry, bilberry, black cohosh, black walnut, blessed thistle, blue cohosh, borage, buchu, burdock root, butcher's broom, caraway seed, cascara sagrada, catnip, cayenne, chamomile, chaparral, chickweed, chlorella, cilantro, cinnamon, clove, comfrey, dandelion, echinacea, eyebright, fennel, garlic, gentian, ginger, ginseng, goldenseal, green tea, hawthorn, hops, horseradish, horsetail, juniper, kelp, liquorice, marjoram, marshmallow, nettle, oat straw, oregano, parsley, peppermint, raspberry leaf, red clover, rose hips, rosemary, sage, skullcap, slippery elm, spearmint, thyme, turmeric, valerian, white oak bark, wormwood, yellow dock.

Legumes: bean (black, red and white), black-eyed peas, carob, garbanzo, kidney bean, lentil, navy bean, peanut

Meats:

Beef: beef: liver

Lake, ocean, river, sea: clams, eggs, clams, fish: fresh water, fish: salt water, halibut, herring, lamb, mackerel, salmon, sardines, tuna.

Lamb: lamb

Pork: lamb

Nuts, Oils & Seeds:

Nuts: almond, Brazil nut, cashew, coconut, hazelnut, pecan, pine nut, pistachio, walnut

Oils: walnut oil

Seeds: chia seed, cacao, mustard seed, sunflower seed

Vegetables: artichoke, asparagus, bean (lima and snap), beet - beet green, broccoli, Brussel sprout, cabbage, carrot, cauliflower, corn, kale, kelp, kohlrabi, lettuce (iceberg), mushroom, mustard green, onion (green and red), parsnips, pea, peppers: bell, potato, pumpkin, radish, rutabaga, spinach, squash, sweet potato, Swiss chard, turnip and turnip greens.

VITAMIN B5 (PANTOTHENIC ACID)

B5 is a very good vitamin for anti-stress. Some B complexes will add additional B5 to the formulas for stress. This vitamin helps to produce the adrenal hormones, our antibodies and helps with the conversion of fats, carbs and proteins. It also helps to turn fats, carbs and proteins into energy. B5 is found in all of our cells and organs and helps with the production of our neurotransmitters. It has also helped with preventing anemia, depression, anxiety and works with our intestinal tracts. The lack of B5 can cause depression, tiredness, tingling in hands and headaches.

Food Sources:
Dairy: buttermilk, goat's milk, milk, whey.

Fruits: apple, apricot, avocado, blackberry, blueberry, cherry, cranberry, date, gooseberry, grape, grapefruit, guava, lemon, lime, mango, orange, papaya, peach, pear, raspberry, rhubarb, Saskatoon, strawberry, tangerine, watermelon.

Grains: buckwheat, oats, rye, wheat, wheat (bran and germ).

Herbs: alfalfa, anise seed, blessed thistle, blue cohosh, catnip, cayenne, cilantro, clove, green tea, hawthorn, horseradish, kelp, liquorice, marshmallow, nettle, oat straw, oregano, parsley, red clover, rose hips, sage, spearmint, thyme, wormwood

Legumes: bean (black, red and white), black-eyed peas, carob, garbanzo, kidney bean, lentil, lima, navy, pinto, soybean.

Legumes: peanut

Meats:

Beef: beef, beef kidney, beef liver

Lake, ocean, river, sea: fish: fresh water, fish: saltwater, halibut, herring, mackerel, salmon, sardines, tuna

Poultry: egg, turkey

Nuts, Oils & Seeds:

Nuts: almond, Brazil nut, cashew, coconut, hazelnut, macadamia, pecan, pine nut, pistachio, walnut

Seeds: sunflower seed

Vegetables: asparagus, bean (lima and snap), beet - beet green, broccoli, Brussel sprout, cabbage, carrot, cauliflower, celery, collard, corn, cucumber, kelp, kohlrabi, lettuce (iceberg and romaine), mushroom, mustard green, onion (green and red), parsnips, pea, potato, pumpkin, rutabaga, spinach, squash, sweet potato, Swiss chard, turnip and turnip greens.

VITAMIN B6 (PYRIDOXINE)

For babies B6 must be in infant formulas if they are not being breast feed. B6 helps to break down amino acids, so they can be absorbed by the cells and protects the liver. Lack of B6 affects the nervous system, and the lack of protein does not allow the brain to develop and function, affects teeth development and causes teeth decay and impress the immune system. Signs of the lack of B6 are greasy scaling dermatitis around the eyes, ears, nose, mouth and thighs, inflammation of the oral area, convulsions and nerve tissue degeneration. Use of oral contraceptives may deplete the B6 and cause depression. B6 has been used to help with arthritis, numbness, burning sensations in extremities, fingers that go to sleep, swollen joints, reduced sensation in joints and leg cramps. B6 has been used in children for convulsions, hyperactivity and children who are unsettled.

Food Sources:
Dairy: yogurt, whey

Fruits: apple, apricot, avocado, banana, blueberry, cantaloupe, chokecherry, cranberry, currant, date, fig, gooseberry, grape, grapefruit, guava, kiwi, lemon, mango, orange, passion fruit, pineapple, plum, raspberry, strawberry, tangerine, watermelon.

Grains: barley, buckwheat, cereal grain, corn, millet, oats, quinoa, rice: brown, rice (white), rye, spelt, wheat, wheat(bran and germ).

Herbs: alfalfa, anise seed, blessed thistle, blue cohosh, catnip, cayenne, chlorella, cilantro, clove, fennel, fenugreek, ginger, hawthorn, horseradish, kelp, liquorice, marshmallow, oat straw, oregano, parsley, red clover, rose hips, spearmint, thyme, wormwood.

Legumes: bean (black, red and white), black-eyed peas, carob, garbanzo, kidney bean, lentil, lima, navy, peanut, pinto, soybean.

Meat:

Beef: beef

Lake, ocean, river, sea: fish: fresh water, fish: saltwater, halibut, herring, mackerel, salmon, sardines, tuna.

Pork: pork

Poultry: chicken, egg, turkey

Nuts, Oils & Seeds:

Nuts: Brazil nut, cashew, coconut, hazelnut, macadamia, pecan, pine nut, pistachio, walnut

Seeds: cacao, flaxseed, hemp seed, mustard seed, sesame seed, sunflower seed

Vegetables: artichoke, asparagus, bean (lima and snap), beet - beet green, broccoli, Brussel sprout, cabbage, carrot, cauliflower, celery, collard, corn, garlic, kale, kelp, kohlrabi, lettuce (iceberg and romaine), mushroom, mustard green, onion (green and red), parsnips, pea, peppers (bell), potato, pumpkin, radish, rutabaga, spinach, squash, sweet potato, Swiss chard, turnip and turnip greens.

Caution: Too much B6 will cause pins and needles, burning feeling in extremities, numbness or lack of coordination. Anyone who is using L-dopa should not take pyridoxine or any B vitamin supplement and should consult their doctor.

VITAMIN B12 (CYANOCOBALAMIN)

B12 is also known as Cobalamin. B12 contains a metal called cobalt and is essential to activate folate for the structure and function of the nervous system. Vegetarians tend to have pallor due to the lack of B12, as meat is one of the greater sources of cobalt is red meat. Without B12, the red blood cells are halted and are not developing right. This can also affect the nervous system, small intestine and eye colour perception can be effected.

Symptoms of B12 deficiency are weakness, sore and inflamed tongue, numbness and tingling in extremities, pallor, weak pulse, irritability, depression, hallucinations and diarrhea. The lack of B12 has been associated with mental health patients, to the level of being deficient. Now doctors at mental institutions require that patients are tested for vitamin levels, mainly for B12.

Food Sources:
Dairy: cheese, buttermilk, goat's milk, milk, whey, yogurt

Fruits: tangerine.

Herbs: alfalfa, angelica, blessed thistle, blue cohosh, catnip, chlorella, clove, ginseng, hawthorn, horseradish, kelp, liquorice, marjoram, oat straw, oregano, red clover, rose hips, spearmint, thyme, white oak bark, wormwood

Legumes: soy bean

Meat:

Beef: beef: kidney, beef: liver

Lake, ocean, river, sea: clams, fish: fresh water, fish: saltwater, halibut, herring, mackerel, salmon, sardines, tuna

Lamb: lamb

Pork: pork

Poultry: egg

Nuts, Oils & Seeds: Nuts: cashews, pecan

Vegetables: bean (lima and snap), dulse, kelp, mushroom, mustard greens, parsnips, rutabaga, spinach, turnip

BIOTIN

Another part of the B complex. Biotin is necessary for the syntheses of protein and fatty acids, and the metabolism for carbohydrates. Biotin is needed for blood sugar regulator, cell development in the fetus, hair, to relieve muscle pain, nerve tissue and skin. Deficiency of Biotin causes anemia, blood sugar that is too high, depression, hair loss, inflammation of skin, insomnia, nausea and a sore tongue.

Food Sources:
Dairy: butter, goat milk, milk.

Fruit: strawberry

Grains: barley, buckwheat, cereal grain, corn, millet, rice (brown and white), rye, wheat.

Legumes: peanut, soybeans.

Meats:

Beef: beef: calf liver, beef kidney, beef liver

Lake, ocean, river, sea: fish: salt water, halibut, herring, mackerel, sardines

Poultry: egg yolks

Nuts, Oils & Seeds: Nuts: walnut

Vegetables: carrots, cucumber, lettuce (romaine).

Caution: It is advised that nursing mothers consult their doctors about taking extra biotin. SIDS has been linked to the lack of biotin in both animals and humans.

CHOLINE

Choline has been used in the treatment of Alzheimer's, dementia, Friedreich's Ataxia, Gilles de la Tourette's disease, Huntington's disease, manic depression and Tardive dyskinesia. Studies are showing differences in muscle spasms and memory improvement, and it assists in treating some of the diseases. Choline is not recognized as a vitamin. It helps to offset other vitamins.

Food Sources:
Fruits: avocado, blackberry, grapefruit, passion fruit, peaches.

Dairy: cheese, buttermilk, goats milk, milk

Grains: buckwheat, cereal grain, corn, wheat, wheat: bran

Legumes: bean (black, red and white), carob, garbanzo, kidney bean, lentil, lima, navy, pinto, soybean

Meats:

Beef: beef liver

Lake, ocean, river, sea: fish: fresh water.

Poultry: egg yolk, turkey

Nuts, Oils & Seeds: Oils: almond oil

Vegetables: asparagus, broccoli, Brussel sprout, cabbage, cauliflower, collard, cucumber, mushroom, pea, spinach, Swiss chard, turnip

Suggested Requirements: Choline is basically non-toxic, but it has made some people depressed when used as a prescription drug.

FOLATE (FOLACIN, FOLIC ACID)

Folate is important for our brain, energy production and the formation of our red blood cells and white blood cells. Our DNA and RNA require folate as a coenzyme for the proper cell division and replication. It also helps with protein metabolism, treats folic acid anemia, for depression, anxiety, the uterine function and lessens the hardening of arteries.

Folate works well with B6, B12 and vitamin C. Lack of folate during pregnancy is linked to some infant deformities and preventing of spina bifida and premature birth. Folate aids in the growth of bone marrow, hair, fingernails and the immune system. Signs of the lack of folate are inflamed and sore tongue, tingling in hands and feet, indigestion, diarrhea, depression, irritability, pallor, fatigue, and slow pulse. Folate is used to maintain a normal blood sugar level, helps with psoriasis, gingivitis and pregnancy.

Food Sources:
Dairy: cheese, buttermilk, goats milk, milk

Fruits: avocado, blackberry, blueberry, cantaloupe, chokecherry, currant, date, gooseberry, grape, grapefruit, guava, kiwi, lemon, lime, mango, orange, papaya, passion fruit, peach, pear, pineapple, plum, raspberry, rhubarb, Saskatoon, strawberry, tangerine.

Grains: bran, buckwheat, couscous, oats, quinoa, rice (brown and white), spelt, wheat, wheat (bran and germ)

Herbs: alfalfa, amaranth, fennel, garlic, oatstraw, olive leaf, parsley

Legumes: bean (black, red and white), black-eyed peas, carob, folate, garbanzo, kidney bean, lentil, lima, navy, pinto, soybean

Meats:

Beef: beef, beef liver

Lake, ocean, river, sea: salmon, sardines

Lamb: lamb

Pork: pork

Nuts, Oils & Seeds:

Nuts: almond, Brazil nut, coconut, hazelnut, pecan, pine nut, pistachio, walnut

Seeds: mustard seed, sunflower seed

Vegetables: artichoke, asparagus, bean (lima and snap), beet - beet green, broccoli, Brussel sprout, cabbage, carrot, cauliflower, celery, collard, corn, garlic, kale, kohlrabi, lettuce (iceberg and romaine), mushroom, mustard green, onion (green and red), parsnips, pea, peppers (bell), potato, pumpkin, radish, rutabaga, spinach, squash, sweet potato, Swiss chard, turnip and turnip greens

Caution: Cancer and epileptic patients must use caution in using folic acid. It is said that nursing mothers should be careful with their intake of folate. Consult your doctor. Folate is essential for fetus development.

INOSITOL

Inositol is another B complex factor. Inositol is needed for the skeletal and heart muscles, blood, brain, liver, lungs and for hair growth.

It is used for its calming effects. It helps to reduce cholesterol and to stop the hardening of arteries. Inositol aids in removing fats from the liver. The lack of this vitamin can cause constipation, hair loss, irritability, skin sores and mood swings. Inositol has been used in high dosages for depression, compulsive disorders and anxiety.

Food Sources:
Dairy: buttermilk, goat's milk, milk, yogurt.

Fruits: apple, apricot, avocado, banana, blackberry, blueberry, cantaloupe, cherry, chokecherry, cranberry, currant, date, fig, goji berry, gooseberry, grape, grapefruit, guava, kiwi, lemon, lime, mango, orange, papaya, passion fruit, peach, pear, pineapple, plum, raspberry, rhubarb, Saskatoon, strawberry, tangerine, watermelon.

Grains: barley, buckwheat, cereal grain, corn, couscous, millet, quinoa, wheat.

Legumes: bean (black, red and white), carob, garbanzo, kidney bean, lentil, lima, navy, pinto, soybean.

PABA (PARA-AMINOBENZOIC ACID)

PABA is a part of the compounds of folate. Pantothenic acid is created with the help of PABA, and PABA can be converted to folate by our intestinal bacteria. PABA is used in sunscreens to block the sun's harmful rays. It has been used for the treatment of skin diseases, Peyronie's disease, scleroderma and chronic discoid lupus erythematosus. It is good for the formation of the red blood cells, aids in intestinal flora and helps to reduce grey hair caused by stress. PABA can help to protect our bodies from ozone, smoke and inflammation from arthritis. Lack of PABA can cause grey hair, tiredness, patches of white skin, digestive troubles and depression. Our PABA levels can be depleted by the use of sulfur drugs.

Food Sources:
Grains: barley, corn, couscous, millet, quinoa, rice (brown and white), rye, wheat.

Meats: Beef: beef kidney.

Vegetables: mushroom, spinach.

Caution: Do not take PABA supplements when taking sulfa drugs.

VITAMIN C (ASCORBIC ACID)

Vitamin C is used to activate cleansing enzymes in the colon and liver. It improve the immune system and fights against colds, allergies, infections, back trouble, heart disease, mental illness, arthritis, infertility, fatigue, heat and cold stress, diabetes, bone disease, toxic effects of pollution and cancer. It is also used to treat glaucoma (eyes), improve healing time for wounds and after surgery, smooth skin and stronger tissue. It helps to increase iron absorption, metabolism and reduction of cholesterol balance estrogen levels. Vitamin C is greatly reduced from our systems from smoking, the use of oral contraceptives, menopause drugs, barbiturates, tetracycline and aspirin. Signs of vitamin C deficiency: scurvy, delayed healing of wounds, separation of longer bones, loosened teeth, anemia, weakness, weight loss, irritable, aches and pains in joints, extremities, and muscles. Easy bruising and bleeding, drying of tear glands, depression, hypochondria and hysteria.

Food Sources:
Dairy: whey, yogurt.

Fruits: apple, apricot, avocado, banana, blackberry, blueberry, cantaloupe, cherry, chokecherry, cranberry, currant, fig, goji berry, gooseberry, grape, grapefruit, guava, kiwi, lemon, lime, mango, orange, papaya, passion fruit, peach, pear, pineapple, plum, raspberry, rhubarb, Saskatoon, strawberry, tangerine, watermelon.

Herbs: alfalfa, aloe vera, amaranth, anise seed, barberry, bayberry, bearberry, bilberry, birch, bistort, black cohosh, black walnut, blessed thistle, blue cohosh, borage, burdock root, butcher's broom, calendula, caraway seed, cascara sagrada, catnip, cayenne, chamomile, chaparral, chickweed, chlorella, cilantro, cinnamon, clove, comfrey, cramp bark, dandelion, echinacea, eyebright, fennel, garlic, gentian, ginger, ginseng, goldenseal, green tea, hawthorn, hops, horseradish, horsetail, Irish moss, juniper, kelp, liquorice, lobelia, marjoram, marshmallow, nettle, oat straw, oregano, parsley, Pau d'arco, peppermint, plantain, raspberry leaf, red clover, rose hips, rosemary, sage, skullcap, spearmint, thyme, turmeric, valerian, white oak bark, witch hazel, wormwood, yarrow, yellow dock.

Legumes: bean (red and white), black-eyed peas, kidney bean, lentil, peanut, navy.

Nuts, Oils & Seeds:

Nuts: Brazil nut, hazelnut, macadamia, pecan, pine nut, pistachio, walnut

Seeds: flaxseed, hemp seed, mustard seed, sunflower seed

Vegetables: artichoke, asparagus, bean (lima and snap), beet - beet green, broccoli, Brussel sprout, cabbage, carrot, cauliflower, celery, collard, cucumber, dulse, garlic, kale, kelp, kohlrabi, lettuce (iceberg and romaine), mushroom, mustard green, onion (green and red), parsnips, pea, peppers (bell), potato, pumpkin, radish, rutabaga, spinach, squash, sweet potato, Swiss chard, turnip and turnip greens.

Caution: Nursing mothers should be really careful of their intake of vitamin C. Some babies get severe cramps from the high vitamin C in mother's milk.

VITAMIN D

Vitamin D is known as the sunshine vitamin. Vitamin D is for the enhancement of intestinal absorption of calcium and phosphorus, to maintain adequate blood levels for the calcification of bone and cartilage. Signs of deficiency are kidney disease, Rickets and Osteoporosis. A deficiency can cause a higher than normal blood levels of lead. Lack of vitamin D cause irritability, restlessness, deformed bone structure, early teeth decay, neuromuscular hyper, irritability, spasms of wrist and foot, convulsive seizures, muscle cramps, burning and tingling and numbness. Vitamin D levels can be affected with the use of liquid paraffin, anticonvulsant drugs, hypnotic glutethimide and corticosteroids. The signs of too much vitamin D are a loss of appetite, thirst, urgency of urination, vomiting, headache and diarrhea.

Food Sources:
Dairy: butter, buttermilk, goat's milk, milk, yogurt

Grains: oats

Herbs: alfalfa, aloe vera, basil, dandelion eyebright, Irish moss, kelp, nettle, oregano, raspberry, rose hips, thyme

Legumes: bean (red), kidney bean

Meats:

Beef: beef: liver

Lake, ocean, river, sea: fish: oils, halibut, herring, mackerel, salmon, sardines, tuna

Poultry: eggs,

Nuts, Oils & Seeds: Seeds: chia seed, hemp seed

Vegetables: mushroom, sweet potato, Swiss chard

Caution: If you are taking different vitamin supplements, make sure that vitamin D is not in all of them, as some supplements duplicate vitamin D. Some doctors are recommending 1000 per day, when there is evidence of osteoporosis. Vitamin D3 is the natural source, and D2 is a synthetic form.

VITAMIN E

Vitamin E helps to fight against cardiovascular disorders, acts like an antitoxin, protects the fatty acids (oils) against oxidation (scientists believe this protects our bodies from many diseases and symptoms of aging). Signs of vitamin E deficiency are diminished function of the pituitary-thyroid, degeneration of the skeletal - striated and cardiac muscles, degeneration of the endocrine glands, peripheral vascular system and the nervous system. There doesn't seem to be any signs of vitamin E deficiency, like rashes or anything. There does seem to be a connection with vitamin C, E and cancer. Vitamin E is used for raising the levels of sex hormones and adrenal sex hormones, used to decrease symptoms of PMS, improve the mental health in elderly women, protect against the oxidation of cells during stress, boosts the immune system, in the healing of wounds and burns, used for cardiovascular patients, ulcers of the leg, early gangrene of the extremities, angina, rheumatic fever and decrease blood clotting.

Food Sources:
Dairy: buttermilk, goat milk, milk

Fruits: avocado, blackberry, blueberry, cherry, chokecherry, cranberry, fig, grape, grapefruit, guava, kiwi, lemon, mango, orange, papaya, passion fruit, peach, raspberry, rhubarb, Saskatoon, strawberry, tangerine

Grains: buckwheat, oats, quinoa, rice (brown and white), spelt, wheat, wheat: bran, wheat (germ)

Herbs: alfalfa, aloe vera, angelica, anise, bilberry, birch, blue cohosh, borage, burdock, calendula, cayenne, chickweed, chlorella, cilantro, cramp bark, dandelion, eye bright, ginseng, Irish moss, kelp, liquorice, nettle, oat straw, oregano, parsley, peppermint, pokeweed, primrose, raspberry leaf, red clover, rose hips, skullcap, slippery elm, witch hazel, yarrow

Legumes: bean (black), black-eyed peas, carob, kidney bean, lentil, lima, peanut, pinto, soybean

Meats:

Beef: beef: calf liver, beef kidney, beef liver

Lake, ocean, river, sea: clams, fish: fresh water, fish: saltwater

Poultry: egg

Nuts, Oils & Seeds:

Nuts: almond, Brazil nut, cashew, coconut, hazelnut, macadamia, pecan, pine nut, pistachio, walnut

Oils: almond oil, coconut oil, cotton seed oil, grapeseed oil, hazelnut oil, hemp seed oil, olive oil, sesame seed oil, Siberian pine nut oil, walnut oil

Seeds: chia seed, cacao, flaxseed, hemp seed, mustard seed, pumpkin seed, sesame seed, sunflower seed

Vegetables: asparagus, bean (lima and snap), beet - beet green, broccoli, cabbage, carrot, collard, corn, dulse, kale, kelp, kohlrabi, lettuce (iceberg and romaine), mustard green, onion (green and red), parsnips, pea, peppers: bell, potato, pumpkin, rutabaga, spinach, squash, sweet potato, Swiss chard, turnip

Caution: Vitamin E doesn't appear to be a toxin but can slow metabolism rate and affect the thyroid. Those who have bleeding disorders, should see their doctor before taking vitamin E.

VITAMIN K

Vitamin K helps the blood to clot and for proper bone mineralization. Lack of vitamin K causes increased bleeding from wounds or surgery. Antibiotics and sulfa drugs with prolonged use can lower vitamin K and cause a deficiency. Epileptic mothers taking barbiturates or phenytoin cause the newborn to have a deficiency too. Those with bleeding disorders may have to get vitamin K shots, before surgery or oral surgery. Antibiotics can interfere with the absorption of this vitamin.

Food Sources:
Dairy: yogurt.

Fruits: apple, apricot, avocado, blackberry, blueberry, cantaloupe, cherry, cranberry, currant, date, fig, grape, guava, kiwi, mango, orange, papaya, passion fruit, peach, pear, raspberry, rhubarb, strawberry.

Grains: buckwheat, oats, rye, wheat, wheat: bran.

Herbs: agrimony, alfalfa, cilantro, parsley, plantain, slippery elm, witch hazel, yarrow.

Legumes: bean: (red and white), black-eyed peas, garbanzo, kidney bean, lentil, navy, soybean.

Meats:

Beef: beef liver

Poultry: egg yolk

Nuts, Oils & Seeds:

Nuts: coconut, hazelnut, pine nut, pistachio, walnut

Oils: almond oil, coconut oil, olive oil, sesame seed oil, Siberian pine nut oil

Seeds: mustard seed

Vegetables: artichoke, asparagus, bean (lima and snap), beet - beet green, broccoli, Brussel sprout, cabbage, carrot, cauliflower, celery, collard, cucumber, garlic, kale, kelp, lettuce (iceberg and romaine), mustard green, onion (green and red), parsnips, pea, peppers (bell), potato, pumpkin, radish, rutabaga, spinach, squash, sweet potato, turnip

VITAMIN P OR KNOWN AS BIOFLAVONOID

Bioflavonoids are known as vitamin P, even though they really are not a true vitamin. This vitamin and vitamin C should be used together for better results. There are many types of bioflavonoids, and they need to be consumed with your daily diet, as the body cannot produce this vitamin. This vitamin can be used for reducing pain due to injuries like bruises, yet can also help with back and leg discomfort. Bioflavonoids are used for protecting the structure of the capillaries, to improve circulation, for oral herpes and used as an antibacterial agent.

Food Sources:
Fruits: apricot, blackberry, cherry, currant, grape, grapefruit, lemon, orange, plum.

Grains: buckwheat, oats, rye, wheat

Herbs: chervil, dandelion, elderberries, hawthorn berry, horsetail, rose hips, shepherd's purse

Legumes: soybeans

Meats:

Beef: beef: liver

Poultry: egg yolks

Nuts, Oils & Seeds:

Oils: Siberian pine nut

COENZYME Q10

Coenzyme Q10 is a very strong antioxidant and is found in many parts of the body and especially in the tissue. Coenzyme Q10 helps with the immune system, the heart (proven to decrease heart attacks or strokes), provides energy for the cells of the body, provides oxygenation of the tissue and anti-aging effects. Coenzyme Q10 has been used for treatment of asthma, allergies and respiratory problems. It is very helpful for decreasing high blood pressure and is used in conjunction with chemotherapy.

Food Sources:
Legume: peanut

Meats: Lake, ocean, river, sea: mackerel, salmon, sardine

Vegetables: spinach

Oils

Oils are essential for the functioning of our brain, skin, respiratory system, blood circulation and for all of our other organs. There are some oils that our body can produce naturally, so we need assistance from the fatty acids (EFA) from other sources. The two oils that we need to take additionally to what we eat in our foods is the omega-3 and omega-6. These two are extremely important for our brain growth and functioning, our immune system and to help regulate our blood.

OMEGA 3 FATTY ACID (ALPHA-LINOLENIC ACID)

This oil is essential for our brain function. After a brain concussion, it is recommended to start to taking the omega oils to assist in the healing process. Omega-3 also plays a huge role in fighting cardiovascular diseases.

Other benefits from omega-3:

Uses: arthritis, asthma, attention disorders, depression, diabetes, digestion, helps to lower high cholesterol and high blood pressure, osteoporosis and the skin.

Sources:
Dairy: butter.

Grains: buckwheat, oats, wheat, wheat (bran and germ).

Legumes: bean (black, red and white), carob, garbanzo, kidney bean, navy, soybean.

Meats:

Lake, ocean, river, sea: fish: freshwater, fish liver oil, herring, salmon, sardines, tuna

Lamb: lamb

Pork: pork

Poultry: turkey

Nuts, Oils & Seeds:

Nuts: Brazil nut, coconut, hazelnut, macadamia, pecan, pistachio, walnut

Oils: almond oil, cotton seed oil, grapeseed oil, hazelnut oil, hemp seed oil, olive oil, sesame seed oil, walnut oil

Seeds: chia seed, flaxseed, hemp seed, mustard seed, pumpkin seed, sunflower seed

Vegetables: asparagus, collards, dulse, garlic, kelp, lettuce (romaine), spinach, squash, Swiss chard, turnip greens.

OMEGA 6 FATTY ACID (LINOLEIC ACID)

Omega 6 Fatty Acid is best combined with the omega-3 fatty acid. The omega 6 oil works for the same conditions as omega-3. I read an article that suggested that we should consume omega-6 2:1 with the omega-3.

Sources:
Grains: millet, wheat, wheat (bran and germ).

Legumes: bean (black, red and white), carob, garbanzo, kidney bean, navy, peanut

Meat:

Lake, ocean, river, sea: fish: oils

Pork: pork

Poultry: turkey

Nuts, Oils & Seeds:

Nuts: almond, Brazil nut, cashew, coconut, hazelnut, macadamia, pecan, pistachio, walnut

Oils: almond oil, coconut oil, cotton seed oil, grapeseed oil, hemp seed oil, olive oil, sesame seed oil

Seeds: chia seed, cacao, flaxseed, hemp seed, mustard seed, pumpkin seed, sesame seed, sunflower seed

Vegetables: lettuce (romaine), mushroom.

OMEGA 9 FATTY ACID (MONOUNSATURATED OLEIC AND STEARIC ACID)

This oil is produced by the body, and is a non-essential fatty acid. Used to balance our cholesterol levels and the fatty acid strengthens the immune system. This can only happen when the body has consumed enough of omega-3 and omega-6. Our body will acquire additional omega-9 if the other two omega oils have become depleted.

Sources:
Grains: wheat germ

Nuts, Oils & Seeds:

Nuts: almond, cashew, hazelnut

Oils: pine Nut oil, walnut oil

Seeds: chia seed, hemp seed

Vegetables: avocados

EPA & DHA

Our bodies will turn the omega-3 fatty acids in EPA and DHA. These are unsaturated fats that we need for our vision and brain development as babies and infants. We still need the EPA in our bodies as we get older, as it plays a role in our mental health and physically body.

Uses:
Lack of EPA can cause depression. Studies have found that suicides can be prevented if a person consumes the right amount of omega-3.

Lack of DHA can cause Alzheimer disease, attention disorders, cystic fibrosis and other diseases.

Amino Acids

L-Glutamine: is an amino acid that helps with cell repair with the following: sports injuries and training, substance abuse, supplement for burns and tissue healing, along with preventing secondary infections from burns. It is also used for treating the following: arthritis and autoimmune diseases, fibrosis, tissue damage from radiation from cancer treatments, peptic ulcers and intestine problems.

L-Glutamine is known to be a brain food or fuel and turns to glutamic acid when it hits the brain. This glutamic acid is necessary for the functioning of the cerebral system and increases the amount of GABA that we need for proper brain and mental activities. This amino acid is used for many brain related problems such as depression, developmental delays and disabilities. L-glutamine helps the body not to crave sugar as much while it works with the liver. The used of L-Glutamine helps recovering alcoholics as one's craving for the alcohol and sugar goes down. One needs to be cautioned not to use this amino acid when cirrhosis of the liver is present or problems with the kidneys, as it will intoxicate the body more.

Sources

Grains: buckwheat

Herbs: parsley

Vegetables: potato, spinach

L-Lysine: This protein is the building block for all the proteins. Lysine is needed for calcium absorption, bone building for children and maintaining a proper nitrogen balance in adults. This amino acid is very good at fighting cold sores and herpes viruses. Using L-lysine with a vitamin C or using elements that contain bio-flavoids can be used to avoid or prevent herpes outbreaks. Acute alcohol intoxication has been treated with the L-lysine. Other conditions that can occur when the body is deficient of L-lysine are as follows: hair loss, anemia, red eyes, lack of concentration, irritable, reproductive disorders and weight loss.

Sources:

Dairy: cheese, buttermilk, goat's milk, milk.

Grains: buckwheat.

Legumes: lima beans.

Meats:

Beef: beef

Lake, ocean, river, sea: fish: freshwater, fish oil, fish: saltwater, halibut, herring, mackerel, salmon, sardines, tuna

Poultry: egg, egg yolk

Vegetables: potatoes.

L-Taurine: This amino sulfonic acid is found more in the animal proteins. Taurine is partly found in our blood cells and heart muscles, the nervous system and our skeletal muscles. We require the Taurine in our bile so that we can easily digest fats, absorb vitamins and help to control the serum cholesterol levels in our body. With the proper Taurine levels the calcium, magnesium, sodium and potassium that we consume is better utilized and not stored wrongly to cause health issues. Patients with hypertension, hypoglycemia, edema and heart disorders benefit from the use of Taurine. Other treatments used with L-taurine are dehydration, seizures, hyperactivity, anxiety and epilepsy. Zinc and Taurine are both connected with proper brain function and the lack of both can cause the seizures or the brain not to develop properly. Vegetarians should make sure that they have a supplement of L-taurine in their diet.

Sources:
Dairy: milk.

Grains: buckwheat.

Meats:

Beef: beef

Lake, ocean, river, sea: fish: freshwater, fish oil, fish: saltwater, halibut, herring, mackerel, salmon, sardines, tuna.

Pork; pork

Poultry: egg, egg yolk

L-Tyrosine: This amino acid is derived from phenylalanine. This one is very important in order for our overall metabolism and nervous system to work properly. L-tyrosine is essential for the adrenaline, the neurotransmitters and the dopamine to be properly regulated. When there is not enough tyrosine, it can lead to depression, as the brain is not producing enough norepinephrine. The tyrosine also is a mild antioxidant, which can suppress hunger, and it helps to reduce body fat. The amino acid helps in the function of the thyroid, pituitary and adrenal glands. When the body is lacking in L-tyrosine, it results in a low body temperature, low blood pressure and also restless legs. This amino acid is also used to relieve Parkinson's, chronic fatigue and narcolepsy.

Sources:
Dairy: cheese, buttermilk, goat's milk, milk, whey, yogurt

Fruits: bananas

Legumes: lima beans

Meats:

BeefLake, ocean, river, sea: fish: freshwater, fish oil, fish: saltwater, halibut, herring, mackerel, salmon, sardines, tuna

Poultry: egg, egg yolk,

Nuts, Oils & Seeds:

Nuts: almonds, cashews

Seeds: pumpkin seed, sesame seed

Vegetables: potatoes

Enzymes

An enzyme is a protein that becomes a catalyst to bring chemical changes with the other substances within our body. Enzymes are needed to help us digest our food better so that it can be properly absorbed. For example, when a female is pregnant, her body may need additional digestive enzymes for her digestion such as a pineapple enzyme. Enzymes have three categories: digestive enzyme, food enzyme and metabolic enzyme.

Pepsin and Trypsin enzyme: These break down the proteins in our digestive tract, and that converts the food into amino acids. Enzymes are the organic part of the amino acids that our body requires.

Another example of an enzyme is the Coenzyme Q10, listed in the minerals of this chapter. Coenzyme Q10 is a very strong antioxidant and is found in many parts of the body and especially in the tissue. Coenzyme Q10 helps with the immune system, the heart (proven to decrease heart attacks or strokes), provides energy for the cells of the body, provides oxygenation of the tissue, and anti-aging effects. Coenzyme Q10 has been used for treatment of asthma, allergies and respiratory problems. It is very helpful for decreasing high blood pressure and is used in conjunction with chemotherapy.

Again, if we are consuming the proper amount of EPA and DHA as in the amino acid section, our body can produce the right amount of enzymes and amino acids that we need.

Sources:
Fruit: the bromelain in the pineapple

Proteins

Proteins contain the following: amino acids, carbon, hydrogen, nitrogen, oxygen, and sometimes phosphorus and sulfur. Proteins help to form the structure of most of our organs. These proteins contribute to making the enzymes and hormones that our body needs to function. Our body needs to the proper intake of food or supplements for the proteins to be synthesized from the amino acids.

Sources:

Legumes: bean (black), carob, garbanzo, kidney bean, lentil, lima, navy, peanut, pinto, soybean

Meats:

Lake, ocean, river, sea: clams

Lamb

Poultry: turkey

Nuts, Oils & Seeds:

Nuts: almond, Brazil nut, cashew, coconut, hazelnut, macadamia, pecan, pine nut, pistachio, walnut

Oils: almond oil, coconut oil, cotton seed oil, sesame seed oil

Seeds: chia seed, cacao, flaxseed, hemp seed, pumpkin seed, sesame seed, sunflower seed

Vegetables: artichoke, asparagus, bean (lima and snap), beet - beet green, broccoli, Brussel sprout, cabbage, carrot, cauliflower, collard, corn, cucumber, garlic, kale, kelp, kohlrabi, lettuce (iceberg), mushroom, mustard green, onion (green), parsnips, pea, black-eyed pea, peppers (bell), potato, pumpkin, spinach, sweet potato, Swiss chard, turnip and turnip greens

Antioxidants.

Our bodies also require antioxidants. Antioxidants protect our cells against free radicals. Free radicals are the chemicals that our bodies absorb from toxins that are in the environment. Some of these products are perfumes, colognes, air fresheners, gasoline fumes, glues from carpets, chipboard, fumes, radiation, tobacco smoke, tires and carpet underlay. Chemicals cause damage to the neurological system and our muscles. These chemicals can also damage the organs such as the liver, lungs, kidneys, heart and skin.

There are many foods that help our bodies by providing the antioxidants that our blood needs to fight off cancers, colds and the flu. They help to keep the immune system stronger. One thing to keep in mind is that you want to know more about where your food is grown and what is used on it while growing and being harvested. Try to buy organic food, and if you are not able to afford organic foods, it is better to buy produce that is locally grown. What can you grow in your own home or yard? What is your local farmer growing? All it takes is one pot of soil and some heritage seeds. Grow the fruits, herbs and veggies that are higher in antioxidants.

Antioxidants include vitamins A, C, and E, beta-carotene, lutein, lycopene, pycnogenol and selenium. Beta-carotene helps increase the disease-fighting powers of antioxidants and can be found in several fresh fruits as well. When foods are consumed raw and uncooked, the nutrients are at a higher level than when they are cooked or processed.

Antioxidants can be found in the following foods. Please do keep in mind that when I was preparing these notes, most of the food sources were what I could find in the local area around the region of Calgary, Alberta. I encourage you to do the research for what you have in your region.

Fruit: With the berries, the darker the berry the higher the antioxidant content, like blackberries, blueberries, cranberries and Saskatoon berries.

- apple, apricot, avocado, blackberry, blueberry, cantaloupe, cherry, chokecherry, cranberry, currant (Red), date, fig, goji berry, gooseberry, grape / raisin, grapefruit, guava, kiwi, lemon, lime, orange, papaya, passion fruit, peach, pear, pineapple, plum / prune, raspberry, rhubarb, Saskatoon berry, strawberry, tangerine, tomato, watermelon

Grains: Grains are lower in antioxidants, but they are a valuable source of the immunity-boosting compounds. When buying grains, choose 100 percent whole grains vs refined or processed grains. The nutrient content is higher in the whole grains.

- barley, buckwheat, cereal grain, corn, couscous, millet, oat, quinoa, rice (brown), rye, spelt, wheat, wheat bran, wheat germ.

HERBS

Herbs have amazing healing properties and are more powerful than the chemicals sold on shelves for ailments.

- amaranth, Ashwagandha, balm of Gilead, basil, bilberry, burdock, cannabis, chamomile, chlorella, cilantro, cloves, fennel, ginger, green tea, hawthorn, holy basil, lemongrass, lobelia, marjoram, milk thistle, oregano, peppermint, reishi mushroom, rose hips, spearmint, thyme, turmeric, white oak bark, yellow dock

LEGUMES

Legumes are also an amazing source of protein, vitamin E and antioxidants. Legumes are a great replacement for those who eat little meat or no meat.

- bean (red), carob, garbanzo bean, kidney bean, lentil, lima bean, navy bean, pinto bean, soybean

NUTS, OILS, SEEDS

Nut: almond, Brazil nut, cashew, coconut, hazelnut, macadamia nut, pecan, pine nut, pistachio, walnut

Oil: almond oil, avocado oil, coconut oil, grapeseed oil, hazelnut oil, hemp seed oil, olive oil, sesame seed oil, Siberian pine nut oil, walnut oil

Seed: chia seed, cacao, hemp seed, pumpkin seed, sesame seed, sunflower seed

VEGETABLES

Many green vegetables are loaded with antioxidants.

- artichoke, asparagus, beet, beet greens, broccoli, Brussel sprouts, cabbage, carrots, cauliflower, celery, collards, corn, cucumber, dulse, garlic, kale, kelp, kohlrabi, lettuce(iceberg and romaine), mushroom (white), mustard greens, onion (Red), pea, pepper (bell), potato, radish, rutabaga, spinach, squash, sweet potato, Swiss chard, turnip

We also have the essential oils that we can use, and some of the meat can provide antioxidant properties for us.

CHAPTER 5

Mother Earth's Foods and Medicines

MOTHER EARTH AND MOTHER NATURE BRING US SO MANY BLESSINGS FOUND IN THE foods that we will be covering and medicines that are grown around the world. This planet, Mother Earth, has the conditions to grow a variety of food and the produce. What we do grow depends on the climate and the soil. When we consume the foods that are grown in our region and store some for the winter, we can have a very healthy lifestyle and have fulfilling, tasty dishes all year round.

In each part of the world, there are seeds for almost any edible plant: fruit, herbs, vegetables, legumes, grains and nuts. We can collect our seeds each year during harvest for the following year. With these plants growing in our yard, one would be very healthy and have fresher food right at our doorstep. When we grow in our own yard and neighbourhood, we can ensure that unsafe and unnatural pesticides and herbicides are not being used. Any little space of lawn or balcony could produce lettuce for a salad, raspberry bush, herbs, bean plants and even herb plants like horse radish or sage. As the produce is enjoyed over the summer, one can start to store some of the bounty to use over the winter.

Our food is our medicine. When we eat for health, we can enjoy amazing meals of fruit and vegetables with the use of our herbs, nuts, seeds and oils as condiments. With the combination of the amino acids, vitamins, minerals, proteins and oils that we receive from our food, we also get the benefit of all the other healing properties for our body. With our herbs, the healing properties can be very powerful, and when used properly, the body would rarely get sick. It is time again to start growing our own food and eating for health.

The rest of this book is about the nutrition and healing properties in different food categories. It has been a lot of fun learning what our foods provide for our bodies and also experiencing the results of good eating and adding herbs as additional medicine in the four seasons of the year. We can obtain our food from around the world, and have a variety to use on the table. All the food categories will have the nutrition factors, healing properties and some ideas for preparing the food.

The chapters with cover the following foods:

Dairy	(Chapter 6)
Fruits	(Chapter 7)
Grains	(Chapter 8)
Herbs	(Chapter 9)
Legumes	(Chapter 10)
Meats	(Chapter 11)
Nuts, Oils & Seeds	(Chapter 12)
Vegetables	(Chapter 13)
Essential Oils	(Chapter 14)

Please note that even though the dairy and meat are not really a product of Mother Earth such as the other food we can grow, there are benefits to consuming them if our bodies can digest the foods. I am not a vegetarian or vegan, but I do limit the amount of meat I eat and rarely is it found on my plate. My body does let me know if I am lacking in the iron. I will make sure I buy the veggies I need for the iron, and at the same time maybe make a small pot of beef to last a meal or two.

GENETICALLY MODIFIED ORGANISM (GMO), ORGANIC, NOT ORGANIC

With the use of the internet and the social media groups, we get to learn a lot more about what is being put into our food and how it is being grown. We can learn what nutritional values are in the foods and how they can heal the body. We can learn about GMO food and organic food.

GMO seeds are not what you want in the gardens. These seeds have been genetically modified to provide higher yields, but the creation of these seeds can cause toxic effects around the world and in our bodies.

Farmers have been forced to plant the seeds and end up with failing crops. The produce from the seeds are causing toxic effects in humans and animals. There has been an uprising worldwide trying to put an end to the chemical company who has tried to take over the produce industries, including developing toxic fertilizers and pesticides. This company also has their hand in many products on the grocery shelf.

WHAT CAN WE DO?

We can order seeds from companies that have had their seeds tested to prove that they are not GMO seeds. We can buy our produce from local farmers who are obtaining a higher level of integrity with their crops and cattle.

WHAT IF I CAN'T AFFORD THE ORGANIC PRODUCE?

Social media can also put the fear into a person stating that all food is contaminated and that there are no nutrients left in what we are buying. This is a fearful energy that can be true, BUT it can also be false. This kind of message can make a person feel that no matter what they eat, they will get sick. I am not going to fall into this trap of uncertainty. I purchase both organic food and non-organic food. I can personally feel what is toxic when I buy the food. My body can and will go into a toxic sweat while carrying the food home. I will apply Reiki energy to the produce and products to help detox and change the vibration of the food. If you are unsure how to apply energy to your produce, just allow yourself to send lots of love towards it while you are preparing your meals. You will see a difference in the taste and how you feel afterwards.

Something else to keep in mind is that the quality of produce can go down as the produce ages by the day. There are a few options for storing the produce to prolong the aging effect and retain the nutrition. The faster we consume or preserve the food, the more nutrients the food will have.

Eating food that is locally grown and processed food can make a difference in the age of the food and what chemicals are in it, and it has a lot less impact on the environment. I only like shopping in grocery stores that let you know what country the food comes from. An example of this, though I may have a tight budget I will only buy garlic that is grown in the area that I am living in. I will not purchase it if the garlic came from overseas.

Chapter 16 will provide information on the best ways of preserving the abundance of produce you have from your gardens and the local markets for the leaner months.

I hope you have fun reading the next few chapters and getting a good idea of what you are eating and how it can heal and maintain a healthy body for you.

We need to learn how to live with Mother Earth again!

CHAPTER 6

Dairy

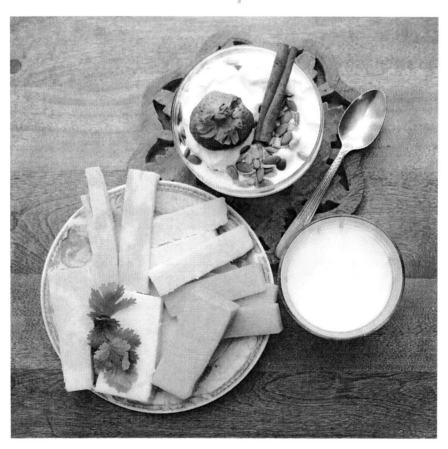

DAIRY PRODUCTS ARE CONSUMED AROUND THE WORLD. YET THERE ARE SOME COUNtries where some of the population do not consume dairy products due to beliefs and upbringing. Dairy and meat production is a large part of the farming industry in America, Australia and Europe.

Over the years the regulations have changed, chemicals have been added to the products such as chlorine (bleach) for sterilization and hormones for larger production. The lack of proper attention to cleanliness lead to dirty stalls and barns and brought on disease in the cattle, and this has also led to heavy sterilization. The industry or corporations looking for larger output of dairy products from the cattle have increased the hormones that have been added to the cows, goats and sheep.

A story I personally remember, is about a friend that remembers when the dairy industry made the dairy farmers in Canada start using chlorine to sterilize everything. This fellow could taste the chlorine in the bottled milk. Over the years, we hear more stories about how we as humans are having a harder time consuming dairy products. Many are lactose intolerant and are moving towards soy products. Yet studies are showing that soya products really are not that healthy and are causing health problems too. Were our bodies really made to consume milk?

Our bodies do need the vitamins, minerals, enzymes and proteins for all of our organs to function properly. If our body cannot digest the dairy products properly, there is the option of using digestive enzymes beforehand. Sometimes our body can digest one product such as cheese better than milk or maybe yogurt is easier on your body.

Being a person with a sensitive stomach, over the years, I found what dairy that I needed to stay away from and also learned that the dairy products go through different processes. I can eat a bit of cheddar cheese and feel okay, yet milk and ice cream will give me a sore stomach. Something to also keep in mind is that I found that in Canada, there is yellow food colouring added to a lot of the cheese which is a chemical that can harm the body. This is especially hard on the kids and can be found in a lot of processed foods. The yellow and red dyes are toxic. I found that in Australia most of their cheese is white and does not have the yellow food dye in it.

If you cannot digest any of the dairy products from cows, goat milk and goat cheese is lactose free. This is a much healthier option for the sensitive tummy (and Mother Earth) than the soy products. Another option is almond milk, which can be found in grocery stores. There are many vegetables and herbs that have a lot of natural calcium and proteins in them. Broccoli is loaded with calcium and you will find the other food products in Chapter 4. There are many people who have lived very healthy lives without dairy, and many that love their dairy and their body needs it. If you are concerned about the dairy and want to consume it, there are a lot more farmers who are farming organically and the products a lot easier to digest.

The main nutrients in the dairy products are as follows:

A: adrenal glands, anemia, infections, bone growth, eyes (night vision), teeth growth.

B2: adrenal glands, birth defects: preventative, blood, eyes, detox, growth, metabolism, nerves, respiratory, skin, thyroid, weight loss

B5: For our adrenal hormones, anti-stress, immune system, metabolism of carbs, fats and proteins and for our neurotransmitters.

B12: anemia, mental health, nervous system, small intestine, red blood cells.

Choline: For helping the other vitamins to work properly. It works with our memory and muscles. It is also used to help treat Alzheimer's, dementia, Friedreich's Ataxia, Gilles de la Tourette's disease, Huntington's disease, manic depression and Tardive dyskinesia.

D: Better absorption of calcium, kidneys, osteoporosis, rickets, teeth

Choline: For helping the other vitamins to work properly. Works with our memory and muscles. It is also used to help treat Alzheimer's, dementia, Friedreich's Ataxia, Gilles de la Tourette's disease, Huntington's disease, manic depression and Tardive dyskinesia.

Folate: For our arteries, bone marrow, brain, DNA, energy production, fingernails, hair, immune system, metabolism, red blood cells, RNA and white blood cells.

Calcium: Anti-cancer, blood (clotting), blood pressure (lower), bones (growth), cholesterol (lowers it), DNA, gums, heart, heartbeat, muscle growth, RNA, and teeth.

Chromium: Kidney support, liver support, regulate the sugar levels, reducing body fat, help the fetus develop properly.

Phosphorus: For the blood: to help clot, bone formation, heart, kidneys, teeth formation. Helps our body process food so that we utilize the vitamins.

L-Lysine: bone development, cold sores, concentration, building block for proteins, hair loss, herpes.

L-Tyrosine: depression, metabolism, nervous system, thyroid gland, pituitary gland, restless legs, weight control.

Interestingly, the B12 is needed to activate the folate in our food, and the lack of this vitamin is also what creates the pallor in vegetarians who are not eating properly. B12 is also needed for our mental health, and a lack of it can cause severe depression.

So many of the nutrients of milk are related to the bone and brain health. Take a good look at the nutrients and see what other food groups can help you to replace these, if you are sensitive to the dairy products. All the food groups are listed under B12. Another way of supplementing your vitamins and minerals is by getting them at the health store. When we are going through a more stressful period in our life, we can get vitamin B supplements or even calcium. Something to keep in mind is that we also need magnesium to assist in the absorption of the calcium. Make sure you talk to qualified staff or your herbalist or naturopath to see what your body requires.

BUTTER

Butter is made from the fat of the fresh milk.

Benefits:
- adrenal glands, bones: health (better absorption of calcium), bone growth, bones/joints/cartilage, nervous system, teeth, thyroid.

Contains:
Vitamins: biotin, D

Minerals: calcium, phosphorous

Other: L-Tyrosine

BUTTERMILK

Buttermilk is made from the liquid that was left over after the butter was churned out of the cream. The sour taste in the milk is from the lactic acid bacteria.

Benefits:
- anti-cancer, antioxidant.

- Other benefits: colon cancer prevention, heart support, immune system, stroke prevention.

Contains:
Vitamins: A, B2 (riboflavin), B3 (niacin), B5 (pantothenic acid), B6 (pyridoxine), B12, choline, folate, inositol, D, E

Minerals: calcium, chromium, magnesium, phosphorous, sodium, zinc

Other: L-lysine, L-tyrosine

CHEESE: COW

When you buy your cheese, try to get the white cheese, as it has no colour additives.

Benefits:
- antibacterial

- Other benefits: adrenal glands, anemia, blood support, bone growth, eyes (night vision), infections (bacterial), mental well-being, metabolism, teeth growth, thyroid.

Contains:
Vitamins: A, B2 (riboflavin), B3 (niacin), B12, choline, folate

Minerals: calcium, chromium, magnesium, phosphorous

Other: L-lysine, L-tyrosine

CHEESE: GOAT

Goat cheese is lactose free and easier for the tummy to digest.

Benefits:
- antibacterial, nervine, relaxant
- Other benefits: adrenal glands, anemia, blood (support), bone growth, DNA, eyes (night vision), hair, infections: bacterial, mental well-being, metabolism, teeth growth, thyroid.

Contains:
Vitamins: A, B1 (thiamin), B2 (riboflavin), B3 (niacin), B5 (pantothenic acid), B6 (pyridoxine), B12, folate, E

Minerals: calcium, iron, magnesium, manganese, phosphorous, potassium, selenium, sodium, zinc

Other: L-lysine, L-tyrosine, omega-6, protein

MILK: COW

Cow's milk has more nutrients than the cheese from the cow.

Benefits:
- antioxidant, nervine, relaxant.
- Other benefits: adrenal glands, anemia, blood, bone growth, eyes (night vision), hair, infections (bacterial), mental well-being, metabolism, teeth growth.

Contains:
Vitamins: A, B2 (riboflavin), B3 (niacin), B5 (pantothenic acid), B12, biotin, choline, folate, inositol, D, E

Minerals: calcium, chromium, magnesium, phosphorous

Other: L-lysine, L-taurine, L-tyrosine

MILK: GOAT

Goat milk can be easier to digest than cow's milk and is lactose free

Benefits:
- antidepressant, antioxidant, relaxant.

- Other benefits: adrenal glands, anemia, blood support, bone growth, DNA, eyes (night vision), hair, infections (bacterial), mental well-being, metabolism, teeth growth, thyroid.

Contains:
Vitamins: A, B2 (riboflavin), B3 (niacin), B5 (pantothenic acid), B12, biotin, choline, folate, inositol, D, E

Minerals: calcium, chromium, magnesium, phosphorous

Other: L-lysine, L-tyrosine

WHEY

Whey is a valuable protein that is now being used in health products such as protein bars and powder formulas for sports and active living lifestyles. Whey is the liquid from the milk that is extracted when making cheese and is also the liquid found on top of the yogurt when you open it up.

Raw milk has two types of proteins when it is first gathered. The proteins are casein and whey. Whey is 20% of the two proteins and found in the watery part of the milk. When the milk is being made into cheese, the whey is what is separated from the cheese and is usually thrown out.

Benefits:
- anti-cancer, antidepressant, anti-inflammatory,

- Other benefits: AIDS, blood pressure (too high), blood sugar (regulate), bone growth, cancer prevention, depression, energy, muscle (inflammation), muscles (support).

Contains:
Vitamins: A, B1 (thiamin), B2 (riboflavin), B3 (niacin), B5 (pantothenic acid), B6 (pyridoxine), B12, C

Minerals: calcium, iron, magnesium, phosphorous, potassium, sodium, zinc

Other: L-tyrosine, protein

YOGURT

Yogurt is best served with no sugar and no fruit. The sugar upsets the floral in our stomach and can contribute to creating more yeast in the body, along with putting stress on the pancreas and blood sugar levels. Yogurt is an excellent food to help correct the bacterial level in our body. Use of man created antibiotics will destroy both the good and bad bacteria in our bodies. The yogurt puts the good bacteria back into the stomach and intestines.

Benefits:
- Other benefits: bone growth, stomach: digestion, yeast infections (probiotic)

Contains:
Vitamins: A, B1 (thiamin), B2 (riboflavin), B3 (niacin), B6 (pyridoxine), B12, folate, inositol, C, D, K

Minerals: calcium, iron, magnesium, phosphorous, potassium, sodium

Other: L-tyrosine, protein

CHAPTER 7

Fruits

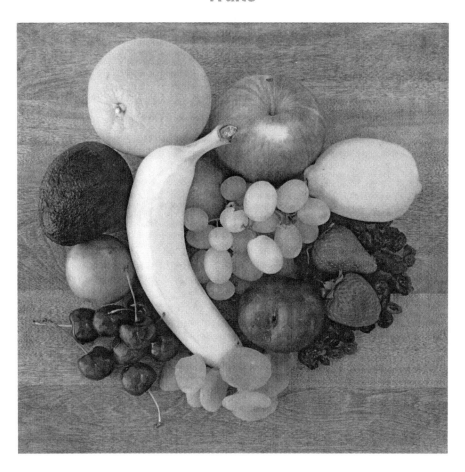

BERRIES ARE A TREASURE CHEST OF ANTIOXIDANTS, ESPECIALLY BLUEBERRIES, CRANBERries and blackberries. Raspberries, strawberries and acai berries are also high on the list. The International Food Information Council points out that many antioxidant-rich foods can be identified by their deep colours, such as the dark red of ripe raspberries or the deep purple of blueberries and blackberries.

FRUIT – BEST WAYS TO CONSUME AND BENEFITS

This winter I started to make a warm drink in the evening, which included some fruit. The odd time it came to mind that drinking a freshly made smoothie with the fruit would be a lot healthier for me. I had just received an email that confirmed what I was thinking. "Don't drink juice that has been heated up. Don't eat cooked fruits because you don't get the nutrients at all. You only get to taste. Cooking destroys all the vitamins." I will be going back to my herbal tea with some honey and ginger in the evening. The fruit smoothies are for in the morning for me.

EATING FRUIT:

We all think eating fruit means just buying fruit, cutting it and just popping it into our mouths. It's not as easy as you think. It's important to know how and when to eat fruit.

What is the correct way of eating fruits? This means that you should not eat your fruits at the end of the meal. Fruits should be eaten on an empty stomach. If you eat fruit first, it will play a major role to detoxify your system, supplying you with a great deal of energy for weight loss and other life activities.

Fruit digests in the stomach a lot faster than the proteins such as meats and breads. If you eat the heavier foods first, the whole meal rots, ferments and turns to acid. The minute the fruit comes into contact with the food in the stomach on top of the other food and digestive juices, the entire mass of food begins to spoil.

So please eat your fruits on an empty stomach or before your meals! You have heard people complaining — "every time I eat watermelon I burp, or when I eat fruit during my meal, my stomach bloats up." None of this should happen if you eat the fruit on an empty stomach. The fruit mixes with the other putrefying food and produces gas, and hence you will bloat! These things can happen when we don't eat the fruit first: greying hair, balding, nervous outburst and dark circles under the eyes.

When you need to drink fruit juice - **include the pulp**. The pulp in the fruit not only provides a fibre for the body, but helps to decrease the sugar high that one can get from drinking just the juice. If you can, with the citrus fruits, try to add the white part (the membrane) as this part of the fruit has the highest content of vitamin C. The pulp also contains a lot of the nutrients we need.

It was interesting to see all the vitamins and minerals in the fruits. The iron was in very low levels, never realizing that iron was in the fruit. Then when I saw that a lot of the fruit had some vitamin K, I was really surprised, as I did not know we had so many options for this vitamin.

FOLLOWING ARE THE MOST COMMON MINERALS AND VITAMINS IN THE FRUIT:

A: adrenal glands, anemia, infections, bone growth, eyes (night vision), teeth growth.

B6: amino acids (better absorption), arthritis: relieves pain, brain support, burning sensations, convulsions, immune system, leg cramps, liver support, nerves.

Folate: arteries, bone marrow, brain, DNA, energy production, fingernails, hair, immune system, metabolism, red blood cells, RNA and white blood cells.

C: allergies, enzyme activation, heart, fatigue, immune system, iron absorption, mental illness, stress, skin (wounds).

K: blood clotting.

Copper: formation of the blood cells, energy, hair, immune support, joints, skin and nerves.

Inositol: For our arteries, bowels, heart muscles, nerves, skeletal muscles and skin.

Iron: blood (red cells), energy and our immune system.

Magnesium: bowels, energy production, heart, insomnia (better sleep), kidneys, muscles and nerves.

Phosphorus: blood (to help clot), bone formation, heart, kidneys, teeth formation. Helps our body process food so that we utilize the vitamins.

Potassium: For our heart, muscles and nervous system.

Zinc: For the immune system, prostate glands, reproductive organs and skin.

FOLLOWING ARE THE FRUITS THAT WE ARE COVERING IN THIS CHAPTER:

apple – apricot - avocado

banana – blackberry - blueberry

cantaloupe - cherry - chokecherry – cranberry – currant (red)

date

fig

goji berry - gooseberry – grapefruit – grape - guava

kiwi

lemon - lime

mango

orange

papaya - passion fruit – peach – pear - pineapple - plum

raspberry - rhubarb

Saskatoon berry - strawberry

tangerine - tomato

watermelon

APPLE

Although an apple has low vitamin C content, it has antioxidants and flavonoids, which enhances the activity of vitamin C. The red delicious, granny smith and gala apples have the highest level of antioxidants in the apple family.

Benefits:
- anti-cancer, antioxidant.

- Other benefits: colon cancer prevention, heart: support, immune system, stroke prevention

Contains:
Vitamins: A, B1 (thiamin), B2 (riboflavin), B3 (niacin), B5 (pantothenic acid), B6 (pyridoxine), inositol, C, K

Minerals: boron, calcium, magnesium, phosphorous, potassium

Other: fibre

Served as:
Apples can be eaten raw, baked, cooked and juiced.

Apples are used in baking, jams, jellies, frozen for the winter and dried as a snack.

Apples are high in pectin that is needed to help jams set.

APRICOT

- Apricots are rich in dietary fibre and antioxidants.

Benefits:
- Antioxidant

- Other benefits: blood cleanse, eyes (mucous membranes and vision), heart support, liver, skin care.

Caution: Those with asthma are warned not to eat dried apricots as they have been treated with sulfite.

Contains:
Vitamins: A, B1 (thiamin), B2 (riboflavin), B3 (niacin), B5 (pantothenic acid), B6 (pyridoxine), inositol, C, K, P

Minerals: calcium, iron, magnesium, manganese, potassium

Other: L-lysine, L-taurine, L-tyrosine, omega-3, omega-6, omega-9, protein

Served as:
Apricots are served raw in salads, dried, baked and preserved in jams, jellies and juices. Apricots can also be frozen to use over the wintertime.

AVOCADO
- Avocado is seen as a vegetable dish, but it does grow on a tree and is a fruit. The vegetable is an amazing source of omega-9. The fat in the avocado is a healthy fat.

Benefits:
- anti-inflammatory, antioxidant.

- Other benefits: blood cleanse and support, bones, heart, skin (care).

Contains:
Vitamins: A, B1 (thiamin), B2 (riboflavin), B3 (niacin), B5 (pantothenic acid), B6 (pyridoxine), choline, folate, inositol, C, E, K

Minerals: calcium, copper, iron, magnesium, manganese, phosphorus, potassium, sodium, zinc

Other: carotenoids, fibre, high fat content, omega-3, omega-6, omega-9

Served as:
Avocado is usually served raw. This fruit is used in Mexican soups.

BANANA
- Bananas are known for their high source of potassium that is good for the heart and helps to lower high blood pressure.

Benefits:
- anti-inflammatory

- Other benefits: blood pressure: too high, bowels, energy, headaches, heart: support, muscle cramps, pesticide (mosquitoes).

Contains:
Vitamins: A, B6 (pyridoxine), biotin, inositol, C

Minerals: copper, iron, magnesium, manganese, phosphorous, potassium

Other: L-tyrosine, fibre

Served as:
Banana can be cooked, baked and eaten raw.

BLACKBERRY

- Blackberries are high in antioxidants, vitamin C and dietary fibre. These properties assist in preventing and reducing the risk of cancer, improve eyesight and reduce heart disease.

Benefits:
- anti-inflammatory, antioxidant, astringent

- Other benefits: anti-aging, autoimmune disease, blood cells (red and white), bone support, breast cancer prevention, cancer fighting, cervical cancer prevention, colon cancer prevention, digestion, estrogen balancing, eyes, heart disease, hot flashes, immune system, menstrual, stomach (gas).

Contains:
Vitamins: A, B3 (niacin), B5 (pantothenic acid), choline, folate, inositol, C, E, K, P

Minerals: calcium, copper, iron, magnesium, manganese, phosphorus, potassium, selenium, zinc

Other: Fibre

Served as:
Blackberries can be served raw in salads, used in fruit drinks, jams, syrups and baking.

BLUEBERRY

- Blueberries are in the top ten for antioxidants that are good for fighting heart disease. This berry has the nutrients to help metabolize carbohydrates, fats and proteins.

Benefits:
- anti-cancer, antioxidant, astringent

- Other benefits: blood sugar: regulate, cancer fighting, diabetes, digestion, heart support, immune support, metabolism.

Contains:
Vitamins: A, B1 (thiamin), B2 (riboflavin), B3 (niacin), B5 (pantothenic acid), B6 (pyridoxine), inositol, C, folate, E, K

Minerals:

calcium, copper, iron, magnesium, manganese, phosphorus, potassium, zinc

Other: fibre, protein

Served as:
Blueberries can be served raw in salads and fruit drinks. This berry can be cooked into sauces, jellies and jams. The berries can be dried or frozen for the winter. Blueberries are used in baking such as in pies and muffins.

CANTALOUPE
- Cantaloupe has a high source of vitamin A (carotenoids).

Benefits:
- Anti-inflammatory, antioxidant.

- Other benefits: bones (support), cancer fighting, eyes, menstruation (irregular periods), metabolism, night vision, skin care, teeth.

Contains:
Vitamins: A, B1 (thiamin), B3 (niacin), B6 (pyridoxine), inositol, folate, C, K

Minerals: copper, iron, magnesium, potassium

Other: fibre

Served as:
Cantaloupe is usually served raw in salads and on its own.

CHERRY
- Cherries are rich in melatonin that reduces the effects of stress and neurological diseases, along with providing a better sleep. The melatonin helps to regulate the blood pressure, lower the heart rate and reduce the chance of a stroke. A powerful antioxidant and cancer prevention.

Benefits:
- anti-cancer, anti-inflammatory, antioxidant

- Other benefits: arthritis, bladder (infection), bladder (support), blood pressure, blood sugar (regulate), bowels (support), brain (memory), breast (support), chronic pain, colon, constipation, fibromyalgia, frozen shoulder, gout, headaches, kidney: support, lung, lupus, muscle (pain), muscle (spasm), neurological system, relaxant, stomach (support).

Contains:
Vitamins: A, B1 (thiamin), B3 (niacin), B5 (pantothenic acid), inositol, C, E, P

Minerals: calcium, copper, iron, magnesium, manganese, phosphorous, potassium

Other: fibre, lutein, protein.

Served as:
Cherries can be eaten raw, place in salads, baked, and preserved in jams and jellies. Cherries can also be pitted and frozen for use over the winter.

CHOKECHERRY
- Chokecherries are high in antioxidants, carotenes, luteins and zeaxanthins. The properties of zeaxanthin can protect us from UV rays and has aided the elderly from age related macular disease in the eyes.

Benefits:
- antioxidant

- Other benefits: bladder (support), eyes (macular disease), kidney infection, kidney (support), skin (care).

Contains:
Vitamins: A, B3 (niacin), B6 (pyridoxine), folate, inositol, C, E, K

Minerals: calcium, iron, magnesium, manganese, potassium

Other: fibre, lutein.

Served as:
Chokecherries can be eaten raw, cooked, baked or preserved in jellies, jams and syrups.

CRANBERRY

- Cranberries are in the top ten for antioxidants that assist with fighting off bacterial infections, cancer, diabetes and inflammation. Cranberries have a large amount of phenolic flavonoid phytochemicals that help the body to fight the aging process and neurological diseases.

Benefits:
- anti-aging, antibacterial, anti-diabetic, anti-inflammatory, antioxidant, antiseptic

- Other benefits: anti-aging, bladder (cleanser), bladder support, blood (regulate HDL, LDL levels), cancer (fighting), diabetes, heart (support), infections (bacterial), inflammation, kidney stones (preventative), liver, neurological diseases, teeth (cavity prevention) (Streptococcus mutants: a negative bacteria), teeth (infections), urinary (infections), urinary support, urinary tract.

Contains:
Vitamins: A, B5 (pantothenic acid), B6 (pyridoxine), inositol, C, E, K

Minerals: calcium, copper, iron, magnesium, manganese, phosphorous, potassium, zinc

Served as:
Cranberries can be used in drinks, fruit cocktails, sauces, jams, jellies, dried as a snack or in salads and sandwich fillers. Used in baking muffins, pies and breads.

Note: Cranberries do not have a long shelf life, but can be frozen to retain the nutrients and used at a later date.

CURRANT (RED)

- The high fibre content of currants helps to reduce cholesterol, and lowers the blood sugar levels. Currants are high in vitamin C and K.

Benefits:
- antioxidant

- Other benefits: blood: clotting, blood sugar (regulate), cancer preventing, cholesterol (lower), heart (cardiovascular), immune system, prostate (support) - cancer preventative.

Contains:
Vitamins: A, B2 (riboflavin), B3 (niacin), B6 (pyridoxine), folate, inositol, C, K, P

Minerals: calcium, copper, iron, magnesium, manganese, phosphorous, potassium, selenium, zinc

Other: fibre, protein

Served as:
Used in baked goods, jams and jellies.

DATE
- Dates are natural source of sugar. The iron found in dates is needed for our red blood cells and increases the oxygen in our blood. High in fibre.

Benefits:
- anti-cancer, antioxidant

- Other benefits: anemia, blood (red blood cells), bowel support, cancer preventative, cholesterol (lower LDL), colon (cancer preventative), colon: support, eyes, heart (support), liver.

Contains:
Vitamins: A, B2 (riboflavin), B3 (niacin), B5 (pantothenic acid), B6 (pyridoxine), folate, inositol, K

Minerals: calcium, copper, iron, magnesium, manganese, potassium

Other: fibre

Served as:
Used in baking, chutney, flavourings, roasted and in vinegars.

Dates are used in raw food balls.

FIG
- Figs are high in fibre, minerals and natural sugars. Figs are high in antioxidant properties: vitamins A, E and K. Even though figs are high in a natural sugar, they help to regulate the blood sugar levels.

Benefits:
- anti-cancer, antioxidant

- Other benefits: blood sugar (regulate), bowel support, cancer fighting, heart (support), liver support.

Contains:
Vitamins: A, B6 (pyridoxine), inositol, C, E, K

Minerals:
calcium, copper, iron, magnesium, manganese, potassium

Other: fibre

Served as:
Used in baking and desserts.

Served with cheese and crackers.

Dates can be roasted and used as a coffee substitute.

Figs were/are used in poultices for tumours, warts and wounds.

GOJI BERRY

- Though goji berries have just become a superfood in the west, research shows that this berry has been used in Chinese medicine for over 6000 years.

Benefits:
- anti-cancer, antioxidant
- Other benefits: blood cleanser, brain support (function), cancer prevention, heart disease prevention, immune system, liver support.

Contains:
Vitamins: A, B2 (riboflavin), inositol, C

Minerals:
calcium, copper, iron, potassium, selenium, zinc

Other: fibre

Served as:
Used in juices, baking, salads and as a dried berry.

GOOSEBERRY

- The gooseberry bush originated in Europe. They are grown in Asia and Africa. Gooseberry should not be planted within 1000 feet of white pines, as the plant can host a deadly virus that affects the white pines.

Benefits:
- anti-cancer, anti-inflammatory, antioxidant

- Other benefits: blood (cleanse and support), cancer prevention, diabetes (blood sugar regulator), hair loss prevention, scurvy, skin care (tone).

Contains:
Vitamins: A, B1 (thiamin), B5 (pantothenic acid), B6 (pyridoxine), folate, inositol, C

Minerals:

calcium, iron, magnesium, potassium

Other: fibre, omega-3

Served as:
Used in juices, pies, and sauces for meat dishes.

GRAPE / RAISIN

- There are three major types of grapes: European, North American and the French hybrids.
- The skin colour of the grape is dependent on the properties. The green to white grapes has more tannins, the catechin, which is an antioxidant. The red-purple grapes are rich in anthocyanins. Both are antioxidants and are found in the skin and seed of the grape.
- The iron level in raisins is high than in the fresh grape stage.

Benefits:
- anti-cancerous, antifungal, anti-inflammatory, antimicrobial, antioxidant
- Other benefits: allergies, Alzheimer's, arteries, arteries (plaque build-up), blood (cleanse and support), colon cancer prevention, heart disease, infections (fungus), nerve disease, prostate support (cancer prevention), stroke prevention.

Contains:
Vitamins: A, B1 (thiamin), B2 (riboflavin), B3 (niacin), B5 (pantothenic acid), B6 (pyridoxine), folate, inositol, C, E, K, P

Minerals: boron, calcium, copper, iron, magnesium, manganese, phosphorous, potassium, zinc

Other: fibre, protein

Served as:
Grapes can be served fresh in salads. They are used as a juice, preserved in jams and jellies. Grapes can be frozen whole or dried to use as raisins.

Grapes are best stored in the fridge.

GRAPEFRUIT

- Grapefruit, lemons, limes and oranges have a high level of bioflavonoids that are found in the white membrane between the fruit and skin. They are very high in vitamin C.

Benefits:
- anti-cancer, antioxidant

- Other benefits: blood pressure (regulate), heart support, immune system.

Caution: If you are on heart medication, you must be careful when eating grapefruit. Consult with your health provider first.

Contains:
Vitamins: A, B1 (thiamin), B2 (riboflavin), B5 (pantothenic acid), B6 (pyridoxine), choline, folate, inositol, C, E, P

Minerals: calcium, copper, magnesium, manganese, phosphorous, potassium, zinc

Other: fibre

Served as:
Grapefruit is served raw, eaten alone or in salads.

This fruit can be used in juices. Make sure you include the pulp.

GUAVA

- Guava is high in vitamin C and good for the immune system.

- A lot of vitamin A (anti-cancer properties), five times more than oranges and high in fibre.

Benefits:
- anti-cancer, antioxidant

- Other benefits: blood pressure (regulate), bowel support, cancer preventative, constipation, heart rate (regulate), prostate support (cancer preventative), skin care, UV ray protection.

Contains:
Vitamins: A, B1 (thiamin), B2 (riboflavin), B3 (niacin), B5 (pantothenic acid), B6 (pyridoxine), folate, inositol, C, E, K

Minerals: calcium, iron, magnesium, manganese, phosphorous, potassium, selenium, zinc

Other: fibre, protein

Served as:
Eaten as a snack, added to salads.

Used in jams, jellies and juices.

Guava has been turned into a cheese or paste.

KIWI
- The kiwi is a tiny but mighty fruit.
- The vitamin C content is five times that of an orange. It is high in vitamin E, magnesium and potassium.

Benefits:
- anti-cancer, anti-inflammatory, antioxidant
- Other benefits: arthritis, blood sugar (regulator), bowel support, colon cancer, digestion, DNA protection, immune system, osteoarthritis, respiratory (discomfort), respiratory (support), rheumatoid arthritis.

Contains:
Vitamins: A, B6 (pyridoxine), folate, inositol, C, E, K

Minerals: calcium, copper, iron, magnesium, manganese, potassium

Other: fibre, protein

Served as:
Kiwi is usually eaten raw, but can be found in some baking and pies.

LEMON
- Lemons have more healing properties than the other citrus fruits.
- Grapefruit, lemons, limes and oranges have a lot of bioflavonoids that is found in the white membrane between the fruit and skin. This is a source that is very high in vitamin C.
- The naringenin in the lemon is an anti-inflammatory, antioxidant and helps to repair any DNA damage.

Benefits:
- antibacterial, anti-cancer, anti-inflammatory, antioxidant, *antiscorbutic*, antiviral, astringent
- Other benefits: arthritis, blood cleanser, cancer prevention, colds, digestion, DNA protection, eye (sight), hearth support, immune system, kidney stones, liver (cleanser), mucous membranes, scurvy, skin (care), skin (infections), weight reduction.

Contains:
Vitamins: A, B1 (thiamin), B3 (niacin), B5 (pantothenic acid), B6 (pyridoxine), folate, inositol, C, E, P

Minerals: calcium, copper, iron, magnesium, phosphorus, potassium, zinc

Other: fibre, lutein

Served as:
- Lemons are best serve fresh and uncooked. Lemons can be sliced up and added to water, used as a garnish with meals.

- The juice is used in many recipes and added as a nice citric tang to sauces.

- If you are using lemon juice for preserving, you need to use the process lemon juice as it has the proper acidic level that is required for safe preserving.

- When using lemon as a juice in drinks it is good to use both the juice and pulp. The pulp adds the fibre we need and also helps to maintain a better blood sugar level.

- The rind of lemons can be used by grating it and adding it to your dishes.

- The oils from the lemon peels can help to soften the hands with its astringent properties.

LIME

- Grapefruit, lemons, limes and oranges have a lot of bioflavonoids that is found in the white membrane between the fruit and skin. This is a source that has a very high amount of vitamin C.

Benefits:
- anti-cancer, ant-oxidant, antiscorbutic

- Other benefits: blood cleanser, immune system, liver cleanser, scurvy.

Contains:
Vitamins: A, B3 (niacin), B5 (pantothenic acid), folate, inositol, C

Minerals:

calcium, copper, iron, magnesium, phosphorous, potassium

Other: fibre, protein

Served as:
Limes are like the lemons and can be used in juices, baking and cooking.

All fruit juices are best used without being warmed up.

MANGO

- Mangos originated in India and a member of the drupe family.

Benefits:
- anti-cancer

- Other benefits: asthma, bone support, breast cancer, colon cancer, diabetes prevention, digestion, eyes (UV rays), hair, heart support, macular support, metabolism, skin (care).

Contains:
Vitamins: A, B1 (thiamin), B2 (riboflavin), B3 (niacin), B5 (pantothenic acid), B6 (pyridoxine), folate, inositol, C, E, K

Minerals: calcium, copper, iron, magnesium, phosphorous, potassium, selenium

Other: fibre, protein

Served as:
Mango can be eaten alone or served in many fruit dishes and juices.

ORANGE

- Grapefruit, lemons, limes and oranges have a lot of vitamin P (bioflavonoids) that is found in the white membrane between the fruit and skin. Oranges have a large amount of in vitamin C.

Benefits:
- anti-cancer, antioxidant

- Other benefits: blood cleanser, cholesterol (lower), colds, colon cancer, heart (support), immune system, kidney: stone, liver.

Contains:
Vitamins: A, B1 (thiamin), B2 (riboflavin), B3 (niacin), B5 (pantothenic acid), B6 (pyridoxine), folate, inositol, C, E, K, P

Minerals: calcium, copper, iron, magnesium, manganese, phosphorous, potassium, selenium, zinc

Other: fibre, protein

Served as:
- When using orange as a juice in drinks it is good to use both the juice and pulp. The pulp adds the fibre we need and also helps to maintain a better blood sugar level.

PAPAYA

- Papaya has received top awards for high vitamin C content, high in antioxidants.

- Papaya has the enzyme called papain. Papain assists with our digestion. Papaya can be found in a digestion enzyme formula.

Benefits:
- anti-inflammatory, antioxidant

- Other benefits: arthritis, blood (cholesterol), *colon cancer prevention,* digestion, eyes, heart *(cardiovascular system),* heart (support), skin (burns).

Contains:
Vitamins: A, B3 (niacin), B5 (pantothenic acid), folate, inositol, C, E, K

Minerals: calcium, copper, iron, magnesium, phosphorous, potassium, selenium, zinc

Other: enzyme, fibre, protein

Served as:
Papaya can be used to make meat tender.

Papaya can be eaten in salads and found in juices.

PASSION FRUIT
- Passion fruit is known for its high amount of fibre.

Benefits:
- anti-inflammatory, antioxidant

- Other benefits: arthritis, asthma, blood circulation, blood cleanser, blood pressure (too high), bone - support (density), bowel support, cancer prevention, digestion, eyesight, immune system, relaxant, skin (care), sleep.

Contains:
Vitamins: A, B2 (riboflavin), B3 (niacin), B6 (pyridoxine), choline, folate, inositol, C, K

Minerals:

calcium, copper, iron, magnesium, phosphorous, potassium, selenium, sodium, zinc

Other: fibre, protein

Served as:
Served on its own or with cheese. Can be used in salads and juice drinks.

PEACH
- Peaches help with treating cancer, cholesterol (lowering), eyesight and immune system.

Benefits:
- anti-aging, anti-cancer, antioxidant, anti-tumour

- Other benefits: blood (support), bone (health), breast cancer prevention, cancer prevention, heart support, hypokalemia (lack of potassium), muscle support (muscular system), nerves - support (nervous system), neurodegenerative diseases, skin (care), teeth, tumours.

Contains:
Vitamins: A, B1 (thiamin), B2 (riboflavin), B3 (niacin), B5 (pantothenic acid), choline, folate, inositol, C, E, K

Minerals: calcium, copper, iron, magnesium, manganese, phosphorous, potassium, zinc

Other: fibre, protein

Served as:
Peaches are served fresh, in baking, as juices and in pies.

PEAR
- The skin of the pear contains three to four times phenolic phytonutrients than the flesh of the fruit. These nutrients include anti-cancer, anti-inflammatory and antioxidants.

Benefits:
- anti-cancer, anti-inflammatory, antioxidants
- Other benefits: blood cleanse, bowels (support), diabetes 2, digestion, heart (support), liver, muscle inflammation.

Contains:
Vitamins: A, B3 (niacin), B5 (pantothenic acid), folate, inositol, C, K

Minerals: boron, calcium, copper, iron, magnesium, manganese, phosphorous, potassium, zinc

Other: fibre, protein

Served as:
Pears can be used in a variety of salads, served with cheese, in juices and canned for the winter.

PINEAPPLE
- The core of the pineapple contains bromelain, a digestive aid for our stomach. Pineapple is a good for reducing the effects of arthritis.

Benefits:
- antibacterial, anti-cancer, anti-inflammatory, antioxidants
- Other benefits: arthritis, blood circulation, bones (health), colds, coughs, digestion, eyes, heart (support), immune system, muscle (inflammation), parasites, respiratory (support), weight (reduction).

Contains:
Vitamins: A, B1 (thiamin), B6 (pyridoxine), folate, inositol, C

Minerals: calcium, copper, iron, magnesium, manganese, potassium

Other: fibre, enzymes, protein, omega-3, omega-6

Served as:
Pineapple is served alone, in salads and in juices.

PLUM / PRUNE

- Black plums are high in antioxidants and good for the immune system and for fighting cancers. Plumes help our body to absorb the iron from our food better.

Benefits:
- anti-aging, anti-inflammatory, antioxidant

- Other benefits: aging, anemia, bowels, cancer prevention, constipation, immune system, mental well-being, muscle (inflammation).

Contains:
Vitamins: A, B1 (thiamin), B3 (niacin), B5 (pantothenic acid), folate, inositol, C, E, K, P

Minerals: calcium, copper, iron, magnesium, phosphorous, potassium, zinc

Other: fibre

Served as:
Plums, like the other fruits, can be eaten solo or in salads.

Prunes are the dried plums and make an excellent travel snack.

RASPBERRY

- Raspberries are in the top ten for being high in antioxidants and large amount of vitamin C.

Benefits:
- anti-inflammatory, antioxidant

- Other benefits: arthritis, blood (cleanse), blood pressure (regulate), blood sugar (regulate), cancer prevention, diabetes, digestion, energy, eyes, heart (cardiovascular support), heart (support), immune system, liver (cleanse), menstrual cramping, skin (care), weight reduction.

Contains:
Vitamins: A, B3 (niacin), B5 (pantothenic acid), B6 (pyridoxine), folate, inositol, C, E, K

Minerals: calcium, copper, iron, magnesium, manganese, phosphorous, potassium, zinc

Other: fibre, protein

Served as:
Raspberry can be found in many baking dishes and pies. Used in juices, sauces, syrups and vinegars.

RHUBARB

- Rhubarb is considered as a vegetable, but in America it is used as a fruit. The leaves are high in oxalic acid that can make us very sick. The higher level of vitamin K provides support for the brain cells and helps with our cognitive skills. This helps to prevent Alzheimer's disease.

Benefits:
- anti-cancer, antioxidant

- Other benefits: Alzheimer's disease, blood circulation, bone health (protection), bowels, brain cells (cognitive skills) constipation, digestion, heart (cardiovascular), heart: support, metabolism - stimulate (to reduce weight gain), stomach (gas).

Contains:
Vitamins: A, B3 (niacin), B5 (pantothenic acid), folate, inositol, C, E, K

Minerals:

calcium, germanium, iron, magnesium, manganese, phosphorous, potassium, selenium, zinc

Other: fibre, lutein, protein

Served as:
Rhubarb can be made into a juice. Being bitter one needs a bit of a sweetener.

Used in baking and pies.

SASKATOON BERRY

- The trees are found in British Columbia, Alberta, Saskatchewan and Manitoba in Canada, from the riverbanks to the hills. The fruit has a taste like almonds, almost nutty tasting, yet with a distinct taste that can be detected when a small amount is mixed with other berries.

- Studies have found that the anthocyanins, the antioxidant pigments from fruit and veggies, have a fighting compound against fat cells. This can be used in the prevention of weight gain.

- This fruit is more powerful than blueberries, raspberries and strawberries.

Benefits:
- anti-aging, anti-inflammatory, antioxidant

- Other benefits: arthritis, blood sugar (regulate), cholesterol level (reduce), colon, heart (cardiovascular), immune system, muscle (inflammation), muscle (pain).

Contains:
Vitamins: A, B2 (riboflavin), B5 (pantothenic acid), folate, inositol, C, E

Minerals: calcium, iron, manganese, potassium, sodium, zinc

Other: fibre, protein

Served as:
Saskatoon berries can be made into beer, cider, juice and wines. This berry can be eaten in cereals, trail mix and pemmican. For the winter the berry can be processed into jams and jellies and used in pies and other baking.

-The fruit has a taste like almonds, almost nutty tasting, yet it has a distinct taste that can be detected when a small amount is mixed with other berries.

STRAWBERRY

- Strawberries are one of the fruits that you should try to get organic. This fruit is sprayed more for pesticides and herbicides. Try to buy organic. - Strawberries have the highest total antioxidant power among major fruits and protect the body from cancer.

Benefits:
- antioxidant

- Other benefits: blood cleanser, blood sugar level (regulate), cancer prevention, heart (cardiovascular support), heart (support), immune system.

Contains:
Vitamins: B3 (niacin), B5 (pantothenic acid), B6 (pyridoxine), biotin, folate, inositol, C, E, K

Minerals: calcium, copper, iron, magnesium, manganese, phosphorus, potassium, selenium, zinc

Other: fibre, protein, omega-3

Served as:
Strawberries can be found in a lot of dishes. Raw in salads and solo. Used in baking and preserves..

TANGERINE

- Tangerines are known for their fresh citric aroma.

- Tangerines added to the bath water will help your hair. Eating tangerines (B12) will slow down the greying of your hair. Tangerine oil is a good antiseptic for wounds.

Benefits:
- anti-aging, antioxidant, antiseptic, antispasmodic, relaxant

- Other benefits: anxiety, bone health, depression, diabetes prevention, digestion, eye health, hair (grey), heart support, immune system, skin cancer, skin care (natural collagen), skin (regenerative), skin (wounds), weight (reduction).

Contains:
Vitamins: A, B1 (thiamin), B2 (riboflavin), B3 (niacin), B5 (pantothenic acid), B6 (pyridoxine), B12, folate, inositol, C, E

Minerals: calcium, copper, iron, magnesium, manganese, phosphorous, potassium, zinc

Other: fibre, protein

Served as:
Eaten raw, in salads and juices.

TOMATO

- Tomato is a fruit, as it grows on a tree. The combination of the vitamin C and E is what makes tomatoes an excellent support for the heart and cardiovascular system. Tomatoes are high in antioxidants and known for their lutein content. High in C, Biotin, Molybdenum and K.

Benefits:
- anti-cancer, anti-inflammatory, antioxidant

-Other benefits: Alzheimer's, blood (cleanser/support), bones (support), breast cancer, cancer prevention, cholesterol (lower), eyes, heart (cardiovascular), kidney (support), liver (cleanse/support), lung: cancer, prostate cancer, prostate support.

Contains:
Vitamins: A, B1 (thiamin), B3 (niacin), B5 (pantothenic acid), B6 (pyridoxine), biotin, folate, C, E, K

Minerals: calcium, copper, iron, magnesium, manganese, molybdenum, phosphorous, potassium, zinc

Other: fibre, protein

Served as:
Tomatoes can be eaten raw and cooked. Even though the tomato plant is a fruit, it is used in many vegetable dishes.

WATERMELON

- Coolest thirst quencher as it is 92% water.

- Watermelon has a lot of glutathione, which helps boost our immune system.

- The watermelon is also a key source of lycopene, which is the cancer fighting oxidant.

Benefits:
- anti-inflammatory, antioxidants

- Other benefits: blood cleanser, bones (support), cancer prevention, heart (support), immune system, kidney support, liver (cleanse and support)

Contains:
Vitamins: A, B1 (thiamin), B3 (niacin), B5 (pantothenic acid), B6 (pyridoxine), inositol, C

Minerals: calcium, copper, iron, magnesium, manganese, phosphorous, potassium, selenium, zinc

Other: protein

Served as:
Watermelon has always been a fun summer treat in salads or alone.

Fruit is an amazing food that can be added to just about any dish.

Mother Earth has provided us with a food that can be both sweet and sour.

CHAPTER 8

Grains

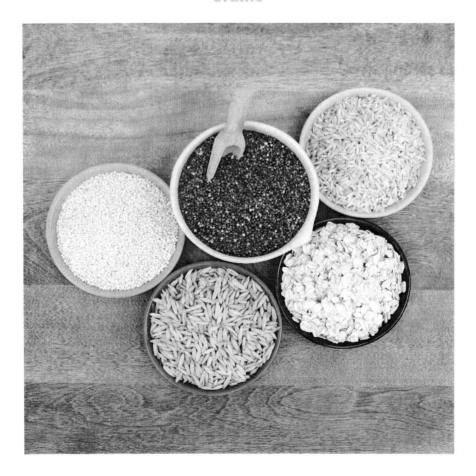

GRAINS HAVE BEEN A STAPLE FOR A THOUSAND YEARS. QUINOA HAS BEEN FOUND IN archeological dig sites. Grains are used in baking, breads, cereals for breakfast and with other recipes. The Natives used the ground flour from the local grains to bake bannock. The Europeans did a lot of baking. Grains are used as a staple in breads, cereals and in meals such as rice and quinoa.

Many of the grains have a lot of the B Vitamins: B1 is a great antioxidant, used for building the blood and blood circulation, brain function, digestion, energy, metabolism and muscle tone.

B2 is for the blood to build the red cells, enhances the anti-body growth, and helps to restore the blood. It also helps with carpal tunnel, syndrome, eyesight, hair, metabolism, nails, pregnancy (for the baby) and skin.

B6 is for the blood (red cell formation), brain function, cholesterol (lowers it), DNA repair, enzyme activation, immune system, mental health, nervous system, physical health, RNA repair, water retention and so much more.

The other vitamins that were in most of the grains:

Biotin: For the adrenal glands, metabolism, nervous system, reproductive tract and skin. Absorption of protein and fatty acids.

Folate: For our arteries, bone marrow, brain, DNA, energy production, fingernails, hair, immune system, metabolism, red blood cells, RNA and white blood cells.

Inositol: For our arteries, bowels, heart muscles, nerves, skeletal muscles and skin.

PABA: For reducing arthritis inflammation, grey hair (stress), intestinal flora, red blood cells, skin (reduces effects of sun rays), skin diseases and toxins from the environment.

E: This is good for cardiovascular disorders, endocrine glands, fatty acid protection, healthy heart, immune system, nervous system, PMS and healing the skin.

An interesting fact about the grains is that they have a lot of the minerals that our bones need and the iron for our blood.

Boron: Used for our bones, brain function and mental alertness. Boron helps the body to metabolize calcium, phosphorus and magnesium. It also helps to derive energy from the fats and sugar.

Iron: Good for blood (red cells), energy and our immune system.

Magnesium: Good for bowels, energy production, heart, insomnia (better sleep), kidneys, muscles and nerves.

Manganese: For blood sugar regulation, bone growth, cartilage, joints, immune system, metabolism (protein and fats) and for our nerves (calming).

Phosphorus: For the blood (to help clot), bone formation, heart, kidneys, teeth formation. Helps our body process food so that we utilize the vitamins.

Potassium: For our heart, muscles and nervous system.

Zinc: For the immune system, prostate glands, reproductive organs and skin.

Today, a lot of people have a have a hard time digesting some of the grains. Some need to use oat flour in their baking or non- gluten flour products. There are two theories about why some cannot digest the wheats. The first is that the gluten is what causes the bloating and stomach cramping. The other is that this is happening because of all the toxic chemicals that are being used for pesticides, the GMO seeds and the fertilizers that are being applied. Again, if we can buy organic or find the grains that our belly is happy with, we are able to add another amazing food group to our table.

BARLEY

Barley is high in antioxidants.

Benefits:
- antibacterial, anti-cancer, anti-inflammatory, anti- oxidant

- Other benefits: anemia, blood support, candida, herpes, leprosy, prostate gland, syphilis and tuberculosis.

Contains:
Vitamins: B1 (thiamin), B2 (riboflavin), B6 (pyridoxine), biotin, folate, inositol, PABA

Minerals: boron, chromium, copper, iron, magnesium, manganese, phosphorous, potassium, vanadium, zinc

BUCKWHEAT

Buckwheat can be used in place of oatmeal or rice. Even though buckwheat is not a true cereal, it is treated like a grain. This plant is a fruit that is related to rhubarb. Buckwheat is good for those who are sensitive to the wheat or protein glutens.

Benefits:
- anti-inflammatory, antioxidant

- Other benefits: adrenal glands, arteries, blood clotting, blood pressure (too high), blood sugar (regulate), bone: support, bowels, cholesterol (to lower), gall bladder, gall stones (preventative), hair, heart (cardiovascular support), immune system, liver, muscle (inflammation), nerves (calming), prostate (support).

Contains:
Vitamins: B1 (thiamin), B2 (riboflavin, B5 (pantothenic acid, B6 (pyridoxine), biotin, choline, folate, inositol, E, K, P

Minerals: boron, calcium, copper, iron, magnesium, manganese, phosphorous, potassium, selenium, vanadium, zinc

Other: L-glutamine, L-lysine, L-tyrosine, omega-3, fibre, lutein, rutin

CEREAL GRAIN

From what I understand, the cereal grain is a mixture of grains. The following nutrients are common with all of them.

Benefits:
- anti-inflammatory, antioxidant

- Other benefits: arteries, blood support, bowel support, cholesterol (to lower), DNA, heart (support).

Contains:
Vitamins: B1 (thiamin), B2 (riboflavin). B6 (pyridoxine), biotin, choline, inositol

Minerals: boron, chromium, iron, manganese, molybdenum, vanadium, zinc

CORN

Corn is a vegetable that is fun to eat and is found in many dishes. This vegetable is eaten around the world and comes in many colours. Corn is used whole as a cooked vegetable and can be use dried and ground up for flour. Corn produces a variety of antioxidants, depending on the variety.

Caution: Corn, along with pork, can be hard for the body to digest. Some of the varieties of corn have been changed (GMO) to produce bigger crops and bigger heads of corn.

Benefits:
- anti-inflammatory, antioxidant

- Other benefits (blood support), bowels, heart, liver, muscle inflammation, nerves.

Contains:
Vitamins: B1 (thiamin), B2 (riboflavin), B6 (pyridoxine), biotin, folate, inositol, PABA

Minerals: boron, chromium, copper, iron, magnesium, manganese, phosphorous, potassium, vanadium, zinc

Other: fibre, lutein

COUSCOUS

Couscous is a tiny grain and is mostly used in salads and soups. The origin of it is unknown, yet evidence shows that it was used in cooking back as far back as 238 B.C.

Benefits:
- anti-inflammatory, antioxidants

- Other benefits: arteries, arthritis, blood support, bones, DNA, hair, muscle relaxant, skin care.

Contains:
Vitamins: folate, inositol, PABA

Minerals: chromium

MILLET
Millet is high in antioxidants

Benefits:
- anti-inflammatory, antioxidant

- Other benefits: adrenal glands, arteries, blood support, bone (support), bowels, hair, heart (support), liver, muscles (inflammation), muscle support, nerves, skin care, UV Ray protection.

Contains:
Vitamins: B1 (thiamin), B2 (riboflavin), B6 (pyridoxine), biotin, inositol, PABA

Minerals: boron, chromium, iron, magnesium, manganese, phosphorous, potassium, vanadium, zinc

OAT / OATMEAL
Oats are high in antioxidants. Oatmeal is used to help reduce the effects of skin inflammation due to chicken pox, dry skin and eczema. Oats is also another good grain for those who are glutton sensitive.

Benefits:
- antibacterial, anti-inflammatory, antioxidant

- Other benefits: adrenal glands, arteries, blood cleanse and support, blood clotting, bone support, bowels, eczema, hair (support), heart (cardiovascular support), liver, muscle (inflammation), muscle (support), nerves, prostate support, skin care, skin (eczema), skin (infections).

Contains:
Vitamins: B1 (thiamin), B2 (riboflavin), B6 (pyridoxine), biotin, inositol, PABA, E, K, P

Minerals: boron, calcium, chromium, copper, iron, manganese, phosphorous, potassium, selenium, vanadium, zinc

QUINOA
Quinoa is known as one of the ancient grains.

Benefits:
- anti-inflammatory, antioxidant

- Other benefits: adrenal glands, arteries, blood (support), bone (support), bowels, hair (support), heart (cardiovascular support), liver, muscles (inflammation), nerves, skin care.

Contains:
Vitamins: B1 (thiamin), B2 (riboflavin), B3 (niacin), B6 (pyridoxine), folate, inositol, PABA, E

Minerals: boron, calcium, copper, iron, magnesium, manganese, phosphorous, potassium, selenium, sodium, zinc

RICE: BROWN

Brown rice is healthier than the white rice. The starch level is lot lower than the white rice.

Brown rice has a protein but not a complete protein. To make it a complete protein, you would combine the brown rice with beans, nuts, seeds or wheat.

Benefits:
- antioxidants

- Other benefits: adrenal glands, arteries, blood support, bowels, hair (support), heart (support), liver, muscle (support), nerves (support), skin care.

Contains:
Vitamins: B1 (thiamin), B6 (pyridoxine), biotin, folate, PABA, E

Minerals: boron, chromium, iron, magnesium, manganese, phosphorous, potassium, selenium, silicon, vanadium, zinc

Other: protein

RICE: WHITE

White rice, white flour, white potatoes and sugar all are products that are not healthy for the human body as it is harder to break down properly along with being starchy foods.

Benefits:
- adrenal glands, arteries, blood support, bone (support), hair: support, heart (support), skin care.

Contains:
Vitamins: B1 (thiamin), B6 (pyridoxine), biotin, folate, PABA, E

Minerals: boron, chromium, iron, magnesium, manganese, phosphorous, potassium, silicon, vanadium, zinc

RYE & RYE FLOUR

Rye grain and rye flour is loaded with nutrients and one of the healthiest grains.

Benefits:
- anti-cancer, anti-inflammatory, antioxidant

- Other benefits: adrenal glands, arteries, asthma, blood sugar regulator, bone support, bowels, breast support, cancer prevention, diabetes 2, gall stones (prevention), hair, heart (cardiovascular) support, liver, muscles (inflammation), nerves (calming), post menopause, prostate (inflammation), prostate support, skin care, UV ray protection.

Contains:
Vitamins: B1 (thiamin), B2 (riboflavin), B5 (pantothenic acid), B6 (pyridoxine), biotin, PABA, K, P

Minerals: boron, chromium, copper, iron, manganese, phosphorous, potassium, vanadium, zinc

SPELT

Spelt is known as a wheat. Research shows that this grain has been used since 5000 B.C.

Benefits:
- anti-inflammatory, antioxidant

- Other benefits: adrenal glands, arteries, blood support, bone support, bowels, hair support, heart (cardiovascular support), liver, muscles (inflammation), nerves (calming), skin care.

Contains:
Vitamins: B1 (thiamin), B2 (riboflavin), B3 (niacin), B6 (pyridoxine), folate, E

Minerals: boron, calcium, copper, iron, magnesium, manganese, phosphorous, potassium, selenium, sodium, zinc

WHEAT

Wheat has a protein that our body needs, but it is not a complete protein. To make it a complete protein, you would combine the wheat with beans or rice.

Wheat bran is known for its high fibre content and high level of magnesium.

Benefits:
- anti-inflammatory, antioxidant

- Other benefits: adrenal glands, arteries, blood support, bone support, bowels, hair, heart (cardiovascular support), depression, liver, muscles, nerves (calming), prostate support, skin care.

Contains:
Vitamins: B1 (thiamin), B2 (riboflavin), B3 (niacin), B5 (pantothenic acid), B6 (pyridoxine), biotin, choline, folate, inositol, PABA, E, K, P

Minerals: boron, calcium, chromium, iron, magnesium, manganese, phosphorous, potassium, vanadium, zinc

Other: fibre, protein

WHEAT BRAN

Wheat bran is known for its high fibre content and large amount of magnesium.

Benefits:
- anti-inflammatory, antioxidant

- Other benefits: adrenal glands, arteries, blood support, bone (support), bowels, hair (support), heart (cardiovascular support), liver cleanse, muscles, nerves (support), skin care.

Contains
Vitamins: B1 (thiamin), B2 (riboflavin), B3 (niacin), B6 (pyridoxine), choline, folate, E

Minerals: calcium, iron, magnesium, manganese, phosphorous, potassium, selenium, zinc

Other: fibre, protein

WHEAT GERM

Wheat Germ is the embrio of the wheat seed.

Benefits:
- anti-inflammatory, antioxidant

- Other benefits: adrenal glands, arteries, blood support, bone (support), bowels, brain, hair (support), heart (cardiovascular support), liver, muscles, nerves (support), skin care.

Contains:
Vitamins: B1 (thiamin), B2 (riboflavin), B3 (niacin), B6 (pyridoxine), B12, folate, E

Minerals: calcium, chromium, copper, germanium, iodine, magnesium, manganese, phosphorous, potassium, selenium, sodium, zinc

Other: omega-3, omega-6

CHAPTER 9

Herbs and Other Healing Plants

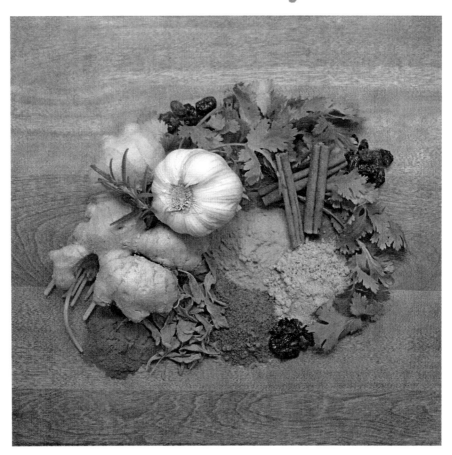

I HEARD MANY YEARS AGO THAT NO MATTER WHERE YOU ARE ON THE PLANET WE CALL Mother Earth, we should have the medicine for any toxin that presents itself.

Many years ago, my cousin introduced me to the power of herbs. I loved to cook healthy meals, but did not realize how amazing these tasty herbs I was using were for healing your body. Herbs that were growing in my gardens and yard, plants found in the forest, out in the prairie, they are everywhere. Hopefully we have covered most of the herbs that you use for cooking, along with providing some amazing information on other plants that can bless our home and table.

This chapter is about herbs, some that I use in my own home and some that are well known for their healing properties. A person can spend a lifetime studying herbs. This is only some of the herbs that are available to us. I suggest that you do research for what is available in your own region.

agrimony - alfalfa - aloe vera – amaranth – angelica - anise seed and oil - arnica - Ashwagandha - astragalus

balm of Gilead - barberry - basil - bayberry - bearberry (uva-ursi) - bilberry - birch - bistort

black cohosh – black walnut – blessed thistle – blue cohosh -borage – buchu – burdock – butcher's broom

calendula – cannabis - caraway seed – cascara sagrada - catnip - cayenne - chamomile - chaparral – chickweed - chlorella - cilantro - cinnamon - cleaver – clove – comfrey- cramp bark - cranes bill

dandelion

echinacea - eucalyptus - eyebright

fennel – fenugreek

garlic - gentian - ginger - ginseng - goldenseal - gravel root - green tea

hawthorn - holy basil - hops - horseradish - horsetail hyssop

Irish moss

juniper

kelp

ladies slipper - lavender – lemon balm - lemongrass - licorice - lobelia

mandrake - marjoram - marshmallow - meadow sweet - melaleuca - milk thistle - mullein - myrrh

nettle

oatstraw - olive Leaf - oregano and oregano oil

parsley - Pau d'arco - peppermint - Peruvian bark - plantain - pleurisy root – poke weed – prickly ash - primrose

raspberry - red clover - reishi mushrooms - rosemary

sage - sassafras - senna - skullcap - slippery elm - spearmint

thyme - turkey rhubarb - turmeric

valerian

white oak bark - white pond lily – white popular – wild indigo - witch hazel – worm wood

yarrow - yellow dock

Disclaimer: I do not personally guarantee any of the following information or that it can cure any disease. I am sharing information that I found in several herbal and healing books.

AGRIMONY (AGRIMONIA EUPATORIA)

Contains:
Vitamins: A, B1 (thiamin), B3 (niacin), K

Minerals: iron

Plant:
A perennial flowering plant. Can grow from 05 – 2 metres tall with yellow flowers on a spike.

Therapeutic action:
anti-parasitic, antiviral, astringent, relaxant

Uses:
Blood: To clean the blood and used to treat jaundice. Provides vitamin K to help stop the bleeding from wounds.

Gall bladder: Used in repairing the gall bladder.

Kidney: Helps to reduce the size of the kidney stones and used to prevent them.

Liver: Helps to cleanse the blood and clean the liver

Lungs: Agrimony will help soothe sore lungs from colds and pollutants.

Skin: Helps to heal external wounds and reduce skin acne.

Spleen: Used to help repair the spleen.

Stomach: Used for the intestines, gastric disorders and stops diarrhea. Agrimony kills parasites in the stomach and intestines.

Other uses and information:
- Used as a flower essence to help dispel mental worry and reduce exhaustion. Helps to stabilize the mood and also helps those who hide their true emotions and discomfort.

- Used for a hair wash, fevers, hemorrhoids, internal bleeding, rheumatism, splinters and sprains.

ALFALFA (MEDICAGO SATIVA)

It is well known as a blood purifier (antifungal and alkalize) along with its healing properties for arthritis.

Contains:
Vitamins: A, B1 (thiamin), B2 (riboflavin), B3 (niacin), B5 (pantothenic acid), B6 (pyridoxine), B12 (cobalamin), folate, C, D, E, G, K

Minerals: calcium, chlorine, copper, iron, magnesium, phosphorous, potassium, silicon, sodium, sulfur, zinc

Other: alpha-carotene, beta-carotene, beta-sitosterol, chlorophyll, courmarin, cryptoxanthin, daidzein, fumaric acid, limoneme, lutein, saponin, stigmasterol, zeaxanthin

Plant:
Alfalfa can be sprouted and eaten as young plants or as grown plants.

Parts used: the flowers, leaves and petals.

Therapeutic action:
anti-inflammatory, relaxant, stomachic

Uses:
Appendix: Alfalfa is used as a natural treatment known to help reduce problems with the appendix.

Blood: Used to help lower high blood pressure, lower blood sugars, lower cholesterol levels, and to treat jaundice as it is a blood purifier. Alfalfa can assist with anemia and diabetes. Useful in preventing blood cancers.

Bones: The bones, skin and joints are the beneficiary when this herb is used, and it can help with arthritis.

Diseases: Used for alcoholism, allergies, arthritis, bursitis, cancer and hemorrhages.

Gland: Known to help with the pituitary gland (overstressed or too much anxiety) and to reduce ulcers

Immune system: As a blood purifier, alfalfa helps to strengthen the immune system.

Kidney: Alfalfa is a good kidney cleanser, gout and urinary problems.

Nose: This herb will aid in lessening nose bleeds.

Stomach: Healing of the bowels, reducing cramps, an appetite stimulant and for reducing nausea. For the intestinal tract, alfalfa can help with digestion.

Other: For mothers who are nursing, alfalfa will aid with lactation.

ALOE VERA

Aloe Vera is a household plant that is used for cuts and burns.

Contains:
Vitamins: A, B1 (thiamin), B2 (riboflavin), B3 (niacin), folate, C, D, E

Minerals: calcium, germanium, iron, magnesium, phosphorus, potassium, sulfur, zinc

Other: acemannan, amino acids, beta-carotene, beta-sitosterol, campesterol, cinnamic acid, courmarin, lignin, p-coumaric acid, saponin

Plant:
This plant is a cactus that can be grown in homes.

Parts used: The leaves are cut or broken off to squeeze out the pulp for usage. The pulp can be used in a drink like a liquid.

Therapeutic action:
antibacterial, anti-inflammatory, antiviral, astringent, demulcent, emollient, expectorant, pectoral, stomachic

Uses:
Blood: Aloe Vera helps the blood to regenerate and helps to improve the blood circulation in the lower parts of the body.

Bowels: Used as a laxative and to expel tapeworms.

Heart: Aloe Vera helps to lower the cholesterol level in the blood and keeps the blood pressure down.

Immune: Working with the liver and blood, aloe vera works at boosting the immune system.

Liver: Helps to cleanse the liver. Adds the iron that the blood requires to prevent anemia, tuberculosis and leg ulcers.

Lungs: For the lungs, aloe vera can help with asthma, and allergies.

Pituitary Gland: Helps to repair the pituitary gland and becomes stronger for the other glands that it oversees.

Skin: The fresh pulp can be used on the skin for abrasions, acne, burns, cuts, insect bites and sunburns. Being an antibacterial plant, aloe vera has been effective for poison ivy and oak. Used on infected skin areas and for psoriasis. Used to cure ringworm. Stops the wrinkling of the skin. Adds the estrogen to the skin.

Stomach: The stomach, colon, digestive system and to stop heartburn.

Other uses and information:
- Aloe Vera can be used as a gel extracted from the leaf.

-It is also made into a juice that can be drank, especially for those with asthma.

Caution: Try a tiny bit on the skin before applying to a large area to check for reaction. Pregnant mothers are advised not to use this herb internally.

AMARANTH

Amaranth is high in antioxidants

Contains:
Vitamins: B1 (thiamin), B2 (riboflavin), B3 (niacin), C

Minerals: calcium, iron, magnesium, manganese, phosphorous, potassium, zinc

Other: fat, fibre, protein

Plant:
The amaranth plant is similar to the wheat plant and has been cultivated for over 8000 years and used in the Aztec culture. The plant has been growing in the USA since the 1970s.

Therapeutic action:
Antioxidants, antiseptic astringent, demulcent.

Uses:
Bowels: The flower and leaves of the plant are good for dispelling parasites and worms from the digestive tract. Also for stopping diarrhea.

Menstruation: The flowers and leaves are used to slow down heavy menstruation.

Mouth: The flowers and leaves are used to stop the gums from bleeding.

Nose: The flowers and leaves are used to stop and prevent nose bleeds.

Skin: The plant parts are used to heal canker sores, skin ulcers and wounds.

Other uses and information:
- Amaranth is grown in Mexico to make a candy for use at festival times.

- India: Amaranth is mixed with honey after it has been popped. The popped grain is used for snacks, especially in schools since it contains iron and is a good energy source.

- Pressed Seed Oil: This seed oil is used in cooking and salad dressings.

- The seeds can be eaten raw, is used in soups and as a rice dish.

ANGELICA (ANGELICA ATRIPURPUREA)

Contains:
Vitamins: B12 (only in parts of the plant), E

Minerals: Calcium

Plant:
This plant is native to the Northern Hemisphere. The plant can grow from 1m – 3m (10 ft. tall). It has large leaves and white to greenish flowers.

Part used: The root of the plant is used. The juice of the plant is used for eyes and ears.

Therapeutic action:
anti-inflammatory, carminative, demulcent, emetic, nervine, pectoral, tonic.

Uses:
Ears: Good for increasing hearing.

Eyes: Good for increasing the eyesight.

Head: Used to reduce headaches.

Joints: Angelica is used to relief the pain and discomfort of rheumatism and arthritis. Helps to reduce back aches.

Lungs: Angelica assists with healing bronchitis, colds and coughs.

Menstrual: Used to reduce menstrual cramps.

Mouth: Good for reducing toothaches.

Muscles: Angelica is a good muscle relaxant.

Prostate: This herb has assisted with healing prostate discomforts.

Skin: Used for cleaning the wound and healing sores.

Stomach: Angelica is an aid in stimulating the appetite and will also help with digestion and heartburn. Great for relieving gas. This is great to use for stomach cramps (colic).

Ulcers: Angelica is known for its ability to heal ulcers.

Other uses and information:
- This is a great herb for colds, coughs and fevers.

- This herb has been used to help recover from exhaustion, will increase the mental health and well-being.

Caution: This herb should not be used by those who are diabetic as it increases the blood sugar level. It should not be used by women who are pregnant.

ANISE SEED & OIL

The seeds and oil smell and taste like licorice.

Contains

Vitamins: A, B1 (thiamin), B2 (riboflavin), B3 (niacin), B5 (pantothenic acid), B6 (pyridoxine), C, E,

Minerals: calcium, iron, magnesium, manganese, phosphorus, potassium, zinc

Other: alpha-pinene, apigenin, bergapten, chlorogenic acid, eugenol, limonene, rutin

Plant:
This plant is native to South-west Asia and the Mediterranean region. The plant has a star-like flower that produces the anise seed. The flowers are white. The seeds need to be planted as soon as the soil warms up and should not be moved till after it is harvested.

Part used: The seed and the oil of the seed is used.

Therapeutic action:
antibacterial, anti-convulsion, anti-infectious, anti-inflammatory, carminative, expectorant

Uses:
Blood: This herb can be used to treat blood infections.

Heart: Slows convulsions and epilepsy.

Immune: Used for pneumonia.

Lungs: Helps to soothe the lungs and clears the mucus. Aids in respiratory problems

Nose: Used for sinusitis.

Stomach: Anise seed is a good intestinal purifier and aids in digestion for gas and colic and stimulates the appetite.

Throat: Anise seed helps to soothe the throat. For cough (hard and dry). Provides a coating for the throat when coughing a lot.

Other uses and information:
- Used as a breath sweetener and used in baking and cooking.

- Used by nursing mothers to promote milk production (lactation)

ARNICA (ARNICA MONTANA)

Known as leopard's bane, mountain arnica, mountain tobacco and wolfsbane.

Contains:
arnicin, lutein, volatile oils.

Plant:
Arnica grows from 30 – 60 cm tall, bright yellow flower heads that can manifest singly in numbers. The leaves are opposite and toothed. The root stalk grows horizontal and is hair-like with white or brown bristles. This plant is found in North America.

Parts used: Flower head

Solvent: Boiling water and alcohol.

Therapeutic action:
anti-inflammatory, diaphoretic, diuretic, emollient, expectorant

Uses:
Bones: Used to help heal fractions, for swollen joints.

Eyes: Good for strengthening the eyesight.

Head: Arnica is used for headaches and concussions.

Mouth: Reduces inflammation in the gums.

Muscles: As an anti-inflammatory, it is used a lot by athletes to reduce bruises, sprains and torn ligaments. Used for rheumatic pain.

Skin: Fast healing of bruises, irritation and wounds.

Throat: Reduces inflammation from harsh coughing and sore throats.

Other uses and information:
- Used in trauma situations to help reduce mental and physical shock. Arnica provides better recovery than morphine. Doctors have used arnica for internal bleeding.

- Arnica is used in lotions, salves, tinctures, homeopathy tablets. Dilute tenfold if applied to open wound.

- Used in poultice or compress. Compress placed on stomach to relieve abdominal pains.

Caution: Tinctures should only be taken under the direction of your herbalist.

Do not use on open wounds or leg ulcers.

ASHWAGANDHA (WITHANIA SOMNIFERA)
Known as Indian ginseng and winter cherry.

Contains:
Vitamin: choline

Other: alkaloids, amino acids, beta-sitosterol, chlorogenic acid, fatty acids, withaferin

Plant:
Ashwagandha is part of the tomato family but is said to have the healing properties of the ginseng. The plant produces white flowers, is a shorter plant and the leaves are oval and pointy at the end like the sage plant. The flowers become a red berry. Traditionally found in the Middle East, Africa and India in the arid regions. The plant now grows in the USA.

Part used: The root of the plant is used.

Therapeutic action:
anti-aging, antibacterial, antidepressant, anti-Inflammatory, anti-malarial, antioxidant, relaxant, stimulant.

Uses:
Blood: Good for stabilizing the blood sugar. Lowers the blood cholesterol.

Brain: used to improve the memory, learning and reaction time with tasks. Ashwagandha has been proven to reduce the brain cell degeneration.

Immune System: Lab results have shown that Ashwagandha can regulate and stimulate the immune system. Ashwagandha has anti-malarial properties.

Muscles: Ashwagandha is an anti-inflammatory for the muscular system.

Nervous System: This herb helps a person to relax more as it calms down the nervous system. Useful for stress related lives and disorders. The herb helps to slow down the depletion of vitamin C and cortisol in the body during stressful times. Has aided with reducing depression and does not create the effects that chemicals create.

Thyroid: This herb helps to regulate the thyroid.

Other uses and information:
- Used to help boost the physical endurance.

- Can be used to improve sexual function.

Caution: Should not be used during a pregnancy. Ashwagandha should not be used with other medication. Using too much can cause diarrhea, nausea and sore stomach.

ASTRAGALUS (ASTRAGALI MEMBRANACEUS)
Astragalus is also called Huang Qi or milkvetch

Contains:
Vitamin: choline

Minerals: calcium, iron, magnesium, manganese, potassium, zinc

Other: essential fatty acids

Plant: Astragalus is part of the legume family. It has pale coloured flowers.

Part used: The root of the plant is used.

Therapeutic action:
antibacterial, anti-cancer, anti-inflammatory, antiviral, diaphoretic.

Uses:
Blood: Good for cleaning the blood when cancer, AIDS and tumours are present. Helps to build up the immune system. Fights off bacterial infections, purifies the blood and regulates the blood sugar levels.

Diseases: Used to reduce the common cold, chronic fatigue, fibromyalgia, influenza and ulcers. Known to help reduce arthritis.

Glands: Helps to repair the adrenal glands.

Heart: Helps to heal edema. Used in Chinese medicine to heal heart disease. Works at reducing high blood pressure and works with the cardiovascular system.

Immune system: Astragalus is used to increase the interferon in the body, to build up the immune system.

Liver: Cleans and supports the liver.

Lungs: Helps to heal emphysema, pneumonia, chronic coughs. Also helps to repair the lungs.

Spleen: Astragalus has been used to build up the spleen.

Stomach: Used for dispelling cysts. Great for the digestion and aids in increasing the metabolism

Uterus: Used to stop bleeding in the uterus.

Other uses and information:
- Helps to fight off viral infections.

- Used as a dietary supplement.

- Used as an energy tonic and as a tonic to build up the immune system. Astragalus has the good fatty acids that our body requires

Caution: If you have MS or a fever, it is safe to use astragalus. Do not use if using other immune suppressing drugs or if pregnant or nursing.

BALM OF GILEAD (POPULUS BALSAMIFERA SPP.)

Known as balsam poplar, cottonwood, popular, tacamahac

Contains:
bisabolene, bisabolol, cineole, humulene, populine, resins, salicin: salicylates, volatile oil

Plant:
Balm of Gilead comes from the bud of the popular trees. The name came from the story that when Moses found that the buds of the popular tree it was good for healing wounds and as a pain reliever. The Blackfoot nation used the inner bark of this tree for smoking meats and it was also used to feed the horses. This tree can grow to 25 metres tall. Fragrant resinous matter that covers the buds is separated in boiling water. The terpene from the resin is therapeutic.

Therapeutic action:
analgesic, antibacterial, anti-inflammatory, antioxidant, antiseptic, astringent, cathartic, demulcent, diuretic: mild, emollient, expectorant, stimulant, stomachic, tonic.

Uses:
Bladder: Support for the bladder.

Blood:

Balm of Gilead is used to cleanse the blood and eliminates scurvy.

Bones: Used for rheumatoid arthritis.

Bowels: Used for chronic constipation: cleansing, soothing, stimulating and toning for the lower bowel area. Used for regenerating and healing the intestines. Balm of Gilead helps to relax the muscles of the bowels.

Eyes: Used for when mucous membranes have become dry.

Head: Balm of Gilead can be used to rub into your temples to reduce headaches.

Kidneys: Balm of Gilead is good as a diuretic. It works with both the bladder and kidneys.

Lungs: Effective for bronchitis and clears the mucous from the lungs and chest.

Muscles: Balm of Gilead can turn into an aspirin effect when applied to the body.

Skin: Used to heal bruises, burns, cuts, frostbite, pimples, rashes, skin irritations, sunburns and wounds. Balm of Gilead can help to get rid of dark spots on the skin and for skin diseases. Works well with psoriasis. Excellent for pain relief from cuts.

Throat: Balm of Gilead can be used in a cough syrup to reduce coughing.

Other uses and information:
- Bud resin is soluble in alcohol, olive oil and other oils, but not in cool water. Used as an anti-cancer solution.

- Balm of Gilead has a salicin that our body can convert to aspirin to help reduce pain. The liquid extract from the bark is used for coughs: for dry cough or sore throat and in cough syrups. The oily resin has major cathartic effects.

- When it is made into compounded ointment or oil, it is very valuable for any skin disease. If expulsive action is too fast, add ginger root to the mixture.

BARBERRY (BERBERIS VULGARIS)

Contains:
Vitamins: B1 (thiamin), B2 (riboflavin), B3 (niacin). High in vitamin C.

Minerals: calcium, iron, magnesium, manganese, phosphorous, potassium, selenium, silicon, zinc

Other: berbamine, berberine, beta-carotene, caffeic acid, kaempferol, lutein, quercetin, sinapic acid, zeaxanthin

Plant:
The plant is known as an evergreen and is found in subtropics and temperate regions, except for Australia. Africa, Asia and South America, good regions, but can also be found in Europe. The leaves are small but thick. The yellow or orange flowers turn into oblong shaped red or dark blue berries. The plants and the colours vary from region to region. The barberry plant is invasive and aids in the growth of some fungi. The plant is forbidden in some regions. The plant is very spiny and is used in hedges to prevent burglars from entering yards and homes. The berries are high in vitamin C and can be eaten, though they are a bit tart.

Part used: The bark, berries and the root of the plant are used.

Therapeutic action:
antimicrobial, antiseptic, antispasmodic, stimulant

Uses:
Blood: Barberry is used to increase the blood vessels to help reduce high blood pressure. Barberry is also effective in cleansing the blood.

Bowels: Barberry can be used to stop diarrhea and reduce constipation.

Gall Bladder: Helps to heal the gall bladder.

Heart: Barberry helps to reduce a fast heart rate.

Intestines: Used to help improve the movement of the intestines.

Liver: Barberry helps the liver to move the bile better. Used to clear jaundice from the liver.

Lungs: Helps to slow down the breathing and works with the bronchial passages.

Mouth: Barberry is used in mouthwashes and is good to gargle with to get rid of bacteria and prevents gum disease.

Skin: Used to kill the bacteria on the skin.

Stomach: Barberry can help the bowels and stomach to remove morbid matter. Helps to reduce indigestion and ulcers.

Throat: Helps to clear and heal the throat.

Other uses and information:
-Used for reducing fevers.

- Reduces inflammation from arthritis.

- Used to prevent or treat dyspepsia.

Caution: Barberry should NOT be used during pregnancy.

BASIL (OCIMUM BASILICUM)

Basil is high in antioxidants

Known as Saint Joseph's Wort

Contains:
Vitamins: A, B2 (riboflavin), D

Minerals: calcium, iron, magnesium, phosphorous

Plant:
Basil is an annual plant that has a strong pungent smell, sweet smell and taste. The plant was originally found in India and Asia. There are many varieties of basil: African blue, holy basil, lemon basil, sweet basil, Thai basil and more.

Parts used: The leaves of the plant are used.

Therapeutic action:
antibacterial, antioxidant, antispasmodic, stomachic, tonic.

Uses:
Bladder: Used to treat the bladder.

Bones: Basil has been used to reduce the discomfort of rheumatism.

Bowels: Helps to reduce constipation.

Head: Used for headaches. Helps to relax the muscles.

Kidney: Helps to treat the kidneys.

Lungs: Helps to treat colds, coughs, respiratory troubles and whooping cough. `

Menstruation: Good to use to reduce cramping.

Skin: Used to treat insect and snakebites. Basil helps to draw out the poison.

Stomach: Used for indigestion and nausea. Used to stop vomiting and stops stomach cramps. Expels worms.

Other uses and information:
- Use to reduce fevers and for nervous conditions.

- Basil is used in many dishes around the world in soups, dressings, salads, sauces and more.

BAYBERRY (MYRICA CERIFERA)
Known as wax-myrtle, waxberry myrtle

Contains:
Vitamins: B1 (thiamin), B2 (riboflavin), B3 (niacin), C

Minerals: calcium, iron, magnesium, manganese, phosphorous, potassium, selenium, silicon, zinc

Other: acrid resin, astringent resins, flavonoids, gallic acid, myricic acid, palmitin – containing wax, saponin triterpenes

Plant:
Bayberry is a dense evergreen shrub, stands 2 – 4 feet tall. It has a greyish bark that peels away to reveal an underlying reddish-brown layer. Shiny dark leaves are lanceolate entire. The flowers are borne in catkins. It is one of the most useful herbs in herbal medicine.

Parts used: Root bark and sometimes the leaves.

Solvent: Bayberry is prepared in boiling water.

Therapeutic action:
alterative, antibacterial, antimicrobial, astringent, diuretic: mild, stimulant, tonic.

Uses:
Blood: Good for improving the circulation. Helps to stop bleeding.

Eyes: Good for the eyes and eyesight.

Diseases: Used to stop dropsy and scarlet fever.

Liver: Bayberry helps with the immune system. Helps to clean and strengthen the liver while reducing jaundice.

Lungs: Used as a decongestant. Bayberry has a major healing effect on the mucous accumulation in the alimentary and respiratory tracts. Used to heal bronchial and pulmonic diseases

Menstrual: Helps to reduce heavy menstrual bleeding.

Mouth: Bayberry helps to stop the gums from bleeding. Used for cankers, both internal and external and for spongy gums.

Skin: Used for minor cuts.

Stomach: Used for to stop diarrhea. Helps soothe indigestion and reduce ulcers.

Throat: Used for sore throats,

Uterus: Used for stopping uterus hemorrhaging. Used to heal a prolapsed uterus.

Other uses and information:

- Bayberry is good to soothe ulcers. Used to heal the body from scurvy, which is a lack of vitamin C.

- The wax from the berries can be used to scent candles. The berries are very waxy and were used by settlers as wax replacement.

- Composition Powder: This should be part of every household. This powder can be used in all cases of the flu, colds, fevers, helping to promote free perspiration. Bayberry has cleared up cases of the flu within twenty-four hours. The tonic must be made personally since the suppliers quit making composition powder due to the high cost.

BEARBERRY (ARCTOSTAPHYLOS UVA-URSI)

Known as: uva- ursi, kinnikinnick, arbutus

Contains:
Vitamins: B1 (thiamin), B2 (riboflavin), B3 (niacin), C

Minerals: calcium, iron, magnesium, manganese, phosphorous, potassium, selenium, zinc

Other: arbutin, beta-carotene, beta-sitosterol, ellagic acid, ericinol, gallic acid, hydroquinones, hyperin, isoquercitrin, methyl-arbutin, myristicin, oleanolic acid, quercetin, quercetrin, tannic acid, ursome, ursolic acid

Plant:
Bearberry is a trailing green plant that forms mats 5 to 10 cm in length. The flowers are a pale pink to a white. Its evergreen leaves are oval, leathery and thin. The branches lose their rusty bark in shreds. The berries are red and not very juicy. The leaves from the plant are used for medicinal purposes. Bearberry is grown in North America.

Parts used: The leaves from the plant are used for medicinal purposes.

Solvent: Alcohol and water

Therapeutic action:
antibacterial, antiviral, astringent, diuretic, tonic

Uses:
Bladder: Used for inflammation of the bladder and kidneys. Used as diuretic to cleanse the bladder and kidney.

Blood: Good for lowering the blood sugar and fighting bacteria.

Bowels: Bearberry is used to stop chronic diarrhea.

Diseases: Used for treating AIDS, herpes and gonorrhea

Heart: Helps to strengthen the heart muscles.

Kidney: Used as a diuretic and for inflammation of the bladder and kidneys. It has been used to help stop bed-wetting. Bearberry is one of the strongest diuretics. Used to dissolve sand, gravel and stones.

Liver: Bearberry cleanses and supports the liver.

Lungs: Been used to help with bronchitis and lung congestion.

Menstruation: Used to lessen heavy menstruation periods.

Mouth: Bearberry assists in treating canker sores and sore gums.

Pancreas: Helps to strengthen the pancreas and lower blood sugar.

Skin: Used to treat the skin from poison oak exposure and used in solutions to help treat rashes and skin infections.

Spleen: Used to help strengthen the spleen

Urinary tract: Good for ulceration of the membrane of the urinary tract. Helps to strengthen the urinary passages. Used to help break down the calculi deposits in urinary tract and as an urinary antibiotic (rids urinary tract of infections).

Uterus: Bearberry has been used to help slow down hemorrhaging after childbirth and can help to reduce the contractions after delivery.

Other uses and information:
- Used for soothing arthritis and nephritis

- The berries are mealy and tasteless when raw, but quite palatable when cooked.

- The A. alpine and A. rubra bearberries are better tasting berries.

Caution: Overuse can prove to be toxic and can cause ear ringing, vomiting, convulsions and collapsing. It is not good for use in cases of severely weak kidneys. Do not use during pregnancy, or while nursing. Not for use by children under the age of twelve.

BILBERRY (VACCINIUM MYRTILLUS)
Bilberry is well known for being a powerful antioxidant and for healthy eye function.

Contains:
Vitamin: B1 (thiamin), B2 (riboflavin), B3 (niacin), C, E

Minerals: calcium, inositol, iron, magnesium, manganese, phosphorus, potassium, selenium, silicon, sodium, sulfur, zinc

Other: anthocyanosides, beta-carotene, bio flavonoids, caffeic acid, caryophyllene, catechin, chlorogenic acid, ferulic acid, gallic acid, hyperoside, lutein, quartering, quercitrin, ursolic acid, vanillic acid

Plant:
Bilberry is native to Europe and can be found growing in North America. This is a perennial shrub plant that grows wild.

Part Used: The leaves, dried fruit and ripe fruit are used.

Therapeutic action:
anti-infectious, anti-inflammatory, antioxidant, diuretic, antiviral.

Uses:
Blood: Bilberry aids as a blood thinner, helps circulation and lowers the blood sugars (diabetes) and cholesterol levels. Used to treat scurvy and typhoid.

Bones: Bilberry has assisted with osteoarthritis.

Bowel: Helps to reduce diarrhea.

Eyes: This herb is known for promoting healthy eye function. It works with the eyes to improve night vision and heal light sensitivity. Used to treat cataracts and renal disorders.

Heart: Bilberry works with the heart and the arteries and varicose veins.

Immune system: Strengthens the immune system as it is an antioxidant.

Kidneys: Strengthens the kidneys, clears urinary tract infections and helps to reduce the effects of gout.

Liver: Being a good antioxidant, this fruit helps to cleanse the blood.

Mouth: Bilberry helps to reduce mouth infections.

Throat: Used to reduce throat infections and inflammation.

Other: Used to treat Reynaud's disease and chronic fatigue.

BIRCH (BETULA)

Contains:
Vitamins: A, B1 (thiamin), B2 (riboflavin), C, E

Minerals: calcium, chlorine, copper, iron, magnesium, phosphorous, potassium, silicon, sodium

Plant: This is a hardwood tree that is grown in the Northern Hemisphere. It is a medium sized tree with simple leaves that grow in pairs. The birch does get flowers that go to seed.

Parts used: It is the inner bark and the buds that are used from the birch tree.

Therapeutic action:
antiseptic, astringent, cathartic, diuretic, stimulant, stomachic, tonic.

Uses:
Bladder: Used for healing the bladder.

Blood: Birch is good for cleaning the blood.

Diseases: Good for working with dropsy and gout.

Kidneys: A tonic has assisted in healing the kidneys and urinary tract.

Liver: Birch supports the liver as it cleanses the blood.

Mouth: Birch can be used as a mouthwash to heal bleeding gums and canker sores.

Skin: When the birch is used in a balm, it can be applied to eczema.

Other: Good for reducing fevers.

BISTORT (POLYGONUM BISTORTA)
Known as snakeweed, adderwort, patient, dock, dagonwort

Contains:
Vitamins: A, B1 (thiamin), B2 (riboflavin), B3 (niacin), B5 (pantothenic acid), B6 (pyridoxine), B12 (cobalamin), C

Other: tannins

Plant:
Bistort is a mountain or northern perennial found west of the Rocky Mountains in Europe and in the Arctic. Grows in damp or wet meadows. The root stock is thick and up to 3.5 ft. long. The root is black on the outside and red inside. The bluish-green basal leaves are on long. Few slim leaves are on short petioles and lanceolate to linear. Flowers are rose red and appear in May to August.

Parts used: root and leaves.

Solvent: water, alcohol.

Therapeutic action:
alterative, anthelmintic, anti-inflammatory, astringent, diuretic

Uses:
Blood: The powder of the root is used to stop bleeding or hemorrhaging. Bistort has worked with diabetes.

Bowels: A tonic can be used to lessen diarrhea and dysentery.

Diseases: Used to heal cholera and leucorrhea. Bistort can help to reduce the discomfort of measles.

Kidney: Using Bistort can help to strengthen the walls of the kidney.

Liver: Bistort helps to cleanse the blood when it has become jaundiced.

Menstruation: Bistort is used to lessen menstrual cramping.

Mouth: A concoction can be made as a mouthwash to use for gum problems and canker sores.

Skin: When bistort is mixed with raspberry leaves, the mixture can be used in a wash for the following skin ailments: fungal rashes, insect bites, pimples, measles and small pox.

Other uses and information:
- Good soothing action to reduce inflammation of the hemorrhoids.

- Seeds were used whole or ground into a flour by the Natives.

BLACK COHOSH (CIMICIFUGA RACEMOSA)
Known as black snake root, squaw root, rattle root and bugbane.

Contains:
Vitamins: A, B1 (thiamin), B2 (riboflavin), B3 (niacin), C

Minerals: calcium, chromium, iron, magnesium, manganese, phosphorous, potassium, selenium, silicon, zinc

Other: beta-carotene, cimicifugin, formononetin, gallic acid, phytosterols, salicylic acid, sulfates, tannic acid, tannin, triterpenes, volatile oil

Plant:
Black cohosh is a perennial that grows in eastern North America and is also cultivated in Europe. The dark brown roots are attached to underground rhizomes. The stem is slender, 1.5 – 2.5 m tall. The plant has compound leaves that have incised leaflets. It flowers from June to July with small white flowers about 20-50 cm long that have a peculiar scent.

Parts Used: the root.

Therapeutic action:
alterative, anti-inflammatory, antispasmodic, diuretic: mild, emmenagogue, expectorant, nervine, tonic

Uses:
Blood: Used to lower high cholesterol levels and used to cleanse toxins from the blood.

Bones: Used for rheumatic pain (especially in pelvic area).

Childbirth: Herbalists have suggested to use smalls amounts of black cohosh two weeks before delivery to induce labour and help with the birthing.

Ears: Used for ear infections.

Head: Good for reducing inflammation from headaches.

Heart: Black cohosh is used for cardiovascular and circulatory problems. Black cohosh has been used as a mild cardiac tonic for fatty hearts as it lowers the heart rate and increases force of pulse and equalizes the circulation.

Kidneys: Used as a diuretic for the kidneys.

Liver: It can also have a stimulating effect on secretion of the liver and spleen.

Lungs: Helps to reduce the effect of asthma and whooping cough. Helps to reduce mucous in the lungs.

Lymphatic System: This herb can be used to help support the lymphatic system.

Menstrual: Black cohosh is good for relieving a delayed menstrual flow. Black Cohosh is found separately or in female formulas for experiencing uterine troubles and menstrual cramps during menstruation or after giving birth. This herb is better to use than hormonal replacement treatments (HRT), as it causes less side effects and will treat the cause. HRT has been found to cause forms of cancers. Black cohosh helps to reduce the hot flashes.

Muscles: Black cohosh is used as an anti-inflammatory and antispasmodic for sore muscles.

Nervous system: This herb is used as a nervine to reduce nervous excitement and epilepsy.

Prostate: Black cohosh has been used to help reduce the growth of prostate tumours.

Uterus: Used for healing uterine ailments.

Other uses and information:
- Used by Natives as an antidote for poison, snake bites and for bad cases of the hiccups.

BLACK WALNUT (JUGLANS NIGRA)

Contains:
Vitamins: B1 (thiamin), B2 (riboflavin), B3 (niacin), C

Minerals: calcium, iron, magnesium, manganese, phosphorous, potassium, selenium, silicon

Other: beta-carotene, ellagic acid, organic iodine, protein, silica

Plant:
The black walnut tree is native to the eastern middle part of the USA to the middle of the States. The black walnut tree may begin to get fruit when the tree is four to six years old and live up to 130 years old. The trees can grow up to 130 ft. The bark is grey to black and rough texture. The male flowers droop and are about 10 cm long. The female flowers are terminal shaped and grow in a group of two to five flowers. These flowers turn to the fruit or nut. The leaves of the tree are long,

up to 60 cm long. The shell of the walnut is a brown to greenish colour and the nut / flesh is brown on the outside, and inside white. The fruit of the tree is ripe in October. The wood of the tree is prized for its rich colour and strength.

Parts used: The leaves and the hulls are used medicinally.

Therapeutic action:
antifungal, anti-parasitic, anti-perspirant, antiseptic, antispasmodic, demulcent

Uses:
Blood: Helps to dispel fatty materials to lower the cholesterol levels and regulate the blood pressure. Black walnut aids in balancing the blood sugar levels, prevent cancer, treating infections and tuberculosis.

Bowels: Black walnut is used in formulas as an aid for a laxative.

Eyes: Good for the eyes, black walnut is used in a formula.

Intestines: Black walnut is used to dispel worms

Liver: Black walnut helps to rid the body of toxins.

Mouth: Helps to heal sores in the mouth and sore throats.

Skin: The iodine in the unripe walnut husk is a good antiseptic for the skin. Used for acne, boils, bruises, eczema, fungal infections, poison ivy, poison oak, ringworm, skin rashes, warts, wounds and herpes. Black walnut's properties make a good anti-perspirant.

Stomach: Used to dispel internal parasites. Helps to improve digestion.

Teeth: Helps to build the enamel on the teeth

Throat: Black walnut helps to ease sore throats and tonsillitis.

Uterus: Black walnut is used to help repair a prolapsed uterus.

Other uses and information:
- Good to stop the lactation for mothers who are ready to stop nursing.

- The hulls from the black walnut can be boiled to get a dye to colour wool.

BLESSED THISTLE (CENTAUREA BENEDICTA)
Known as Carduus, Cardin, holy thistle, St. Benedict's thistle, old lady's thistle

Contains:
Vitamins: A, B1 (thiamin), B2 (riboflavin), B3 (niacin), B5 (pantothenic acid), B6 (pyridoxine), B12, C

Minerals: calcium, iron, manganese, phosphorous, potassium, selenium, silicon, zinc

Other: beta-carotene, beta-sitosterol, ferulic acid, kaempferol, luteolin, oleanolic acid, stigmasterol

Plant:
Blessed thistle is an erect plant with woody-branched stems. The flowers grow flowers from May to June and are 2 – 3 inches long, greyish-green and oblong to lanceolate. Flowers are one inch long and 1 ¾ inches wide.

Parts used: Entire herb: flowers, leaves and stem.

Solvent: Cold to hot water, alcohol.

Therapeutic action:
alterative, antimicrobial, anti-parasitic, antispasmodic, cathartic, diaphoretic

Uses:
Blood: Good for blood circulation and cleansing the blood

Diseases: Works with fevers and dropsy.

Eyes: Good for strengthening the eyesight.

Gall Bladder: Blessed thistle is used help to treat the gall bladder

Head: Used to reduce headaches and helps with our memory

Heart: Helps to strengthen the heart.

Liver: Cleanses the liver as it is used as a blood purifier and dispels the jaundice in the body.

Lungs: Blessed thistle helps to strengthen and heal the lungs and works with respiratory infections.

Menstruation: *Good for menstrual problems and to help level the hormones.*

Stomach: Used for digestion, stimulates the appetite, stimulates gastric secretions and digestive tonic. Also used to dispel parasites in the stomach and intestines.

Other: Used to help increase lactation for nursing mothers.

BLUE COHOSH (CAULOPHYLLUM THALICTROIDES)
Known as squaw root, papoose root

Contains:
Vitamins: B1 (thiamin), B2 (riboflavin), B3 (niacin), B5 (pantothenic acid), B6 (pyridoxine), B12, C, E,

Minerals: calcium, iron, magnesium, manganese, phosphorous, potassium, selenium, silicon, zinc

Other: anagryine, beta-carotene, caulophylline, caulophylio-sapinon, caulosapinon, heragenin, phytosterols, saponin

Plant:
The plant can be a medium to tall plant. The plant has a bluish-green colour. It is a perennial and has bluish-yellow flowers. The fruit of the plant looks like blueberries. The leaves are a long oblong shape. This plant is native to the Eastern United States and Eastern Canada.

Therapeutic action:
antibacterial, anti-inflammatory, antispasmodic

Uses:
Bladder: Blue cohosh is used for treating bladder infection.

Blood: Used to lower high blood pressure and assists with diabetes.

Bones: Good for bringing relief to sore joints.

Bowels: Blue Cohosh has been used as a laxative.

Childbirth: Blue Cohosh is used to promote contractions for childbirth and should only be used at the very end of the pregnancy. The herb has also been used for its abortive abilities and to help prevent conception. The Native Americans were the first to use this herb for these purposes.

Head: Used to help improve memory.

Menstrual: Used to help reduce cramping during menstrual time. Helps to start the menstruation cycle, reduce swelling and cramping before and during the cycle.

Muscles: Blue cohosh helps to treat dropsy, muscle spasms, fits and convulsions. Blue cohosh helps to relax the muscles and stop muscle cramps.

Nervous System: Blue Cohosh aids in nervous disorders and calms down a person. Used to treat epilepsy and fits.

Stomach: Blue Cohosh can be used to treat colic.

Throat: This herb is good for soothing sore throats and for hiccups.

Uterus: Used for helping to bring down the swelling of the uterus, reducing cramps during childbirth.

Other uses and information:
- Good for nervous disorders and helps to relax a person. Has helped with treating epilepsy, leucorrhea and neuralgia.

- Blue cohosh is best used with another herb like black cohosh.

Caution: This herb should not be used during the first two trimesters of pregnancy.

BORAGE (BORAGO OFFICINALIS)
Known for its oilseed

Contains:
Vitamins: A, B1 (thiamin), B2 (riboflavin), B3 (niacin), C, E

Minerals: calcium, iron, magnesium, phosphorous, potassium, zinc

Other: beta-carotene, rosmarinic acid, silicic acid, tannin

Plant:
Borage was first found in Syria. Now it can be found in Asia, Europe South America and in North Africa. The plant can grow to 3 feet high, with flowers that are blue in the triangular shape. Pick the leaves about six weeks after seeds germinate. Pick the flowers just before or after they open.

Parts used: leaves and flowers

Therapeutic action:
antibacterial, anti-inflammatory, antiseptic, astringent, cathartic, emmenagogue, emollient, stimulant, tonic,

Uses:
Diseases: Works with fevers and dropsy.

Eyes: Used for eye inflammation and as an eyewash for sore and tired eyes.

Gall Bladder: Borage is used to treat the gall bladder.

Head: Used to reduce headaches.

Heart: Helps to strengthen the heart.

Hormones: Used as a regulator for the metabolism, hot flashes, PMS, and menopause.

Kidneys: Used for the kidneys and adrenal glands.

Liver: Borage helps to clean the liver when it has become jaundiced.

Lungs: Helps with bronchitis, colds and fever.

Skin: Use to heal rashes, enhance the health of the skin and nails.

Stomach: Borage is good for the digestion and dispels worms from the stomach and intestines.

Other uses and information:
- Used to help increase lactation for nursing mothers, for ringworm, helps with insomnia and to calm the nerves. Borage has been used for recuperating from an illness. Used to help balance the glands and enhance the adrenals.

- Borage has been used to grow with legumes, tomatoes, spinach and strawberries, as it repels the moths.

- Use young leaves in salads. The flowers can be eaten too. The plant tastes like a cucumber, and the flowers have a honey-like taste. Borage is used as a garnish in soups and as a filler for pastas.

BUCHU (BAROSMA BETALINA)

Known as buku, bucco

Contains:
Vitamins: B1 (thiamin), B2 (riboflavin), B3 (niacin)

Minerals: magnesium, manganese, phosphorous, potassium, selenium, silicon, zinc

Other: alpha-pinene, alphaterpinene, barosma-camphor, daisimin, diosphenol, dosphenol, flavonoid, hesperetin, limonene, methone, mucilage, pulegone, quercetin, quercetrin, protein, rutin, volatile oils

Plant:
Buchu grows in South Africa. The leaf has two varieties: long leaf and short leaf. The short leaf plant is more medicinally superior. This plant can grow to about 100 cm tall. The flowers have five petals that are either purple, red, pink or white.

Parts used: The leaves of the plant are used, and they should not be boiled.

Solvent: water and alcohol.

Therapeutic action:
anti-infectious, anti-inflammatory, antiseptic, astringent, carminative, diaphoretic, diuretic (mild), stimulant.

Uses:
Bladder: Buchu makes for a good diuretic and helps to control the kidney and bladder. Used to treat bladder infections. For the urinary tract, Buchu is taken cold, as it increases the quantity of urine (urine will become dark and strong smelling.) When taken warm, it has a gentle diaphoretic action.

Blood: Used to treat the first stages of sugar diabetes.

Bones: Used for rheumatism.

Colon: Buchu helps to soothe the colon and bring any swelling down.

Gall Bladder: Helps to treat gall stones.

Kidney: Buchu makes for a good diuretic and helps to control the kidney and bladder as it absorbs excessive acid. Helps with yeast infections. Used to decrease fluid retention (dropsy).

Menstruation: Used for pre-menstrual bloating.

Mouth: Buchu helps bring down swelling in the mouth and gums.

Pituitary Gland: Used to help the pituitary gland secrete protein that is needed to balance the hormones.

Prostate: When mixed with palmetto, it is used for prostate problems.

Sinuses: This herb helps to heal the sinuses and works as a disinfectant for other mucous membranes.

Stomach: Used to help with digestion, soothing for the stomach, and soothes the pelvic area and pelvis nerves. Soothes the mucous membranes of the stomach.

Uterus: Used for urethritis.

Other uses and information:
- When used with squaw vine or unicorn root, it lessens lower back and loin pains.

- When buchu is mixed with sassafras and made into a tea, the combination will help with hypothalamus.

- Buchu leaves and stalks put into brandy will create a tincture.

- When the leaves and stalks are steeped in vinegar, the remedy can be used for compresses and have been taken internally.

BURDOCK (ARCTIUM LAPPA)

Burdock is known as powerful antioxidant and one of the best blood purifiers.

Known as beggar's button, burr seed, clotbur, cocklebur, hardock, turkey burseed

Contains:
Vitamins: A, B1 (thiamin), B2 (riboflavin), B3 (niacin), C, and E, PABA

Minerals: calcium, iron, magnesium, manganese, phosphorus, potassium, selenium, silicon, zinc

Other: acetic acid, actin (bitter glycoside), amino acids, arctigenin, arctin, beta-carotene, butyric acid, caffeic acid, chlorogenic acid, costic acid, inulin, inulin, isovaleric acid, lauric acid, ligans, mucilage, myristic acid, propionic acid, sitosterol, stigmasterol, sulfates, tannin, triterpenes, ursolic acid, vanillic acid, volatile oil, zeaxanthin

Plant:
Burdock is best picked in the spring of the second year or in fall of the first year. A bi-biannual found in Europe and North America. The root is up to 3 feet long and up to 1 inch thick, fleshy, grey brown on the outside and white inside. It is best picked in the July of the second year or in fall of first year. Stem leaves and flowers appear in the second year. The leaves are oblong, green and hairy on top, downy grey on the bottom. The flowers are purple, loose corymbose clusters from July to September.

Parts used: The root of this plant has been used for medicinal purposes for hundreds of years. Also used are the seeds and young stems.

Therapeutic action:
alterative, antibacterial, antifungal, antioxidant, antiseptic, antispasmodic, antiviral, diuretic, expectorant, stimulant, tonic.

Uses:

Blood: Burdock is an excellent blood cleanser and purifier. It can help to control cell mutation in cancer cells. The inulin in the burdock helps with diabetes and hypoglycemia as it does not provide the spikes in the blood sugar levels.

Bones: Burdock helps to decrease the effects of arthritis.

Gall Bladder: Aids with the functioning of the gall bladder.

Immune system: Burdock helps to fight off infections in different organs in the body.

Kidney: The skin and kidneys are the greatest recipients of this herb, as burdock cleans out excess waste and uric acid from the kidneys. Being an antibacterial and antifungal, burdock is used for healing organs and the body of infections.

Liver: The liver and gall bladder benefits from the increase of bile secretion when this herb is used with other herbs. Burdock contains inulin, a carbohydrate that strengthens the liver. Used to help one recover from hepatitis.

Lungs: The burdock helps with the respiratory system and clears congestion.

Lymphatic System: Helps to rebuild the lymphatic system.

Skin: The skin is the recipient of the healing benefits that the kidney gets from the use of burdock, helping to detoxify the epidermal tissues. Experience has shown how applying the raw root to a bruised area will reduce the pain. Heals boils, eczema, pimples and psoriasis.

Stomach: Burdock has a high inulin and mucilage that aids in the soothing the gastrointestinal tract. Aids with digestion.

Other uses and information:

- Used to treat the following: gonorrhea, gout, sciatica, scurvy and syphilis.

- A recent study showed that burdock blocked dangerous chemicals from causing damage to cells.

- Aids in alleviating distress to the body that is related to chronic fatigue syndrome.

- Burdock can be used with other herbs such as sarsaparilla and yellow dock or alone.

- Stalks can be boiled and eaten like asparagus. The raw stems and young leaves are used in - salads.

- The root can be used as a coffee substitute after it has been chopped and roasted. It has a nutty taste.

Caution: Burdock use does interfere with iron absorption. Overuse can create anemia.

BUTCHER'S BROOM (RUSCUS ACULEATUS)

Contains:
Vitamins: B1 (thiamin), B2 (riboflavin), B3 (niacin), C

Minerals: calcium, chromium, iron, magnesium, manganese, phosphorous, potassium, selenium, silicon, zinc

Other: beta-carotene, chrysophanic acid, glycolic acid, neoruscogenin, rutin, saponin.

Plant: This is a low growing evergreen with spiny looking leaves. It has greenish flowers that grow in the springtime and produce a red berry. The butcher's broom is found in the woods, in the shade and can be found growing in gardens.

Therapeutic action:
anti-inflammatory, antiseptic, anti-inflammatory, catharic, diuretic. stimulant

Uses:
Arteries: Circulation: good for treating Raynaud's disease (constriction of arteries, like the fingers due to long exposure to cold weather). It also helps to keep the blood circulating to the heart and the brain.

Bladder: Butcher's Broom is used for treating the kidneys and bladder.

Blood: Good for treating jaundice, thrombophlebitis and supporting the veins (this is when blood starts to clot in a vein). This herb is used for post-operative blood clotting and lowering the cholesterol levels.

Ears: Good for treating Meniere's disease. (Meniere's disease is ringing in the ears, ear infections, and hearing loss.)

Head: Butcher's broom is used for headaches.

Heart: Helps with the heart if there is a possibility of edema.

Kidneys: Butcher's broom is used for treating the kidneys and bladder.

Liver: Used to treat jaundice.

Menstrual: Butcher's broom aids in treating menstrual discomforts.

Veins: Butcher's broom helps to build up the walls of the veins. Helps to treat varicose veins.

Other uses and information:
- Good treating hemorrhoids. Butcher's broom is good for healing carpal tunnel syndrome, edema (dropsy).

- This herb is also an aid in losing weight.

- Used to help decrease vertigo.

Caution: Best used with vitamin C.

CALENDULA (CALENDULA OFFICINALIS)

Also known as marigold, calandula, garden calendula, garden calandula, holigold, golds, pot marigold, Mary bud, Mary Gowles, bride of the Sun, butterwort

Contains:
Vitamins: A, C, E

Minerals: calcium, phosphorous

Other: Coenzyme Q10

Plant:
Calendula comes from the petals of the marigold plant. This plant can be found growing in flower gardens.

Parts used: The entire plant can be used.

Therapeutic action:
antispasmodic, astringent, demulcent, emollient, pectoral, tonic

Uses:
Blood: Calendula is used for cleansing the blood and reducing anemia and hepatitis.

Ears: Good for reducing ear infections.

Eyes: Good for relieving eye infections.

Gall Bladder: Used to help heal the gall bladder

Heart: The marigold/calendula is excellent for the heart and blood circulation, as it contains Coenzyme Q10.

Liver: Cleanses the blood and strengthens the liver.

Lungs: Helps to soothe the lungs from the effects of bronchitis

Menstrual: Used to regulate the menstrual cycle and reduce cramps.

Mouth: Calendula has been used to reduce toothaches and eliminate canker sores.

Skin: Calendula contains vitamin E and is very soothing for the skin and helps to reduce inflammation. Used for bee stings, burns, diaper rashes, rashes, sunburns and other skin disorders.

Stomach: Used for stopping diarrhea.

Other uses and information: - Good for reducing fevers and hemorrhoids.

- Calendula has been found to be effective in treating varicose veins.

- The marigold plant is grown to keep insects away from other plants in the garden.

- The tea is for fevers and to help regulate the menstrual cycles and soothe swollen tonsils.

- The tincture is for skin ailments, ulcers and muscles spasms. Used in a poultice for bleeding hemorrhoids.

CANNABIS

Known as hemp, marijuana

Contains:
cannabichromenenic acid, cannabichromevarinic acid, cannabidiol, cannabidiolic acid, cannabigerolic acid, cannabigerovarinic acid, cannabidivarinic acid, esters, ethers, ketones, phenols, tetrahydrocannabinol, terpenes, terpenoids, tetrahydrocanabivarinic acid.

Plant: Cannabis (hemp) has been grown for hundreds of years around the world. This plant has been used for its oil, materials, medicinal properties and as a building product. The fibres of the plant can be used as a replacement to trees. The plant grows fast and has a much lower impact on the earth. The plant can grow higher than 5 feet and about 3 feet wide. Each leaf can have up to seven parts to it, and they fan out. The first leaves of the plant are small. The plant grows flower buds that produce the seeds.

Part used: The whole plant can be used: stalk, leaves, seeds.

Therapeutic action:
anodyne, anti-cancer, anti-inflammatory, antispasmodic, anti-emetic, nervine, stimulant, stomachic, tonic

Uses:
Blood: Good for cleansing the blood, treating AIDS and cancer.

Bowels: Good for bringing relief to constipation.

Diseases: Used for Crohn's disease

Head: Used to reduce the effects of painful headaches.

Liver: Cannabis helps to fight off cancerous cells.

Menstruation: Used to bring relief to painful cramping.

Muscles: Used as a muscle relaxant.

Nerves: Cannabis can help provide a relaxing effect and help with sleep. The cannabidiol in the cannabis is the chemical that helps the brain to relax and lessen epileptic attacks. The cannabidiol does not provide a high and has a powerful medicinal effect. The herb has assisted with treating Dravet's Syndrome, multiple sclerosis and PTSD.

Stomach: Used for helping with increasing the appetite and aids with digestion.

Other uses and information:
- This plant can be used in food, as an oil, smoked or vapourized.
- The tetrahydrocannabinol is the compound that provides the pain relief.

Caution: This plant can cause short-term memory loss. Studies have shown that this herb should not be smoked by those under the age of twenty-one. The smoking effect can cause problems with schooling, the ability to concentrate and damage the brain cells. Other side effects are anxiety, dry mouth, increased heart rate and lack of motor skills. Daily use for recreation can cause addiction.

Mothers who are pregnant should not smoke cannabis during the pregnancy. It can affect the unborn child.

CARAWAY SEED (CARUM CARVI)
This seed is known for its aromatic flavour.

Contains:
Vitamins: A, B1 (thiamin), B2 (riboflavin), B3 (niacin), C

Minerals: calcium, cobalt, copper, iodine, iron, magnesium, prosperous, potassium, silicon, sodium, zinc

Other: carvacrol, carvone, ketone, terpene

Plant:
The seeds are used. This plant is a biennial that is found growing in north and central Europe, West Asia and in the Himalayan area. The plant has slender stems, fleshy root and feather shaped leaves. It grows white flowers that turn to a fruit.

Part used: When the fruit dries, the seeds are found in the long pods.

Therapeutic action:
antihistamine, anti-inflammatory, antimicrobial

Uses:
Blood: This herb helps to cleanse the blood and the liver.

Eyes: Caraway seed used for better eye vision and to clear eye infections.

Glands: Caraway seeds help keep the glands active.

Kidney: Used for cleansing and strengthening the kidney.

Liver: This herb helps to cleanse the blood and strengthen the liver.

Lungs: Its antihistamine abilities help in healing the lungs from bronchitis.

Mouth: Good to use for bad breath.

Skin: Scabies can be eliminated with caraway tea.

Stomach: Used to help calm the stomach, especially in babies with colic. The herb is a muscle relaxant and has the antimicrobial properties that can help in the digestion and for irritable bowel syndrome. Caraway seeds have anti-nauseating effects that help the body to be more comfortable when using other medications. Known for eliminating hookworms.

Urinary tract: Used to get treat candida.

Other uses and information:
- Due to the aromatic flavour of the caraway seed it is used in baking, cheeses, meats, as a pickling spice and in teas.

CASCARA SAGRADA (FRANGULA PURSHIANA)
Known as sacred bark, California buckthorn

Contains:
Vitamins: B1 (thiamin), B2 (riboflavin), B3 (niacin), C

Minerals: calcium, iron, magnesium, manganese, phosphorous, potassium, selenium, silicon, zinc

Other: aloe-amyrin, anthraquinones, chrysophanic acid, chrysophanic acid, emodin, frangulin, linoleic acid, malic acid, tannin

Plant:
The tree is 15 to 25 feet tall, with a reddish-brown bark that is often covered in lichen. The leaves are alternate, dark green, ovate and round at base. The flowers are small and a greenish colour. They produce black pea size drupes.

Parts used: The aged dry bark is used and the bark should be over a year old.

Therapeutic action:
Alterative, anti-parasitic, hepatic, stomachic, tonic

Uses:
Bowels: Increases secretion of the stomach, liver, pancreas and lower bowel. Helps to lessen constipation and gets rid of parasites.

Gall Bladder: Used for activating the gall bladder and pancreas

Intestines: Cascara Sagrada has active principles that get absorbed through the small intestine, enter the systemic circulation that stimulates the auerbachian plexus. It can be used over long periods of time, but is best used in combination, as it is too strong on its own. It is recognized for having permanent beneficial effect on intestinal tract.

Liver: Increases secretion of the liver.

Pancreas: Increases secretion of the pancreas. Used for activating the pancreas.

Stomach: Used for assisting the bowels to empty properly. Increases secretion of the stomach.

Other uses and information:
- Can be used as a tea but tastes very bitter.

CATNIP (NEPETA CATARIA)
Known as catmint, catswort

Contains:
Vitamins: A, B1 (thiamin), B2 (riboflavin), B3 (niacin), B5 (pantothenic acid), B6 (pyridoxine), B12, C

Minerals: calcium, chromium, iron, magnesium, manganese, phosphorous, potassium, selenium, silicon, sulfur, zinc

Other: alpha-humulene, beta-elemene, citral, citronellal, geraniol, myrcene, nepetalacone, piperitone, pulegone, rosmarinic acid, thymol,

Plant:
Catnip grows from 2' to 3' high. The stems are erect, square, hairy, branching. Leaves are opposite and covered with soft down. The underside of the leaf is paler in colour. It has many flowers, white or purplish, set in whorled spikes. The flower is a whitish in colour with dotted red spots.

Parts used: The whole plant is used.

Solvent: alcohol or boiling water. Catnip should always be infused

Therapeutic action:
anti-inflammatory, anti-parasitic, carminative, diaphoretic, emmenagogue, nervine, relaxant, stimulant, tonic

Uses:
Blood: Good for improving circulation.

Colon: Used as enema to relax spastic colons. Used to stop diarrhea.

Intestines: Used for getting rid of intestinal worms.

Lungs: Helps to reduce lung congestion and to treat chronic bronchitis.

Menstrual: Catnip has helped to reduce menstrual cramps and regulate the menstrual cycle.

Muscles: Used to reduce muscle inflammation and cramps.

Nerves: Mild stimulant and relaxant. Used for nervous headaches, hysteria and to reduce the effects of stress.

Pregnancy: Catnip has been used to prevent premature births and miscarriages. Helps to reduce morning sickness.

Skin: Catnip is used to heal skin sores. The bruised leaves can be used in a poultice.

Stomach: Catnip helps to reduce digestive gas and helps with the digestion. Can also be used to stimulate appetite. Safe to use for infant colic.

Other uses and information:
- Used for lowering fevers, for colds and flus and induces sleep.
- Reduces atherosclerotic plaque in animals. Great to mellow out cats.
- Externally, the herb is bruised and applied to piles for two to three hours for pain relief and used to reduce hemorrhoids.
- Has been used to reduce convulsions in children.
- This herb has been an aid in drug and nicotine withdrawal.
- Catnip in the yard will help keep rats away.

CAYENNE (CAPSICUM MINIMUM, C. FASTIGIATUM, C. ANNUM)

One of best stimulants

Known as capsicum, red pepper, bird pepper, African pepper

Contains:
Vitamins: B1 (thiamin), B2 (riboflavin), B3 (niacin), B5 (pantothenic acid), B6 (pyridoxine), C, E

Minerals: calcium, iron, magnesium, phosphorous, potassium, selenium, sulfur, zinc

Other: amino acids, alpha-carotene, ascorbic acid, beta-carotene, beta-ionone, caffeic acid, campesterol, capsaicin, carotene, carvone, caryophyllene, chlorogenic acid, citric acid, cryptoxanthin, hesperedin, kaempferol, limonene, lutein, myristic acid, oleic, p-courmaric acid, quercetin, scopoletin, stigmasterol, zeaxanthin

Plant:
Cayenne is a perennial that grows to 3 feet plus. Its stem has woody bottom and the leaves are ovate. It has a drooping white to yellow flower and grows in twos or threes, with dark coloured anthers. The fruit grows in bunches of two or three and are scarlet red to yellow. The best capsicum is the African bird's eye cayenne (C. fastigiatum).

Parts used: the fruit and the oil from the seeds

Therapeutic action:
antispasmodic, astringent, carminative, diaphoretic, stimulant, tonic

Uses:

Blood: Good for the circulatory system, feeding cells and giving them elasticity. Cleanses the blood system. Lowers the cholesterol and triglycerides in the blood to lower the LDL/HDL ratio. Decreases platelet aggregation. Helps to dilate the arteries. Stops internal bleeding from ulcers.

Bones: Cayenne is beneficial for easing arthritis and rheumatism.

Diseases: Used to stop alcohol addictions and will reduce dilation of blood cells.

Heart: Helps with circulation of the blood. Used to equalize high and low blood pressure.

Kidneys: Cayenne helps with the kidneys.

Lungs: Helps to heal the lungs.

Nose: Used to clear the sinuses.

Pancreas: Used for healing the pancreas and spleen.

Skin: Used to stop wound bleeding and also helps to heal frostbite,

Stomach: Used to treat stomach problems and ulcers. Aids in digestion.

Throat: Helps with sore throats.

Other uses and information:
- Use at beginning of cold/flu, not at end.

- Cayenne has been used with lobelia for the nervous system

Caution: Avoid getting cayenne near the eyes.

CHAMOMILE (MATRICARIA RECUTITA OR MATRICARIA CHAMOMILLA)

This herb is known for its relaxing properties.

Contains:
Vitamins: B1 (thiamin), B3 (niacin), C

Minerals: calcium, chlorine, potassium, selenium, zinc

Other: apigenin, azulene, borneol, caffeic acid, chlorogenic acid, farnesol, gentisic acid, geraniol, hyperoside, kaempferol, luteolin, p-courmaric acid, perillyl alcohol, quercetin, rutin, salicylic acid, sinapic acid, umbelliferone

Plant:
Annual that grows to .3 - .6 m tall. It is branched with smooth, solid, striated greenish stems. The leaves are 5 cm long, and are green smooth small linear leaflets. The flower is white and yellow and flowers from May to August. The odour is pleasant with an aromatic bitter taste.

Parts used: mainly the flower, sometimes the whole herb. Should be kept in sealed container.

Therapeutic action:
antimicrobial, antioxidant, antispasmodic, diuretic, carminative, diaphoretic (hot), emmenagogue, nervine, stimulant, stomachic, tonic.

Uses:
Blood: Chamomile is good for our blood circulation.

Bones: Chamomile has been used to bring down inflammation of arthritis.

Hemorrhoids: Helps to reduce the inflammation of hemorrhoids, but must be applied in a tincture or lotion.

Lungs: Used to reduce congestion.

Menstruation: In a tea, can help to reduce menstrual cramps and slow down the flow.

Mouth: As a mouthwash, chamomile will heal minor mouth infections and heal the gums.

Nerves: Chamomile in a tea is a great way to relax in the evening for a better sleep and to treat insomnia. Used for anxiety, nerves and to release the effects of stress.

Skin: Soothes and softens the skin. Good for washing with and in ointments. Used to help reduce eczema and other rashes.

Stomach: Chamomile is used for healing the weaker stomach and to help stimulate the appetite. Used for colitis. Helps in the digestion of foods. A cold infusion is soothing for the stomach. Add a bit of ginger, helpful for flatulent colic, heartburn, loss of appetite and sluggish intestinal canal.

Other uses and information:
- Been used to reduce fevers and pains.

- Chamomile has been tested and shown properties that help to fight cancer.

- Used for ridding one of nightmares, child who is cranky, and for one who wakes up from a bad dream.

- German Chamomile is antifungal and antibacterial.

- Used in teas for calming in the evening and as a tonic/lotion for hemorrhoids.

- Chamomile tea is good for nursing mothers who have colicky babies.

Caution:
Do not use chamomile for long periods as it can cause an allergy towards rag weed.

Should not be used with other sedatives or alcohol.

Pregnant mothers should not use chamomile as there have been cases of the herb causing uterine contractions that have led to miscarriages.

CHAPARRAL (LARREA TRIDENTATE, L. DIVERICATA)

Known as creosote bush, greasewood, black bush, grease bush

Contains:
Vitamins: B1 (thiamin), B2 (riboflavin), B3 (niacin), C

Minerals: calcium, magnesium, selenium, sulfur, zinc

Other: alpha-pinene, amino acids, beta-carotene, borneol, camphene, flavonoids, gossypetin, limonene, protein, volatile oil

Plant:
Chaparral belongs to desert group of Artemisia. It grows in southwestern USA and is about 4 – 8 feet tall. The stems and leaves are dark green (pale of yellow in drought), and the leaves are strongly scented. The flower is bright yellow with five petals. The flower lower appears in spring or winter. The fruit is rounded, covered with white hair and grows to 4" long.

Parts used: leaves and stems.

Solvent: hot water

Therapeutic action:
alterative, anti-inflammatory, antiseptic, carminative, demulcent, diuretic: mild, expectorant, pectoral, tonic

Uses:
Blood: Chaparral helps to fight the free radicals and removes the heavy metals from the body. Used for cleansing the blood and fighting off disease such as HIV, cancer, leukemia, and tuberculosis. Helps the body to fight off exposure to radiation.

Bones: Used by Mexicans for rheumatism and arthritis.

Bowels: Used to help in bowel elimination. Used to reduce diarrhea and to heal gastroenteritis

Eyes: Good for improving the eyesight.

Kidneys: Used to help treat and support the kidney

Liver: Slows down production of LDL cholesterol and inhibits lipid peroxidation in the liver.

Lungs: Helps to heal the lungs of tuberculosis and influenza.

Lymphatic: Used to help heal the lymphatic system.

Menstruation: Chaparral helps to reduce menstrual cramping.

Muscles: Used for back problems and sore muscles.

Prostate: Used to help with prostate gland troubles.

Skin: Chaparral can be used for skin problems: acne, eczema, itches, scabies, snake bit, sores. Used to get rid of dandruff and promotes hair growth. Chaparral also helps the skin when damaged by sun exposure.

Other uses and information:
-Chaparral has been used in the treatment of cancer and venereal disease.

- Used for weight reduction. Used for purging hallucinogens from the system.

- Used to reduce tumours.

- In 1992, the use of chaparral was stopped by the USA government due to six cases (no solid evidence presented) of liver toxicity.

- Chaparral had been banned in the USA and Canada, but is still being used in households.

Caution: Recommended for external use only. If chaparral is taken internally but with caution, in large doses and for prolonged periods, it can cause liver damage.

CHICKWEED (STELLARIA MEDIA)
Known as starweed, stitchwort, scarwort

Contains:
Vitamins: A, B1 (thiamin), B2 (riboflavin), B3 (niacin), C, E

Minerals: calcium, iron, magnesium, manganese, phosphorous, potassium, selenium, silicon, sulfur, zinc

Other: beta-carotene, fibre, high in protein, rutin

Plant:
Annual herb with trailing stem which mats. The leaves are ovate 1 – 3 cm long while the upper leaves are sessile. Flowers are solitary or in few flowered cymes.

Part Used: the whole plant

Solvent: This herb is mixed with water and/or alcohol.

Therapeutic action:
alterative, anti-inflammatory, antiseptic, diuretic, demulcent, emollient, pectoral

Uses:
Blood: Chickweed is used as a cleanser for the blood and for blood poisoning, and it works with circulatory problems.

Bowels: Used to help stop bleeding in the bowels.

Breast: Used for breast inflammation during lactation.

Heart: Used for pulmonary problems.

Lungs: Chickweed can help to stop bleeding in the lungs and heals bronchitis, coughs and nasal congestion.

Muscles: Helps to lessen muscle cramps, tightened and contracted sinews.

Skin: Used in ointments and cleansers for the skin and in babies for rashes. Chickweed can be used in poultices to heal skin abscesses, athlete's foot, breast inflammation, candida, carbuncles, genital rashes, infections, ulcers and warts. This herb works on the cellular level of the skin.

Stomach: Used in a tea to strengthen the stomach.

Testicles: Chickweed has been used to reduce swelling of the testicles.

Other uses and information:
- Used for internal and external inflammation.

- Chickweed has also been useful in weight loss as it helps to suppress the appetite.

- Used to reduce the size of tumours

- Cooking: Used in salads and soups.

- Skin Ointment: Used for all types of skin problems: skin ulcers, carbuncles, external abscesses.

- Baths: for soothing effect.

CHLORELLA

Contains:
Vitamins: A, B1 (thiamin), B2 (riboflavin), B3 (niacin), B6 (pyridoxine), B12, C, E, PABA

Minerals: calcium, copper, iodine, iron, magnesium, zinc

Other: amino acids, carotene, chlorophyll, inositol, pantothenic acid

Plant:
Chlorella is a naturally grown fresh water one cell algae. This plant/algae has been part of the earth's living structure since the beginning. Records have shown the use of chlorella since 3000 B.C. Pure chlorella has 13% DNA / RNA factors compared to spirulina that has 4.5%.

Therapeutic action:
antibacterial, antimicrobial, antioxidant, nervine

Uses:

Blood: This herb as an antioxidant will help to detoxify the liver and blood along with removing heavy metals and toxins from our bodies. DNA / RNA factors to help rebuild cells and as a protection against diseases.

Bowels: Used to help heal and cleanse the bowels and reduce constipation. Chlorella is wonderful for working with the colon and promoting better functioning of the bowels.

Immune: As an antioxidant, chlorella will boost the immune system with amino acids such as lysine.

Mouth: Used to heal the gums and teeth as chlorella is antibacterial.

Nerves: Chlorella has a high level of vitamin Bs, which aids in lowering the stress levels and lessening depression.

Organs: This one celled algae is known for its healing abilities for the skin and liver. Used after surgeries to promote healing for organs and tissues.

Other uses and information:

- Also to help eliminate bad breath and underarm odour.

- Chlorella is rich in protein and has more B12 than liver.

- Chlorella is prescribed by many dentists after the old mercury fillings are removed. Its ability to remove heavy metals such as mercury and toxins is well known.

- The production of interferon can be increased with chlorella, and this will help to reduce allergy and cold symptoms.

- Chlorella can be used in the powdered state and put into smoothies or other power drinks. Chlorella can also be found in a compressed pill or placed as a power into capsules.

CILANTRO

Known for its heavy metal cleansing

Contains:

Vitamins: A, B1 (thiamin), B2 (riboflavin), B3 (niacin), B5 (pantothenic Acid), B6 (pyridoxine), C, E, K

Minerals: calcium, iron, magnesium, manganese, phosphorous, potassium, selenium, sodium, zinc

Other: borneol, cymene, epigenin, kaempferol, linalool, phellandrene, pinene, quercetin, terpineol, volatile oil,

Plant:

The oil is very high in antioxidant properties. The leaves are also called coriander. This plant can grow from 9 inches tall to 7 feet tall. It has white or pink flowers that turn to the seeds that are also used.

Parts Used: The leaves, stems and seeds are used.

Therapeutic action:
antifungal, antimicrobial, antioxidant, anti-parasitic, antiseptic, antispasmodic, anxiety, carminative, cathartic, nervine, stimulant, stomachic, tonic

Uses:
Blood: Good for cleansing the blood as it has a high antioxidant level, and it is believe to regulate the blood sugar levels. Cilantro has also been shown to assist in healing Alzheimer's disease, as it cleanses the blood and reduces neuronal damage.

Bones: The vitamin K level in cilantro is very high and essential for keeping our bones healthy and is also a good preventative of osteoporosis disorders.

Diseases: The high level of antioxidants and heavy metal cleansing of cilantro helps to build up the immune system and can prevent diseases.

Heart: Cilantro has been used to help keep the cardiovascular system healthier and stronger. It is believed to reduce the cholesterol level of the blood.

Liver: Cleanses the blood and provides a good support for the liver.

Nerves: Cilantro is high in the B vitamins that can be used for anxiety, depression, insomnia and nervousness. .

Stomach: Cilantro assists in soothing the stomach and aiding in digestion.

Other uses and information:
- Cilantro has a compound that sticks to heavy metals in the body and helps to release the metals from the tissues to which they are attached. This is very beneficial for those who have had mercury fillings in their mouth. Mercury finds a way into the blood stream and slowly can poison the body.

- It is a good source of dietary fibre.

- Cilantro and coriander can be used in both raw dishes and cooked dishes. It is a good addition to black bean dishes.

- The leaves can be made into a tea or other drink.

- The leaves and stems can be used in culinary dishes and teas.

- The seeds are used as flavouring for dishes and used in essential oils.

- The oil from the seeds are extracted to use in an essential oil.

CINNAMON (CASSIA)
Cinnamon is high in antioxidants and is known for its antibacterial properties and lowering blood sugar levels.

Contains:
Vitamins: A, B1 (thiamin), B2 (riboflavin), B3 (niacin), C

Minerals: calcium, chromium, copper, iodine, iron, manganese, phosphorus, potassium, zinc

Other: alpha-pinene, benzaldehyde, beta-carotene, beta pinene, borneol, camphor, caryophyllene, cinnamaldehyde, courmarins, cuminaldehyde, eugenol, farnesol, geranial, limonene, mannitol, mucilage, tannin, terpinolene, vanillan

Plant:
Cinnamon comes from the inner bark of the cinnamon tree. There are several species of this tree. The tree is native to the Mediterranean, Bangladesh, Burma, India and Sri Lanka. This plant is a part of many legends and is highly valued.

Parts used: The parts that are used are the inner bark, essential oil and twigs.

Therapeutic action:
antibacterial, antibiotic, antifungal, anti-inflammatory, anti-stress

Uses:
Blood: This herb is very beneficial towards helping to lower the blood sugar levels for diabetics. Cinnamon helps to increase the blood circulation.

Chest: Cinnamon used in teas or with honey will help the lungs with chest infections. It is well known for its antibiotic properties.

Digestion: Cinnamon helps to soothe the stomach when affected by indigestion. It also helps to stop diarrhea and vomiting.

Immune: Cinnamon is excellent for warding off flus and coughs.

Liver: With the antifungal and antibacterial properties, cinnamon is a great assistant to help cleanse the liver too.

Menstruation: Will help with heavy periods and cramping.

Mouth: Cinnamon will assist in healing infections that cause toothaches.

Nerves: Used to for anxiety, to restore energy, calm the nerves and release stress. Used for neuralgia: pain from damaged nerves.

Stomach: This herb is great to use for colic.

Uterus: Assists in healing infections in the uterus.

Other uses and information:
- Cinnamon can be added to baking, mixed with honey and in tea, placed in water as a mouthwash, as a spice, in essential oils, in massage oils, in a decoction, tincture, powder in capsules and in a compress.

CLEAVER (GALIUM APARINE)
Known as clivers, goose grass, bayriff, goosebill, bedstraw. ** Member of bedstraw genus

Contains:
chlorophyll, starch, gallotannic acid, citric acid, rubichloric acid.

Plant:
This plant is a member of bedstraw genus. Found in river banks, moist woods and cultivated feeds. Can be found in grain crops. Grows annually from 3 to 10 cm long. The leaves are sixes, sevens or eights. Leaves are 1 to 3 cm long. The flowers are few and are greenish-white. The fruit is covered with little bristles.

Solvent: water: do not boil

Therapeutic action:
alterative, antiscorbutic, aperient, diuretic, soothing, relaxing, tonic

Uses:
Bladder: Cleaver assists with both the bladder and kidneys.

Bowels: This herb can be used as a mild laxative.

Breast: This herb assists in treating breast tumours.

Kidney: Cleaver helps with the de-obstruction of the urinary organs when used with broom, uva-ursi, birch and marshmallow. Cleaver can soften stones, gravel, and decrease the size of calculi to help in elimination.

Skin: Cleaver can help to ease the pain of sunburn and reduce freckles, psoriasis and abrasions. Cleaver has helped to treat skin cancer and tumours. This herb can be used in an ointment to apply to the skin.

Other uses and information:
- The juice of cleaver is used as an antiscorbutic.

- Decoct the fresh herb and apply to the area with a sponge or cloth to the skin area.

Caution: Cleaver is a strong diuretic and should not be used with diabetes. It over stimulates the adrenals and inhibits the action of the insulation.

CLOVE (SYZYGIUM AROMATICUM)
Cloves are known as a super herb. It is a powerful herb used to treat viral infections and used as a preventative.

Contains:
Vitamins: A, B1 (thiamin), B2 (riboflavin), B3 (niacin), B5 (pantothenic acid), B6 (pyridoxine), B12, C

Minerals: calcium, iron, magnesium, manganese, phosphorous, potassium, sodium, zinc

Other:
beta-carotene, beta pinene, campesterol, carvone, caryophyllene, chavicol, cinnamaldehyde, ellagic acid, eugenol, gallic acid, kaempferol, linalool, methyleugenol, methylsalicylate, mucilage, oleanolic acid, stigmasterol, tannin, vanillan,

Plant:
Cloves come from the Myrtaceae tree family. This tree grows up to 12 m tall and is native to the Indonesian area. It is the flower buds that produce the cloves. It has large leaves, and the flowers grow in clusters. The flowers are a pale colour that turn to green then to a red colour.

Parts used: flower buds.

Therapeutic action:
antibacterial, anti-emetic, antioxidants, anti-parasitic, antiseptic, antispasmodic, antiviral, stomachic, tonic

Uses:
Blood: Good for increasing the blood circulation and helps with low blood pressure.

Bowels: Cloves can help stop diarrhea.

Colon: Cloves has been used to treat colitis (inflammation of the colon).

Ears: Good for healing earaches.

Mouth: Clove oil can be applied to the area of a toothache and mouth pain. It is an antiseptic and will help to clear infections. The oil can be used to stop bad breath. Usually bad breath is cause by an infection in the mouth or the body.

Muscles: Cloves have assisted in decreasing muscle spasms.

Stomach: Cloves is great to use to help with digestion, reduce gas and has been used to stop vomiting and nausea.

Other uses and information:
- Good for treating epilepsy and palsy.

- The clove oil is best used with olive oil or with distilled water.

- The powder form of cloves can be used in a tea with cinnamon to help stop nausea, ward of bacterial infections and flu bugs.

COMFREY (SYMPHYTUM OFFICINALE)
Known as knitbone, knitback, bruisewort, boneset

Contains:
Vitamins: A, B1 (thiamin), B2 (riboflavin), B3 (niacin), C

Minerals: calcium, copper, germanium, iron, magnesium, manganese, phosphorous, potassium, protein, selenium, sodium, zinc

Other: allantoin, amino acids, aspargine, beta-carotene, beta-sitosterol, caffeic acid, chlorogenic acid, protein, pyrrolizidine alkaloids, rosmarinic acid, sitosteral, stigmasterol, tannin

Plant:
Comfrey is a perennial. The plant has a stout spreading root that can be easily divided for garden propagation. The plant will grow up to 3 feet high. It has coarse lance shaped leaves. Flower is a tubular shape that can be blue, purple, yellow or red.

Parts used: leaves and root

Solvent: water

Therapeutic action:
anti-cancerous, anti-inflammatory, astringent, demulcent, expectorant, tonic.

Uses:
Blood: Good for those suffering from anemia, as comfrey will rebuild the blood while cleansing it. Mucilage of comfrey root is a great cell proliferator, a new cell grower.

Bones: Comfrey is an amazing bone healer. HealComfrey has allantoin, which is excellent when used in a tea to help heal bones. Studies show that the broken bone needs to be set properly before administering the tea. Good for arthritis, broken bones, sprains and fractures.

Kidney Stones: Used for dissolving kidney stones.

Liver: Comfrey will rebuild the blood while cleansing it.

Lungs: Used for coughs, respiratory system, healing hemorrhage of lungs. Used to reduce asthma attacks.

Pituitary gland: Comfrey has a natural hormone that stimulates and restores the pituitary gland. This helps to strengthen the skeletal system of the body.

Skin: When comfrey is used in an ointment or poultice, it can heal the skin fast. There have been cases were the herb has been used in place of stitches to cuts, with no apparent scar later. Used to heal bedsores, bites, bleeding, bruises, burns, cuts, dermatitis, hemorrhoids, psoriasis, rashes, skin ulcers, scabies and sunburn. The mucilage of comfrey root is a great cell proliferator as it stimulates new cell grower.

Stomach: Comfrey has been used to stop diarrhea and aid in digestion.

Other uses and information:
- Due to the banning of this amazing herb by the governments, I will not show any other uses or how it is used. I felt the need to share the information as I saw this herb in almost every garden in my neighbourhood in Alberta, Canada.

Caution: Internal use can cause damage to the liver. Use should be under the supervision of a doctor. Should not be used during pregnancy.

CRAMP BARK (VIBUMUM OPULUS)

Known as highbushes, cranberry, guelder, rose, snowball tree

Contains:
Vitamins: C, K

Other: The bark contains tannin, valerianic acid, vibutin and viburnine.

Plant:
While doing research, it was hard to determine which tree this really came from. Yet a picture I saw resembled the snowball tree. I did some studying with the books that Terry Willard wrote for his herbology classes, and this is some of the information that he shared. Small tree or shrub 1 - 4m tall. The bark is a grey colour and the leaves are lobed. The leaves are ovate and coarsely toothed. The flowers are orange to red (sometimes white) and quite acidic.

Parts used: Bark, inner bark is preferable.

Solvent: water, diluted alcohol

Therapeutic action:
antispasmodic, astringent, diuretic, expectorant, nervine, relaxant, tonic

Uses:
Lungs: Recognized by the National Formulary as an antispasmodic for asthma.

Menstrual: Cramp bark is known for its anti-inflammatory properties that help to reduce menstrual cramping. This herb helps to relax the uterus and quiets excessive ovarian action.

Nerves: Used for convulsions, fainting and fits. Used for neuralgia that is caused by damaged nerves. Recognized by the National Formulary as an antispasmodic for hysteria.

Stomach: Known for its ability to relieve abdominal cramps that are due to intestinal problems.

Uterus: Helps to relax the uterus during menstruation.

Other uses and information:
- Used for lockjaw.

- Used in rituals by the Natives. Used during the different seasons for blessings.

CRANESBILL GERANIUM (GERANIUM MACULATAM)

Known as crowfoot, cranesbill, stork bill, wild alum root, wild geranium

Contains:
Minerals: calcium

Other: gallic acid, gum, pectin, resin, starch, tannins

Plant:
This perennial is found in woodlands in North America. Root stock is stout and produces a hairy stem, which grows from 1 – 2 feet high with long leaves. The white, rose and purple coloured flowers grow in pairs from April to July.

Parts used: Root stock, sometimes the leaves.

Solvent: water and alcohol

Therapeutic action:
astringent, diuretic, tonic

Uses:
Blood: Good for stopping light hemorrhaging. Unicorn root and cranesbill are used together to slow down diabetes. The Blackfoot Nation (Canada) uses the powdered cranesbill for first aid to stop bleeding.

Breast: Used to firm up sore and tender nipples. (Only the nipple should be massaged with the decoction.)

Intestines: Used for cholera, diarrhea and dysentery

Kidney: Unicorn root and cranesbill are used together to treat Bright's disease that is caused by albumin in the urine and high blood pressure.

Mouth: Used for canker sores.

Skin: Cranesbill is a powerful astringent and excellent to use to heal the skin. It reduces wrinkles and closes the skin pores.

Other uses and information:
- Used to treat atonic vagina, hemorrhoids and indolent ulcers.

- Used to draw mercury out of the body, ex: silver amalgams.

- The cranesbill stringent is weaker than white aak but stronger than witch hazel.

- First Nations used cranesbill as birth control. Soaking together cranesbill, wood ash, and water for half hour within first month after delivery would prevent pregnancy for a year. Drinking cranesbill tea would prevent pregnancy.

DANDELION (TARAXACUM OFFICINALE) AND DANDELION ROOT
Known for being a blood purifier.

Contains:
Vitamins: A, B1 (thiamin), B2 (riboflavin), B3 (niacin), C, D, E, G

Minerals: calcium, chlorine, iron, magnesium, manganese, phosphorus, potassium, selenium, sodium, zinc

Other: beta-carotene, beta-sitosterol, caffeic acid, cryptoxanthin, lutein, mannitol, myristic acid, p-coumaric acid, saponin, stigmasterol

Plant:
The plant is considered a weed and is found in many parts of the world. It is used as a salad green when the plant is young, in teas, tablets and capsules.

Parts used: roots, tops, leaves and flowers.

Therapeutic action:
anodyne, antibacterial, anti-cancer, anti-inflammatory, astringent, cathartic, diaphoretic, hepatic, stimulant, stomachic, tonic

Uses:
Bladder: Dandelion is used to strengthen the bladder and kidneys.

Blood: Good to use in a tea after taking pain killers and anesthetic from an operation. Dandelion helps to cleanse the bloodstream and liver: hepatitis and jaundice.

Bones: Used for decreasing the inflammation of rheumatism.

Breast: Dandelion has worked well for treating breast tumours.

Heart: It also helps to lower the serum cholesterol and therefore is good for the heart.

Kidney: Used to treat dropsy.

Liver: Dandelion can be used in capsules or in a tea to help cleanse the liver, (hepatitis and jaundice). Good to use in a tea after taking pain killers and anesthetic from an operation.

Menstrual: Dandelion tea helps to reduce menopausal symptoms.

Mouth: Dandelion has helped with abscesses in the gums.

Pancreas: Dandelion works well to strengthen the pancreas.

Skin: Helps to relieve edema and age spots as dandelion helps to cleanse the liver. Used to treat boils, psoriasis, eczema and other skin diseases.

Stomach: Used to work with the stomach and increases the bile production. This helps to reduce constipation.

Caution: Those with gallstones and biliary tract obstruction are advised not to use dandelion. Do not use with other prescription diuretics.

ECHINACEA (ECHINACEA AUGUSTIFOLIA)
Known as Black Sampson, cone flower, purple cone flower

Contains:
Vitamins: B1 (thiamin), B2 (riboflavin), B3 (niacin), C

Minerals: calcium, iron, magnesium, manganese, phosphorous, potassium, selenium, zinc

Other: alpha-pinene, apigenin, arabinogalactan, beta-carotene, beta-sitosterol, betaine, borneol, caffeic acid, caryophyllene, chlorogenic acid, cynarin, echinacoside, ferulic acid, kaempferol, luteolin, quercetin, rutin, stigmasterol, vanillan, verbascoside.

Plant:
Echinacea is an herbaceous plant with thick black pungent root. The stem is slender to stout stem 2 – 3 feet tall with bristly hairs. The flowers are narrow, 1 – 2" long, rose – purple and rarely white.

Parts used: rhizome and root

Therapeutic action:
analgesic, antibacterial, antimicrobial, antiseptic, antiviral, diaphoretic

Uses:
Blood: Echinacea builds up the white blood cells, and it detoxifies and cleanses the blood. Used as an antiseptic and analgesic and for snake bites. Has an antiviral activity that blocks virus rector sites on the surface of cell membranes and inhibits viruses from infecting the cells.

Liver: This herb is used to clean the blood and will assist in cleaning the liver.

Lymphatic System: Helps to heal the lymphatic system

Skin: This herb is an antiseptic and will heal wounds in the skin.

Throat: Used for bronchitis, coughs and sore throats.

Diseases: Builds the body immunity for viral and fungal infections, typhoid fever and bacteria. Used in cold and flu formulas. Used for prevention of cancer and to inhibit tumours. Used for yeast infections, AIDS, Chronic Fatigue Syndrome and MS.

Other uses and information:
- Echinacea can be bought as a liquid, in tablets and as tea.

Caution:
- Echinacea should be used with caution by people who are allergic to ragweed or to plants from the sunflower family. This herb should not be taken for long periods by people with autoimmune disorders. This herb must be used periodically, (a couple of weeks on and a couple of weeks off). Overuse of this herb can cause stress to your immune system and cause temporary infertility to men.

EUCALYPTUS (EUCALYPTUS GLOBULUS)

Contains:
alpha-pinene, beta pinene, caffeic acid, carvone, ferulic acid, gallic acid, gentistic acid, hyperoside, p-cymene, quercetin, quercitrin, rutin,

Plant:
Native to Australia, this plant is part of the myrtle family. Eucalyptus has over 700 species and is now being grown in many countries, including Canada on Salt Springs Island. It is easy to start from seed. The eucalyptus plant is one of three known gum trees. The other trees are known as angophora and corymbia. These trees exude a lot of sap if the bark breaks or is injured. The eucalyptus plant can grow from 33' to 200' tall. The leaves of the plant are covered with oil glands and at the same time they can convert oxygen into ozone. The leaves look waxy, and they are long in shape.

Parts used: the bark, leaves and oil are used.

Therapeutic action:
antibiotic, anti-inflammatory, antiseptic, antiviral

Uses:
Diseases: Eucalyptus has been used to treat diphtheria, malaria and typhoid.

Lungs: Inhaling the fumes of the oil helps to clear the lungs and sinuses. Used to treat asthma, bronchitis and croup.

Muscles: The oil has been used to reduce swelling and for relief for sore muscles. It has the properties to help increase the blood flow.

Stomach: Used to stop nausea (one small drop under the tongue). Eucalyptus has been used to expel worms.

Skin: The oil is used as an antiseptic to prevent infections in the skin or to stop germs from spreading and heal wounds. You can use the oil, mixed with water as an insect repellant. It has been used to clear up external ulcers

Throat: Eucalyptus can be found in many sore throat lozenges.

Other uses and information:
- Eucalyptus is used to treat paralysis and for treating cancer.

- Veterinarians use eucalyptus oil for distemper in dogs, influenza in horses and for skin parasites or bug bites.

EYEBRIGHT (EUPHRASIA OFFICINALIS)

Known as meadow eyebright, red eyebright

Contains:
Vitamins: A, B1 (thiamin), B2 (riboflavin), B3 (niacin), C, D, E

Minerals: calcium, chromium, copper, iodine, iron, magnesium, manganese, phosphorous, potassium, selenium, zinc

Other: beta-carotene, caffeic acid, ferulic acid, silicone, tannins

Plant:
The plant is native to Europe. The flowers are white or purple or blue with about eight petals and yellow centre.

Parts used: the leaves, stems and parts of the flower are used.

Therapeutic action:
alterative, demulcent, emollient, pectoral.

Uses:
Blood: Eyebright helps to cleanse the blood and the liver.

Ears: Used for earaches.

Eyes: Good for strengthening the eyesight, relieves eye strain or irritation. The tannins decrease the inflammation. Used to treat blepharitis, conjunctivitis and cataracts.

Liver: Eyebright helps to cleanse the toxins from the liver.

Lungs: Used for colds and coughs.

Stomach: Used to soothe the ulcers.

Throat: Used for sore throats.

Other uses and information:
- It is good for allergies that bother the eyes and nose and good for hay fever.

- It has been known to strengthen the brain by improving the memory and is used for vertigo.

- Good for the sinuses.

Caution: For use on the eyes – only use eyebright solutions that are made in a controlled lab. It is suggested that one contact a doctor about using eyebright if they are wearing contacts or have had any eye surgery. Side effects can be itchy or watery eyes, nausea and sweating.

Use during pregnancy is not determined, talk to you health care provided first. .

FENNEL (ANETHUM FOENICULUM)

Fennel is known for its liquorice taste. It is also known to help protect the body during any chemotherapy treatments.

Contains:
Vitamins: A, B3 (niacin), B6 (pyridoxine), C

Minerals: calcium, folate, iron, magnesium, manganese, phosphorous, potassium, selenium

Other: alkaloid, anethol, beta-carotene, flavonoid, fibre, high in protein, phenol, rutin

Plant:
Fennel is a perennial, originally found in the Mediterranean and is a part of the carrot family. This plant grows yellow flowers, and the leaves are long and thin. The base of the plant is bulb shaped and is used in cooking.

Parts used: The leaves, stalk and seed of the plant are used. Pick the leaves as needed, best just before flower blooms. Dry or freeze leaves.

Therapeutic action:
antibacterial, anti-cancer, anti-flatulent, anti-inflammatory, antioxidant, antispasmodic, diuretic, stomachic, tonic

Uses:
Blood: Fennel helps to reduce high blood pressure. This herb helps to treat anemia with its good source of iron. Fennel has a high level of antioxidants to help clean the blood.

Bowels: Fennel can be used as a laxative for the bowels.

Brain: Used to keep the brain healthy and for the memory.

Eyes: Helps to keep the eyes healthy and prevents macular degeneration.

Hair: This herb can assist in decreasing hair loss.

Lungs: Used for bronchitis and coughs and has a soothing effect.

Mouth: Fennel is used in products as a mouth freshener and in toothpaste products. Its antibacterial properties would be beneficial especially during a cold or flu.

Skin: The collagen in fennel helps with repair of skin tissue if damaged.

Stomach: Used for the release of stomach gas, acid reflux, colic and cramps. Its digestive aid helps to maintain the tone of the stomach muscles to helps to fight infection in the gastrointestinal tract. Fennel also helps in the distribution of mucus that we need in our intestinal tract. The seeds can be chewed to suppress a person's appetite.

Other uses and information:
- Assists with dyspepsia and flatulence.

- Fennel assists in the production and secretion of milk for the nursing mother.

- This herb is known to help the body fight breast and liver cancer, as it prohibits tumours from growing.

- Fennel has a lot of vitamin C that assists in warding off colds and viruses.

Caution: This herb can be dangerous if too much is consumed.

FENUGREEK (TRIGONELLA FOENUM)

Contains:
Vitamins: B1 (thiamin), B2 (riboflavin), B6 (pyridoxine),

Minerals: copper, iron, magnesium, manganese, selenium

Other: Fenugreek has a lot of fibre. The plant contains an number of powerful phytonutrients: choline, diosgenin, estrogenic isoflavones, gitogenin, tigogenin, trigonelline, vamogenin.

Plant:
Fenugreek is an annual plant the has three small leaves growing together. The plant is well used in Asia and is now grown in many countries.

Parts used: leaves and seeds.

Therapeutic action:
anti-inflammatory, antispasmodic, diuretic, stimulant, stomachic, tonic

Uses:
Blood: Good for reducing the cholesterol in the blood. Fenugreek helps to regulate the blood sugar levels.

Bowels: Fenugreek has been used to help to ease constipation.

Heart: Helps to reduce the risk of cardiovascular problems.

Kidneys: The herb assists in supporting the kidneys.

Lungs: Used for mucus conditions of the lungs and cleans out the bronchial passages.

Menstrual: Fenugreek can help to reduce the effects of menopause as it has estrogen in it. This chemical helps to reduce cramps, depression, mood swings and unusual hunger swings that go with both menstrual periods and menopause.

Throat: Fennel is used in products to help soothe sore throats.

Caution: Fenugreek is not recommended to use during a pregnancy as it can cause a miscarriage.

GARLIC (ALLIUM SATIVA)

Garlic is high in antioxidants.

Contains:
Vitamins: A, B1 (thiamin), B2 (riboflavin), B3 (niacin), C

Minerals: calcium, copper, germanium, iron, magnesium, manganese, phosphorous, potassium, selenium, sodium, sulfur, zinc

Other: allicen, beta-carotene, beta pinene, beta-sitosterol, caffeic acid, chlorogenic acid, diallyl-disulfide, ferulic acid, geraniol, kaempferol, linalool, oleanolic acid, p-coumaric acid, phloroglucinol, phytic acid, quercetin, rutin,

s-allyl cysteine, saponin, sinapic acid, stigmasterol

Plant:
This plant is grown around the world. The bulb gets bigger each year as it is re-harvested. The bulbs can be from white to a purple.

Parts used: The bulb and young stalk of the plant can be used in cooking. After leaves have died, lift out bulbs, dry in sun or dry room.

Therapeutic action:
alterative, anthelmintic, antiseptic, antispasmodic, diaphoretic, diuretic, expectorant, pectoral, stimulant, tonic

Uses:
Blood: Studies have shown that two to three garlic cloves eaten a day slows the white blood cell activity, helps to detoxify the body and regulate the blood sugar levels. Helps to improve the blood circulation.

Diseases: Garlic is used to inhibit viruses and infectious diseases. Garlic contains anti-cancer preventing properties. Garlic has been used in AIDS treatments.

Ears: Been known to help reduce ear infections.

Eyes: Good for strengthening the eyesight.

Heart: Garlic is used to help with both high and low blood cholesterol levels and leads to helping the heart out by regulating the triglycerides. It improves circulation.

Liver: Garlic helps to detoxify the liver.

Lungs: Used to reduce asthma, bronchial problems and lung congestion. Used as an expectorant causing a person to expel excess phlegm from the lungs.

Skin: Garlic is used in poultice to draw out infection of boils, slivers and wounds. Used as a fungicide for the skin.

Stomach: Used for digestive disorders and is used as an anthelmintic to rid body of pin worms and other parasites. Also an aid for treating candida.

Other uses and information:
- Garlic has been used to help with insomnia.

- Cover the skin area with olive oil first to prevent burning or stinging of the garlic. Next apply the poultice of fresh garlic to the skin.

- Garlic can be used fresh, in tablets, capsules of oil, tincture and syrup.

Caution: Garlic is a blood thinner, so caution is recommended for those who take anticoagulants

GENTIAN (GENTIAN LUTEA)

This herb has been used for over 2000 years to help heal the liver.

Contains:
Vitamins: B1 (Thiamin), B2 (Riboflavin), B3 (Niacin), C

Minerals: calcium, chromium, iron, magnesium, manganese, phosphorous, potassium, selenium

Other: amarogenin, absorbic, caffeic, carvacrol, gentioflavosid, gentiopicrin, gentianine, gentialutine, nicotinic, nixanthones, gentianose, limonene, linalool, pectin, phenolic acids, and voilatile oil.

Plant:
Large perennial herb with a thick stem that is a yellowish green. The leaves are oblong shaped, and about 15 – 30 cm long. The flowers are orange to a yellow. The flowers appear June - August. This plant is a perennial. It has a strong odour with both a slightly sweetish and bitter taste.

Parts used: root.

Solvent: water and alcohol.

Therapeutic action:
anthelmintic, antibiotic, anti-inflammatory, antiseptic, astringent, stomachic, tonic

Uses:
Blood: Good for cleansing the blood to treat hepatitis, jaundice and malaria.

Bowels: Gentian can help with both diarrhea and constipation.

Diseases: Assists with treating dyspepsia.

Heart: Helps to stimulate and strengthen the cardiovascular system.

Kidney: Gentian with its antibiotic action assists with the kidney to help heal discharges, urinary tract infection and vaginal rashes.

Liver: Gentian helps to cleanse the blood and strengthen the liver.

Muscles: Gentian is a good anti-inflammatory for the sore muscles.

Skin: Gentian is good for healing the skin

Stomach: Used as a digestive bitter. Gentian helps to be stimulate the gastric juices, and this helps to promote the digestion of the food that we consume. Gentian can assist with heartburn and nausea.

Other uses and information:
- It is good for improving the appetite when someone is concerned about being anorexic.

- Used to help to stimulate the metabolism.

- The First Nations people use gentian for digestive disorders.

GINGER (ASARUM CAUDATUM, ZINGIBAR OFFICINALE)
Ginger has strong antioxidant properties

Contains:
Vitamins: A, B1 (thiamin), B2 (riboflavin), B3 (niacin), B6 (pyridoxine), C,

Minerals: calcium, iron, magnesium, manganese, phosphorous, potassium, selenium, zinc

Other: alpha-pinene, beta-carotene, beta-sitosterol, caffeic acid, camphor, capsaicin, caryophyllene, chlorogenic acid, citral, curcumin, farnesol, ferulic acid, geraniol, gingerois, lecithin, zingerone

Plant:
Ginger is native to Asia. The ginger plant is a perennial tuberous root. It has erect annual stems and smooth sheathed leaves that are 2 – 3 feet high. The flower is a yellow and solitary, with an inner lobe lip of dark purple.

Parts used: The dried rhizome and roots are used in both root and powder form. The powder form keeps better.

Therapeutic action:
antibacterial, anti-inflammatory (better than ASA and has less side effects), antimicrobial, antioxidant, antispasmodic, anti-pyretic, carminative, diaphoretic (if taken hot), thermogenic

Uses:
Blood: Ginger is good for lowering the cholesterol level and as an antioxidant for the blood. Ginger has been used for poor blood circulation in both hands and feet.

Bones: Ginger brings down the inflammation with arthritis.

Bowels: Ginger had been used to help heal bowel disorders.

Gall Bladder: Helps to heal the bladder

Head: Used for headaches and migraines.

Heart: Ginger helps the blood and provides better circulation for the blood to get to the heart.

Kidneys: Used for the kidneys.

Liver: Ginger cleanses and protects the liver.

Lungs: Helps to diffuse mucus in the lungs.

Menstruation: Used to treat hot flashes. Ginger is great for menstrual cramps and can be used to help slow down excessive menstrual flow when the ginger is used in a hot drink

Skin: Used to bring down inflammation from hives by using ginger in the bath water. Used to treat sores and wounds.

Stomach: Used for morning sickness, motion sickness, nausea and as a digestive aid as it helps to reduce gas. Ginger with its antibacterial properties helps to cleanse the colon and intestines along with protecting the stomach.

Other uses and information:

- It has been used to lower fevers and reduce muscles spasms.

- Wild ginger is considered the better of two gingers, but Jamaican ginger is most often used.

- Ginger is a good base to add other herbs to, to help deliver the herbs to the stomach.

- For a tea: Grate an ounce of ginger root, pour a pint of boiling water on it and let steep for 20 minutes.

- Good for sweating out colds: 1/4 teas in hot water, relieves stomach indigestion.

- Used in baking fruits, beef, beverages, conserves and cooking, fish, lamb, pickles, pork, soups, stewed fruits, veal and vegetables.

Caution: If taking anticoagulants or experiencing gallstones, using ginger is not recommended. Do not use much ginger during pregnancy.

GINSENG

(Panax quinguefolium) wild American Ginseng

(Eleutherococcu) Siberian Ginseng (not a true ginseng and the root is woody).

(Panax shin-seng) Korean Ginseng

Contains:
Vitamins: A, B1 (thiamin), B2 (riboflavin), B3 (niacin), B5 (pantothenic acid), B12 (cobalamin), C, E

Minerals: calcium, chlorine, germanium, iron, magnesium, manganese, phosphorous, potassium, selenium, silicon, zinc

Other: beta-sitosterol, campesterol, cinnamic acid, ferulic acid, fibre, folate, fumaric acid, ginsenosides, kaempferol, oleanolic acid, panaxic acid, saponin, sodium, stigmasterol, sulfur, tin, vanillic acid.

Plant:
Ginseng can be found in Bhutan, Asia (eastern region), China (north-east), Korea, North America and Siberia. There are eleven species of this plant, having different properties.

Part used: root

Therapeutic action:
anti-cancer, anti-emetic, anti-inflammatory, expectorant, hepatic, nervine, pulmonary, stimulant, stomachic

Uses:
Blood: Good for increasing the blood circulation, reduces cholesterol, treats blood diseases. Stops internal bleeding.

Ears: Good for improving the hearing.

Eyes: Good for improving eyesight.

Glands: Ginseng is used to support the adrenal and reproductive glands.

Heart: Helps to prevent arteriosclerosis, regulates the blood pressure and stimulate the heart.

Liver: Used to strengthen and support the liver. Used for anemia, immune system, cleaning the liver of chemicals, drug and radiation poisoning and to treat liver diseases.

Lungs: Used for bronchitis and to strengthen the lungs.

Menstruation: Used to treat menopause and menstruation symptoms.

Muscles: Used to reduce the inflammation in the muscles.

Nerves: Used to reduce the effects of mental fatigue, nervousness, stress and weakness. Helps to stimulate the brain and energize the body. Reduces irritability and increases a sense of peacefulness.

Skin: Used to treat age spots,

Stomach: Used for increasing the appetite, improve digestion, reduce nausea and to stop vomiting.

Other uses and information:
- Used as a sexual stimulant.

- Used to stop cocaine addictions.

- Used in China to slow down the aging process.

- Used to treat ulcers.

- Reduces fevers.

Caution: Should not be used if you have asthma, hypoglycemia (low blood sugar), high blood pressure, heart disorders or insomnia or in pregnant and nursing mothers.

GOLDENSEAL (HYDRASTIS CANADENSIS)

Known as ground raspberry, jaundice root, warnero, yellow root

Known as one of the most powerful herbal remedies: natural antibiotic and cancer fighter.

Contains:
Vitamins: B1 (thiamin), B2 (riboflavin), B3 (niacin), C

Minerals: calcium, copper, iron, magnesium, manganese, phosphorous, potassium, selenium, zinc

Other: berberine, hydratine ($C_{22}H_{23}NO_6$) and the most active ingredient, xanthopuccine. Goldenseal has a green oil, a volatile oil (fragrance) that contains resin, albumin, sugar, starch and fatty resins.

Plant:
Goldenseal is a perennial bush that is native to moist woods and damp meadows. This plant belongs to the buttercup family. The root has strong odour and taste. The stem is 8 – 20 inches tall. The leaves are a dark green and are 4 to 6 inches wide. Flowers are small, solitary, white or rose colour and appear in May and June. The berries are small and look like raspberries.

Parts used: root

Solvent: alcohol, diluted alcohol and boiling water

Therapeutic action:
alternative, antibiotic, anti-inflammatory, antimicrobial, anti-tumour, astringent, stomachic, tonic

Uses:
Blood: Good for lowering sugar levels.

Bowels: Goldenseal can assist with diarrhea and hemorrhoids.

Ears: This herb can be used in an eardrop for earaches.

Intestines: Improves the quality and quantity of the mucus membranes in the GI tract (is called the king of the mucous membranes) and is used as a treatment of gastritis.

Liver: Cleanses the liver, treats liver diseases and alcoholic liver disease.

Lungs: Helps to improve the mucous membranes of respiratory tract, which helps to reduce hay fever and laryngitis.

Mouth: Goldenseal is used for mouth cancer, clearing up gum infections and thrush.

Menstrual: This herb assists with lessening uterine contractions and menstrual problems from excessive periods.

Skin: The Cherokees used goldenseal for skin ulcers and arrow wounds. This herb is used to treat the skin affected by eczema, ringworm, infected sores and wounds.

Stomach: Used for stomach flu and for slight food poisoning.

Throat: Used to relieve sore throats.

Uterus: Goldenseal is good for the uterine and vaginal area, as it strengthens the mucous membranes. Stops uterine hemorrhaging.

Other uses and information:
-Good for reducing swollen glands.

Caution: Breast feeding or pregnant women should not use goldenseal.

If you have high blood pressure, liver disease or are taking any medication, you must consult your doctor first before taking goldenseal.

GRAVEL ROOT (EUPATORIUM PUPUREUM)
Known as Joe Pye, kidney root purple thorough weed, queen of the meadow, tall boneset

Contains:
eurparin, oleoresin.

Plant:
Gravel root grows in North America. Gravel root has a purplish band about 1 inch wide around the nodes. The perennial plant grows from 5 – 6 feet high. It has pale purple to white tubular flowers that bloom in August and September. The leaves are rough and jagged. The roots have a slight bitter aromatic taste, and the plant smells like old hay.

Parts used: root

Solvent: water

Therapeutic action:
anti-inflammatory, anti-parasitic, astringent, diuretic, nervine, relaxant, stimulant, tonic.

Uses:
Bladder: This herb is used for supporting the bladder.

Bones: Gravel root helps with lessening the effects of rheumatism.

Diseases: Used to treat herpes and malaria.

Intestines: Used to expel tapeworms

Nervous System: As a nervine, it influences the entire sympathetic nervous system.

Prostate: Gravel root can be used for healing prostate discomforts.

Urinary Tract: Used for the genitourinary tract. Gravel root supports the bladder and kidneys. This herb relaxes and stimulates the tone of the pelvic viscera. It helps to remove the gravel from the urinary tract and can reduce the effects of gout. Used for bloody urine and irritation in the urinary tract.

Uterus: Gravel root helps to support the uterus.

Other uses and information:
- Good for treating dropsy.

- Gravel root tones the mucous membranes and cleans sediments off the surface area.

- Used to reduce the inflammation of back pain.

- When gravel root is combined with capsicum and juniper, it is used for typhoid fever.

Caution: Can eliminate kidney stones too fast. Gravel root needs to be taken with a demulcent like marshmallow and should not be taken in large quantities.

GREEN TEA (CARMELLIA SINENSIS)
Green tea is high in antioxidants

Contains:
Vitamins: B1 (thiamin), B2 (riboflavin), B3 (niacin), B5 (pantothenic acid), C

Minerals: calcium, iron, magnesium, manganese, phosphorous, potassium, zinc

Other: amino acids, alpha-genine, astragalin, benzaldehyde. Beta-carotene, beta-ionone, beta-sitosterol, caffeic acid, caffeine, carvacrol, catechin, chlorogenic acid, cinnamic acid, , cryptoxanthin, epicatechin, epigallocatechin, eugenol, farnesol, gallic acid, geraniol, hyperoside, indole, isoquercitrin, lutein, lycopene, myricetin, myristic acid, narigenin, polyphenois, procyanidine, quercetin, quercetrin, rutin, salicylic acid, tannic acid, thymol, vitexin, zeaxanthin

Plant:
Green Tea originated in China and is now grown around the world. Green tea does not go through the same process that the other teas go through. It is kept in its natural state.

Parts used: leaf

Therapeutic action:
antihistamine, antioxidant, diuretic

Uses:
Bladder: Green tea is an excellent diuretic for the bladder.

Blood: Green tea is an excellent antioxidant that helps to clean the blood and protect the body from diseases and cancers. It can help to regulate blood clotting and lower the cholesterol level. With the antioxidant properties, green tea will help to strengthen the immune system. It is good for regulating the blood sugar levels.

Liver: Helps to clean the blood so that the liver does not have to work so hard.

Lungs: Green tea assists in reducing asthma.

Prostate: Enlarged prostates can be eased with the use of green tea.

Teeth: Green tea aids in reducing tooth decay.

Other uses and information:
- Green tea has been used for weight loss.

- Best used without any milk. Milk interferes with the body absorbing the nutrients of the green tea.

CAUTION: Drinking green tea should be limited to two cups per day for pregnant mothers, nursing mothers, and those who may have an irregular heartbeat or troubles with anxiety.

HAWTHORN (CRATAEGUS LAEVIGATA) (CRATAEGUS OXYACANTHA)

Contains:
Vitamins: B1 (thiamin), B2 (riboflavin), B3 (niacin), B5 (pantothenic acid), B6 (pyridoxine), B12, C

Minerals: calcium, chromium, iron, magnesium, manganese, phosphorous, potassium, selenium, silicon, sodium, sulfur, zinc

Other: acetylcholine, adenine, adenosine, amino acids, amygdalin, anagryine, anthocyanidins, beta-carotene, beta-sitosterol, caffeic acid, catechin, choline, chlorogenic acid, epicatechin, esculin, hyperoside, pectin, quercetrin, rutin, ursolic acid, vitexin

Plant:
Hawthorn is found in Europe and Northern Asia. This shrub is found in thickets and woods. Grows to 30 feet high. The plant has single seed vessels in each blossom that turn to produce a bright red single berry. The berries look like miniature stony apples. The flowers bloom in May.

Parts used: the flowers, fruit and leaves are used.

Therapeutic action:
anti-inflammatory, antioxidant, antiseptic, tonic

Uses:
Blood: Good for lower the cholesterol level of the blood. Used to decrease anemia and increases the immunity level of the blood. Helps to lower the blood pressure.

Bones: Used to reduce rheumatism.

Diseases: Hawthorn is a good antioxidant and helps to build up the immune system.

Heart: Used for a cardiac tonic, dilating coronary blood vessels. Used for cardiac weakness, cardiac pain, rapid or feeble heart and heart strain due to overexertion. Helps to restore the heart muscles. Used for angina and heart valve defects.

Kidneys: Used as an infusion for dropsy.

Lungs: Helps with respiration.

Nervous System: Hawthorn has a mild sedative act: calms the nerves during depression and is used to decrease insomnia.

Skin: Hawthorn can be used in a poultice to help draw out thorns and splinters.

Throat: Used for sore throats.

Other uses and information:
- Used to increases the enzyme metabolism.
- Used as weight loss tea, as the hawthorn helps to decrease fat deposit levels.

HOLY BASIL
Known in Hindi as tulsi and in Sanskrit as tulasi

Plant:
Holy basil is an aromatic and native plant to India and is now found around the world. It has been used in Ayurveda medicine for a long time and is regarded as a sacred plant in India. This plant is used in cooking, healing and meditations.

Therapeutic action:
anti-inflammatory, antioxidant, antiviral, cathartic, nervine, pesticide, stomachic

Uses:
Blood: Good for purifying the blood, reducing the blood sugar and cholesterol levels. This herb has been used to stop malaria that is caused by mosquito bites.

Head: The anti-inflammatory properties make it good for reducing headaches.

Heart: This herb is wonderful for heart diseases.

Intestines: Assists in repairing intestinal distress.

Kidneys: Holy basil helps to reduce kidney stones.

Liver: As this herb cleanses the blood, it helps to support the function of the liver.

Lungs: Used for the bronchial tubes to remove the catarrhal matter and phlegm.

Mouth: This herb helps with maintaining the teeth.

Nerves: Holy basil is known for its ability to help calm the nerves when a person is experiencing a lot of stress.

Pancreas: Helps to regulate the blood sugar levels.

Skin: Holy basil can be used for the skin to stop ringworm.

Stomach: Holy basil is used to strengthen the stomach lining. This herbs assists with digestion and other stomach ailments.

Throat: Used to soothe sore throats.

Other uses and information:
- Good for enhancing memory and providing clarity.

- This herb can be used to promote perspiration during a common cold and fever.

- Holy basil helps to decrease inflammation and the discomforts from it.

- Holy basil can be used in a capsule form or as a fresh herb.

HOLY THISTLE (CARBENIA BENIDICTA) SEE BLESSED THISTLE

Hops (Humulus lupulus)

Contains:
Vitamins: B1 (thiamin), B3 (niacin), C

Minerals: calcium, chromium, magnesium, potassium, selenium, silicon, zinc

Other: alpha-pinene, alpha-terpineol, beta-carotene, beta-sitosterol, caffeic acid, campersterol, catechin, chlorogenic acid, citral, eugenol, ferulic acid, limonene, p-cymene, piperdine, quercetin, tannins

Plant:
This plant is a perennial. The stem is rough, very long and it twists around supports. The leaves are opposite, serrated and cordate. The flowers are yellowish green in colour.

Parts used: fruit and flowers.

Solvent: boiling water, diluted alcohol

Therapeutic action:
anthelmintic, antispasmodic, diuretic, nervine, stomachic, tonic

Uses:
Bones: Hops has assisted in reducing pain from rheumatism.

Bowels: Used as a gentle enema.

Gall Bladder: Used to reduce stones in the gall bladder.

Heart: Hops Increases the heart action and capillary circulation while it can still induce sleep.

Kidneys: Hops reacts with calculi, dissolving them and increasing the urine production and reduces stones in the kidneys.

Liver: Has assisted with some liver problems and can help to clear up jaundice.

Nerves: Hops is known for its ability to calm the nerves.

Stomach: Hops has been used for relieving pain in the stomach area. Hops aids in bile secretion.

Throat: Used as a cough syrup for soothing the throat.

Other uses and information:
- This herb is soothing and is used for cerebral conditions.

- This herb can be used for excessive sexual desire as an anti-aphrodisiac.

- A pillow made of hops sprinkled with some alcohol can be used for insomnia. A tea and tincture can also be used.

- When hops are mixed with poppy heads and used in a poultice, it can be used for rheumatism.

Caution: If prone to allergies, use rubber gloves when picking. People have had dermatitis on their hands, faces and legs after prolonged exposure to the fresh hops.

This plant should not be used if you are taking any antidepressants.

The volatile oil is a sedative in small doses and can be hypnotic in large doses. When overused, it can be paralyzing.

HORSERADISH (COCHLEARIS AMORACIN, RORIPA AMORACIA, AMORACIA LAPATHIFOLIA)

Known as great railfort, mountain radish, red cole.

Contains:
Vitamins: A, B1 (thiamin), B2 (riboflavin), B3 (niacin), B5 (pantothenic acid), B6 (pyridoxine), B12 (cobalamin), C

Minerals: calcium, iron, magnesium, phosphorous, potassium, sulfur

Other: acetates, acetates, albumin, allyl, gum, isothiocyanate, gluconasturtiin, myrosin, resin, sigrine sugar, starch

Plant:
This plant is a perennial and only the root is used. It grows from 1 – 5 ft. tall. Horseradish has long leaves that are 8 to 12 inches long. The flowers are white with two celled pods. The main root is usually 12 inches long and tapers to a conical shape. The root is yellowish, scaly and has a pungent odour when scraped. Horse radish is a member of the mustard family.

Parts used: the root.

Solvent: apple cider vinegar. Regular vinegar can be used but it is not as healthy as the apple cider vinegar. Once the root is exposed or grated, it will turn yellow/brown unless vinegar is added right away.

Therapeutic action:
antibacterial, antiseptic, diaphoretic, digestive, diuretic, rubefacient, stimulant

Uses:
Bones: Horseradish helps to reduce the inflammation of rheumatism.

Diseases: This herb has helped to clear up scurvy that is due to the lack of vitamin C.

Kidneys: Horseradish is used as a diuretic (promotes production and excretion of urine) and eases the effects of dropsy.

Liver: This herb helps to clean the liver.

Lungs: Horseradish is used as an expectorant, to rid the lungs of stubborn coughs and influenza. When it is mixed with water and sugar horseradish helps with whooping cough and hoarseness

Sinuses: Excellent for clearing the sinuses

Skin: Horseradish is used as a diaphoretic, as it opens the pores to promoting skin sweating and raising body temperature. It also is used to help remove freckles when mixed with white vinegar.

Spleen: This herb helps to help cleanse the spleen.

Stomach: Horseradish helps to increase the digestive system and expel worms.

Other uses and information:
- Used for chilblains (ulcers on the feet), treated with a poultice of horseradish.

Caution: Horseradish should not be used when pregnant.

HORSETAIL (EQUISETUM ARVENSE)
Known as puzzle grass, snake grass

Contains:
Vitamins: B1 (thiamin), B2 (riboflavin), B3 (niacin), C

Minerals: calcium, chromium, iron, magnesium, phosphorous, potassium, selenium, silicone, sulfur, zinc

Other: beta-carotene, beta-sitosterol, caffeic acid, campesterol, equisetonin, ferulic acid, gallic acid, kaempferol, luteolin, paba, p-courmaric acid, tannic acid, vanillic acid

Plant:
Horsetail is reproduced by the spores from the plant also known as a living fossil. Some of the original trees/plants grew to 30m tall.

Parts used: the whole plant can be used.

Therapeutic action:
anti-inflammatory, antiseptic, antispasmodic, astringent, demulcent, diuretic: mild, nervine, stimulant, tonic

Uses:
Bladder: Horsetail is used for the urinary tract as it helps to clear up infections.

Blood: Good to help the blood to coagulate. Adds iron to the blood to reduce anemia.

Bones: The calcium and silica in horsetail helps to strengthen and heal broken bones that have been reset, fractured bones and cartilage. This herb can be found in some anti-inflammatory formulas for arthritis, gout and osteoporosis. Horsetail also helps heal the reconnective tissues to the bones.

Eyes: Good for improving eyesight.

Diseases: Used to heal dropsy, gonorrhea, pulmonary, rickets, tuberculosis.

Gall Bladder: Helps with the gall bladder.

Head: Used to strength and improve the growth of hair.

Heart: Horsetail helps to improve the circulation of the blood and is beneficial for the heart.

Kidneys: Beneficial for the kidneys at it lessens dropsy, clears infections and strengthens the kidneys.

Liver: Helps the liver when it is being overused.

Lungs: Horsetail assists with the airways and clears up bronchitis.

Menstrual: Helps to regulate the menstrual period.

Mouth: The calcium and silica help with the teeth.

Muscles: Good anti-inflammatory for relaxing the muscles and reducing cramps.

Nerves: This herb can help to calm the nerves and promote relaxation.

Nose: Horsetail helps to reduce nose bleeds.

Prostate: Horsetail has assisted with relieving prostate discomforts.

Skin: Horsetail can be used in a poultice to stop bleeding and help heal burns and wounds. It is beneficial for both skin and nails. It can be used to heal skin rashes.

Other uses and information:
- Horsetail is found in several products that are used for the bones, eyes, hair, skin and teeth.

Caution: If horsetail is used for a long time, you may want to take additional vitamin B1 (thiamin) for better absorption of the B1. The horsetail will start to interfere with the absorption of the B1.

HYSSOP (HYSSOPUS OFFICINALIS)
Known as a holy herb

Contains:
Minerals: choline

Other: alpha-pinene, benzaldehyde, beta-ionone, beta-sitosterol, borneol, caffeic acid, camphor, carvacrol, choline, eugenol, ferulic acid, flavonoids, geraniol, hesperedin, hyssopin, limonene, linalool, marrubin, oleanolic acid, pinocamphone, rosmarinic acid, sitosteral, tannin, thymol, ursolic acid

Plant:
Hyssop is native to Europe and part of mint family. It has a square stem and is a shrubby perennial plant. Grows to 2 feet. Hyssop has an nice aromatic odour and a hot, spicy and bitter taste. The flowers are bluish purple and grow on one side of the vertical spike.

Part used: the flowers, leaves and shoots are used.

Solvent: water and alcohol.

Therapeutic action:
antiseptic, antispasmodic, antiviral, carminative, diaphoretic, emollient, expectorant, pectoral, stimulant

Uses:
Blood: Blood regulator, increases blood circulation and regulates the blood pressure.

Kidneys: Helps to cleanse and support the kidneys.

Liver: Helps to cleanse and support the liver

Lungs: Hyssop helps with asthma, bronchitis, chest infections, congestion and improves the breathing when there is a shortness of breath. Brings out the mucus from the lungs and helps to reduce congestion.

Muscles: Hyssop has been used to relieve muscular rheumatism

Nerves: Used to lessen epilepsy

Skin: Hyssop can help to moisturize the skin and is used for cuts and to reduce bruises. Can be used in a poultices. The fresh green leaves are used.

Stomach: Used for grippe water and helps to dispel gas.

Throat: Used for sore throats. Can be used with sage and used as a gargle to soothe the throat.

Other uses and information:
- Good for colds and used as a stimulant. Used to for fevers, herpes, measles and scarlet fever.
- Bruising: Used to remove discolouring from bruises. Place in cheesecloth and soak in boiling water for herb to absorb the water. Apply as poultice.
- Chest and throat: Tonic used for bronchitis, chest disease, hoarseness, irritable tickling cough.
- Rheumatism: Fresh green hyssop tops eaten several times a day can help with rheumatism.
- Skin: Used in baths. Good to combine with marigold flowers (calendula)
- Stomach: Warm infusion of hyssop mixed with horehound improves tone of feeble stomach.

IRISH MOSS (CHONDRUS CRISPUS)

Contains:
Vitamins: A, B1 (thiamin), B2 (riboflavin), B3 (niacin), C, D, E, K

Minerals: calcium, iodine iron, magnesium, manganese, phosphorous, potassium, selenium, sodium, sulfur, zinc

Other: beta-carotene

Plant:
Irish moss is a species of red algae. It grows along the rocky parts of the Atlantic coast of Europe and North America.

Therapeutic action:
anti-cancer, anti-emetic, antiseptic, antispasmodic, astringent, stomachic

Uses:
Bladder: Irish moss is used for healing the bladder.

Blood: Irish moss has been used to treat tuberculosis that affects the blood.

Bones: Good for healing the bones as Irish moss contains calcium, magnesium and vitamin D. It can also help to reduce inflamed joints.

Bowels: Irish moss helps to form the stools after bouts of diarrhea.

Intestines: Used for healing the intestines.

Kidneys: Irish moss helps to reduce the inflamed tissues of the kidneys and assists with treating goitre.

Liver: Helps to cleanse the liver and the blood.

Lungs: Helps to heal the lungs from bronchitis, as it soothes the inflamed tissues.

Skin: This herb is used in lotions to rehydrate the skin, as it works on a cellular level for the organs of the body.

Stomach: Used for treating intestinal discomforts.

Thyroid: The iodine in this herb helps to work with the glandular system.

Other uses and information:
- This plant is an excellent plant to help regain strength after a long illness, as it is high in the nutrients that the body needs to recover.

- Irish moss is used in hair rinse products to bring the moisture back into the hair.

- Irish moss is used for cancer, peptic ulcers and varicose veins.

JUNIPER (JUNIPERUS COMMUNIS AND JUNIPERUS HORIZONTALIS)

Contains:
Vitamins: B1 (thiamin), B2 (riboflavin), B3 (niacin), C

Minerals: calcium, chromium, iron, magnesium, manganese, phosphorous, potassium, selenium, zinc

Other: alpha-pinene, beta-carotene, beta pinene, betuline, borneol, camphor, caryophyllene, catechin, farnesol, glycolic acid, limonene, linalool, menthol, myrcene, penine, rutin, tannin.

Plant:
The bush is usually low lying to spreading shrubs and sometimes the plant will grow to 1 metre high. It has blue-green needle-like leaves. The fruit turns to a pale green to whitish purple berry like cone. The berries take two years to ripen. The first year berries are a green colour, and the second year the berries are purplish. The second year berries are less bitter. The plant is found in North America, but does not grow well in the prairies, unless the bush is maintained in a yard-like environment.

Parts used: Ripe dry berries. These are prepared with boiling water or alcohol. Oil of juniper comes from distilling the fruit berries.

Therapeutic action:
antibiotic, antifungal, antiseptic (berries), antiviral (oil), carminative, diuretic, emmenagogue, stimulant, stomachic.

Uses:
Bladder: The juniper berry is used for increasing urine flow, clearing up bladder infections and helps to strengthen the bladder when mixed with bearberry. This plant also helps the body get rid of uric acid. When the berries are mixed with hydrangea tincture, the mixture is very good for dissolving kidney stones that have gone to the bladder.

Kidneys: The juniper berry is used for increasing urine flow, clearing up kidney infections. This plant also helps the body get rid of uric acid. When the berries are mixed with hydrangea tincture, the mixture is very good for dissolving kidney stones that have gone to the bladder.

Lungs: Used to treat asthma and as a decongestant.

Pancreas: Juniper berries are a natural insulin to regulate the blood sugar levels and works with the pancreas.

Prostate: It has been used to help with prostate disorders

Stomach: It is used to improve digestion and to strengthen weak stomachs. The oil is used in the production of stomach acid.

Other uses and information:
- Juniper berries have helped with colds and flus.

- The berries have been used to grow trust when in the state of fear about moving forward.

- The berries have been used for gout.

- The berries have been known to taste like gin. They can be made into mush and shaped in to cakes. The purple berries (second year berries) are more palatable and more medicinal. Berries can be eaten raw.

- The Cree call juniper "Ka Ka Kau-mini", they made poultices with the bark.

- The Blackfoot call the Juniperous horizontalis "Sik-Si-Nou-Koo" (black and rounded objects). The Blackfoot use the juniper berries on the floor of the sweat lodges, and on Sun Dance floor. They make a liniment by infusing juniper root and poplar leaves for stiff backs or backaches. An infusion from the root is used as a general tonic. The Natives would bathe their horses with juniper root water for healthy gloss in hair. Black beads can be made with the juniper berries. The hides are smoked yellow by smoking greased leaves of juniper.

- Europeans have been using juniper berries as a diuretic, stimulant and carminative for many years. Many herbalists suck on juniper berries while treating patients with infectious diseases. Gargling juniper tea is a disease contagion. Powdered berries have been used to destroy fungi.

- In the Mediterranean, juniper is used in baths for treating neurasthenic neurosis and for scalp psoriasis.

- In Sweden juniper is used to treat wounds and for inflammatory diseases.

Caution: Juniper should not be used by pregnant women, as it can interfere with iron and other mineral absorption. Large amounts should not be taken over long periods of time. The berries should not be boiled as they lose the volatile oils. Even though the berries can help with clearing kidney infections, prolonged use can cause kidney irritation.

Do not use if you do have a kidney disease.

KELP (FUCUS VERSICULOSUS)
Known for its high content in iodine

Contains:
Vitamins: A, B1 (thiamin), B2 (riboflavin), B3 (niacin), B5 (pantothenic Acid), B6 (pyridoxine), B12 (cobalamin), C, E, K

Minerals: chlorine, copper, iodine, iron, magnesium, manganese, phosphorous, potassium, silicone, sulfur, zinc

Other: barium, boron, chromium, lithium, nickel, silver, sodium

Plant:
Kelp is a seaweed and known as brown algae. There are around thirty types of brown algae. The plant grows in the ocean/sea forests but in the shallower waters. The water is above zero, 6 – 14 c. The kelp can grow up to 80m long and is fast growing.

Part used: The whole plant is used.

Therapeutic action:
alterative, anti-flatulent, antiseptic, astringent, carminative, cathartic, stimulant, stomachic

Uses:
Adrenal Glands: Kelps high content of iodine is beneficial for the pituitary, adrenal glands and the metabolism.

Blood: Good for cleansing the blood and reducing diabetes.

Bowels: Kelp works with the bowels, reduces constipation and works with colitis.

Gall Bladder: Kelp helps to support the gall bladder.

Head: Used to reduce headaches.

Heart: Kelp helps to cleanse the arteries and helps to lower high blood pressure.

Kidneys: Kelp helps to support the kidneys.

Liver: Kelp cleanses the blood and assists the liver.

Lungs: Assists with asthma and healing the lungs.

Nerves: Kelp is beneficial for the nervous system and reducing depression.

Pancreas: Used to strengthen the pancreas so that the pancreas can properly regulate the blood sugar levels.

Prostate: Used for toning the prostate.

Skin: The minerals in this plant assist with the skin, clear the complexion and reduce eczema and wrinkles.

Stomach: Used for lessening gas in the stomach, aids in digestion and has been used to reduce morning sickness.

Thyroid: Kelp has a high source of iodine, and this is beneficial for the thyroid. The thyroid is what regulates our metabolism rate and regulates our weight gain or loss.

Uterus: Kelp will help to strengthen the uterus especially after a tough pregnancy and birthing process.

Other uses and information:
- Kelp is a plant from the ocean that contains a large source of minerals and vitamins that our bodies need to function properly.

- Kelp plays a big role during pregnancy and reduces water retention. Used for healing the goitre.

- Kelp can be used in both a powdered form or in capsules.

LADIES SLIPPER ROOT (CYPRIPEDIUM PUBESCENS)
Known as American valerian, moccasin flower, nerve root, Noah's Ark, yellow lady slipper root

Contains:
Vitamins: B1 (thiamin), B2 (riboflavin), B3 (niacin), B5 (pantothenic Acid), B6 (pyridoxine), B12 (cobalamin),

Other: cypripedin, gallic acids, tannic

Plant:
This plant has orchids that are 15 to 25 cm tall with variously coloured, very beautiful flowers. The leaves are alternate and sheath the stem. The roots are thick, creeping and fibrous. This rare plant is found deep in moist wooded areas. This plant can only be used from a cultivated crop.

Parts used: roots

Solvent: boiling water and dilute alcohol.

Therapeutic action:
anodyne, antibacterial, anti-inflammatory, antispasmodic, diaphoretic, diuretic, nervine, pectoral, relaxant, stomachic, tonic.

Uses for:

Diseases: Ladies slipper root is used to treat cystic fibrosis, epilepsy and typhoid fever.

Head: Used to stop the pain and relax the muscles that cause headaches.

Heart: Helps to regulate the heart.

Lungs: Assists with breathing.

Muscles: This gentle but powerful herb is used as an anti-inflammatory to reduce cramping and muscle pain.

Nervous System: This plant is known as one of the best and safest herb to use for the nervous system. It helps to calm the body and the mind. This is one of the few plants that are safe to use with the young children to help them out. Used for hysteria, insomnia, nervousness, restlessness and tremors.

Stomach: Lady's slipper is used for reducing stomach pain and for colic.

Other uses and information:
- Lady's slipper combined with chamomile can be used for depression.

LAVENDER (LAVANDULA ANGUSTIFOLIA)

Contains:
alpha-pinene, beta pinene, borneol, camphor, caryophyllene, coumarin, geraniol, limonene, linalool, luteolin, rosmarinic acid, tannin, umbelliferone, ursolic acid

Plant:
Lavender is part of the mint family. It is found in Africa, Asia, Canary Islands, Cape Verde, Europe and the Mediterranean. Today this plant can be found in flowers gardens and is grown on farms. The plant has toothed leaves with a fine hair. The oil is extracted from the leaves. The flowers are from a blue to a violet colour.

Parts used: It is the flowers that are used. The flowers can be used dried or the essential oils are extracted from it.

Therapeutic Action:
anodyne, anti-convulsive, antidepressant, anti-infectious, anti-inflammatory, antiseptic, antispasmodic, antitoxin, anxiety, relaxant.

Uses:
Blood: Good for lowering blood pressure due to its calming effect.

Bones: Lavender can help to reduce the effects of rheumatism.

Gall Bladder: Helps to dissolve gallstones.

Head: Used to stop dandruff and reduce hair loss.

Lungs: Helps to promote better breathing for the lungs. Aids with treating asthma, bronchitis and influenza. Lavender is also used to treat tuberculosis, a highly contagious disease.

Lymphatic system: Used to help improve the lymphatic system.

Menstrual: Helps to lessen menstrual cramps and both pre-menstruation and menopause symptoms.

Mouth: Used for mouth abscesses and thrush.

Muscles: Helps to relax the muscles.

Nerves: Lavender can be used to relief stress and aids in lessening depression, headaches, hysteria and insomnia.

Skin: Lavender is used in an ointment to heal burns. It is also good for the skin and any skin discomforts like eczema, scars and stretch marks. Lavender can be found in many skin products. This herb is even used in baby products and can lessen diaper rash.

Stomach: Lavender can be used in a tea for better indigestion and to reduce nausea.

Throat: Lavender can be used in a tea for laryngitis, throat infections and whopping cough.

Other uses and information:
- Lavender is great for a sleep aid and has been used for allergies. Used to lessen convulsions.

- Lavender has been used for herpes.

- Lavender can be added to universal oil to blend into feet or hands.

Caution: Lavender should not be used during a pregnancy.

LEMON BALM (MELISSA)

Plant:
Lemon balm is a perennial and a member of the mint family. It is originally found in the Mediterranean and in Europe. This plant is now being grown and cultivated in the United States. This plant has a lemony scent, and it attracts bees and hence the nickname of Melissa. (Melissa meaning of honey)

Parts used: the leaves and extracted oils.

Therapeutic action:
antibacterial, anti-inflammatory, antiviral, stimulant, stomachic, tonic.

Uses:
Diseases: Used to treat colds and flus.

Head: Used to reduce headaches.

Lungs: Lemon balm helps to heal the lungs and chest from colds and chest discomforts.

Nerves: Used for calming the nerves in stressful situations and helps to reduce exhaustion and insomnia.

Stomach: Used for indigestion.

Thyroid: Used for healing the thyroid and Grave's disease. When the thyroid does not work properly, it affects the goitre too.

Other: Lemon balm has antibacterial and antiviral properties that have been used in treatment for the herpes simplex.

Other uses and information:
- Best used as an essential oil for the skin. Lemon balm can be found in essential oils used in aromatherapy, but is usually combined with other oils.

- Used as a tea to calm the nerves.

- It is advised that those using thyroxine, not to consume lemon balm, as the herb will stop the absorption of some thyroid medications.

- Whole leaves or crushed leaves are used in cooking

LEMONGRASS (CYMBOPOGON CITRATUS)
Known as barbed wire grass, cha de Dartigalongue, citronella grass, fever grass, Gavati Chaha, Hierba Luisa or silky heads

Contains:
Vitamins: A, C

Minerals: calcium, iodine, iron, magnesium, manganese, phosphorus, potassium, selenium, zinc

Other: alpha-pinene, beta-sitosterol, caryophyllene, citral, farnesol, geraniol, limonene, luteolin, myrcene, quercetin, rutin, saponin, triacontanol.

Plant:
The plant originated in India, grown in Israel and can also be found in many other countries.

Part used: the leaves and stems are used for teas and fragrances.

Therapeutic action:
antibacterial, anti-cancer, anti-emetic, antifungal, anti-inflammatory, antioxidant, antispasmodic, astringent, pesticide, relaxant, restorative, stomachic, tonic,

Uses:

Bladder: Lemongrass is used to support and treat the bladder.

Blood: This herb is excellent for fighting cancer cells. A study was done at the Ben Gurion University of the Negev discovered last year that the lemon aroma in herbs like lemongrass kills cancer cells in vitro while leaving healthy cells unharmed.

Head: Used to relax the muscles that tighten during stressful times and cause headaches.

Heart: Lemongrass assist in lowering high blood pressure that can affect the heart.

Immune system: This herb helps to reduce fevers and reduce flu symptoms with its antifungal properties. This herb is used a lot with Ayurveda medicine in relieving cough and nasal congestion.

Kidneys: This herb has been beneficial for the functioning of the kidneys.

Liver: Lemongrass' ability to work with the body on a cellular level will help strengthen the liver and cleanse the blood.

Skin: Lemongrass assists in healing the skin when there are wounds, as it causes the skin to draw tight to stop the bleeding. This is great to use for children. Used in sprays and is a safe pesticide in the warmer weather. Used in a warm poultice to heal boils.

Stomach: Lemongrass is used as a digestive aid, reduces colic in the little ones and is good for the intestinal tract.

Other uses and information:

- A study was done at the Ben Gurion University of the Negev last year discovered that the lemon aroma in herbs like lemongrass kills cancer cells in vitro while leaving healthy cells unharmed. The research team was led by Dr. Rivka Ofir and Prof. Yakov Weinstein, incumbent of the Albert Katz Chair in cell-differentiation and malignant diseases from the Department of Microbiology and Immunology at BGU. The citral in the lemongrass is the ingredient that the cancer cells do not like.
- The essential oil can be used for perfumes for its lemony fragrance.

- Steeped in teas for those who are fighting cancer.

- Used in Asian dishes.

LICORICE ROOT (GLYCYRRHIZA GLABRA)

Licorice root is known for its taste that is added to dishes.

Contains:

Vitamins: B1 (thiamin), B2 (riboflavin), B3 (niacin), B5 (pantothenic acid), B6 (pyridoxine), B12 (cobalamin), C, E

Minerals: calcium, iodine, iron, magnesium, manganese, phosphorous, potassium, selenium, silicon, zinc

Other: anethole (what provides the licorice taste), apigenin, benzaldehyde, beta-carotene, beta-sitosterol, betaine, camphor, carvacrol, eugenol, ferulic acid, geraniol, glycyrrhizin (this is what creates the sweetness of the root), kaempferol, lignin, mannitol, phenol, quercetin, salicylic acid, stigmasterol, thymol, vitexin,

Plant:
Licorice is a native plant to some area in Asia and in the southern regions of Europe. The licorice plant is part of the legume family, but it is the root that is being used medicinally. This plant is a perennial that can grow up to 3 feet (1 metre) high. The leaves are long, and the flowers can be from a pale blue white to a purple colour. Licorice root is not harvested until the second or third year.

The glycyrrhizin in the root is what creates the sweet taste. This is up to fifty times sweeter than sucrose. The anethole in the plant is what provides the licorice taste that is also found in the fennel plant and anise seed. The concentrated extract from the plant can be very bitter. In Spain, the plant is grown as a mouth freshener.

Part Used: The root. You can dig up the root, wash it and chew on it.

Therapeutic action:
antibacterial, anti-cancer, anti-inflammatory, antimicrobial, anti-parasitic, anti-spasmodic, antiviral, carminative, cathartic, expectorant, nervine, stimulant

Uses:
Adrenal Glands: Used for stimulating the adrenal glands and reduces adrenal exhaustion (Cushing's disease)

Blood: Good for helping the blood to produce interferon. Interferon is a protein that builds up the body's immune system and helps the body to fight off viral infections like herpes and HIV. The interferon is also a tool to fighting off cancers. The herb also assists in regulating low blood sugar levels (hypoglycemia).

Glands: Used to support the glandular function (Addison's disease)

Heart: This root helps to strengthen the heart muscles.

Liver: Licorice root helps the liver and blood to deter cancer-forming cells that create liver cancer and blood disorders.

Lungs: Used for allergies, asthma, bronchial congestion, emphysema and respiratory discomforts.

Menstrual: The vitamin B in the licorice is beneficial during PMS and reduces menopausal discomforts.

Mouth: Licorice helps to stop the formation of plaque on the teeth and stops bacteria growth.

Muscles: Helps to reduce inflammation of the muscles and muscle spasms.

Prostate: Licorice root reduces prostate inflammation.

Skin: Used for age spots in the skin.

Stomach: Used for cleansing of the colon, used as a laxative and is found in some detox cleanses. Licorice root helps to increase the mucus secreting cells that provide better intestinal cell life.

Throat: Found in teas and lozenges for soothing of the throat during colds and coughing.

Other: Good for cleansing the body of parasites. Decreases inflammation. Also used for depression (good vitamin B source.) and been used to treat lupus, scleroderma, rheumatoid arthritis and animal dander allergies.

Other uses and information:
- Used in throat soothing teas. Licorice candy is generally made with anise seed and does not have the same properties as the real licorice root.

- The spice is used in many Chinese dishes such as in broths for flavouring.

- In Europe, the licorice root was made into little wooden sticks that are chewed on for the flavour.

- In Japan, the licorice root is being used in the treatment and control of chronic viral hepatitis.

- In China, tuberculosis is being treated with this root.

- Licorice root has also assisted in drug withdrawal.

Caution: Overuse of licorice can cause estrogen or progesterone effects that cause change to pitch of the voice.

The herbal licorice should not be used for those who have glaucoma, severe menstrual problems, high blood pressure or history of strokes or during a pregnancy. Licorice should not be used for more than seven days in a row, as it can affect the blood pressure, decrease the potassium levels and cause water retention.

LOBELIA (LOBELIA INFLATA)
Known as puke weed, this plant has no harmful effects.

Contains:
Vitamins: C

Minerals: copper, iron, selenium, sodium, sulfur,

Other: cobalt

Plant:
Lobelia is a small shrubby plant that is hardy and can survive in different habitats. The flowers can be found in a variety of colours. This plant is used as an ornamental garden plant.

Part used: The whole plant.

Therapeutic action:
anti-emetic, anti-inflammatory, antioxidant, antiseptic, antispasmodic, astringent, relaxant, stomachic, tonic, vermicide

Uses:
Blood: Good for cleaning the blood from poisons that have entered it. Helps to improve blood circulation. Used to treat hepatitis, syphilis and tetanus.

Bones: Lobelia helps to ease the discomforts of arthritis and rheumatism.

Bowels: This herb reduces constipation,

Ears: This herb is used for earaches and ear infections.

Diseases: Lobelia assists in treating rabies and the fear of water that is caused by the rabies. Also works with palsy to reduce the spasms and tremors. Used for scarlet fever and tonsillitis.

Head: Used to reduce headaches.

Heart: Helps to strengthen the heart.

Intestines: Lobelia is used to dispel worms from the intestines.

Liver: Cleanses the blood when affected by hepatitis and syphilis

Lungs: Helps to heal the lungs by lessening the congestion from bronchitis. It eases asthma, catarrh, coughs, croup, pneumonia and whooping cough.

Menstruation: Lobelia reduces cramping during the menstrual period. Used for hormonal control.

Mouth: Used for lockjaw as it relaxes the muscles. Also used to strengthen the teeth and for toothaches.

Muscles: This herb helps to relax the muscles and stop the spasms.

Nerves: Lobelia helps to relax the body and mind and reduce nervousness.

Skin: This herb is used for eczema, symptoms of poison ivy and poison oak, ringworm and skin wounds.

Stomach: Used for food poisoning. Been used for colic, stomach spasms and reduces vomiting.

Other uses and information:
- Good to use to reduce convulsions that are caused by epilepsy.

- Used to reduce allergies and assists with childhood diseases.

- Used as a natural pain reducer and for shock.

- Lobelia can be used with slippery elm and soap to heal abscesses and boils.

- Used in a tincture for earaches, ear infections and lockjaw.

MANDRAKE (PODOPHYLLUM PELTATUM)

Known as May apple, raccoon berry, low apple, devil's apple.

Mandrake is a very powerful herb and must be used with caution.

Contains:
gallic acid, glycoside, podophyllinic acid, podophyllotoxin, quercetin.

Plant:
Mandrake grows in rich wood thickets in Canada and the USA. The stem grows to 1 foot long and is pale green. The white flowers grow in May and the fruit is a yellowish berry that is 1-2 inches long.

Parts used: root

Solvent: alcohol, partly boiling water

Therapeutic action:
alterative, cathartic, diaphoretic, emetic, hepatic, nervine, tonic, vermicide

Uses:
Blood: Mandrake is used for lead poisoning that affects the blood and the organs.

Bones: Used for rheumatism.

Bowels: Works mainly on the duodenum and increases intestinal secretion and bile flow when taken in small doses. It is used with other supporting herbs. Used to decrease constipation and to reduce diarrhea.

Diseases: This herb when used with other herbs can be used to treat cancer.

Gall Stones: Mandrake will reduce gallstones and reduce the painful effect they have on the gall bladder.

Glands: Mandrake helps to stimulate the glandular system.

Head: Used as a pain killer for headaches.

Intestines: Used for dispelling worms.

Liver: This herb works with chronic liver disease and jaundice. It is used with other supporting herbs.

Lungs: Assists with asthma that is caused by hay fever and allergies.

Nerves: Used to calm the nerves.

Skin: Used to retard the growth of warts, especially venereal warts.

Stomach: Used for digestion and to stop vomiting.

Uterus: Mandrake helps to clear uterine disorders.

Other: Good to use for chronic pain.

Other uses and information:
- Mandrake is used to reduce fevers and typhoid fever.

Caution:
Use with care. This plant is being studied in the use of cancer treatments.

Should not be used during pregnancy.

Should not be used with other strong cathartics.

Large dose will cause watery stool, griping and nausea. Rarely used alone.

MARJORAM (ORIGANUM VULGARE)
Marjoram has antioxidant properties.

Contains:
Vitamins: A, B1 (thiamin), B2 (riboflavin), B3 (niacin), B12 (cobalamin), C

Minerals: calcium, iron, magnesium, phosphorous, potassium, silicon, sodium, zinc

Plant:
Marjoram is part of the same family as the oregano plant. This plant does not like cool weather and grows like a shrub. The plant can have a citrus to a pine taste. The leaves are smooth with fine hairs and only grow to about 1.5 cm long.

Part used: the entire plant

Therapeutic action:
antioxidant, antispasmodic, carminative, diuretic, pulmonary, stimulant, stomachic.

Uses:
Bladder: Used to help stop bed-wetting.

Bowels: Marjoram helps to reduce diarrhea.

Head: Used to stop headaches caused by nervousness.

Intestines: Strengthens the intestines.

Kidneys: Used for water retention that causes dropsy.

Liver: Marjoram helps to cleanse the liver.

Lungs: Marjoram is used for asthma and to stop violent coughing. Sweet marjoram can be used in tea to relieve chest congestion.

Mouth: Marjoram oil is used for toothaches.

Nose: Used to relieve hay fever and blocked sinuses.

Stomach: Used for colic and to stop cramps, improve digestion, slow down gastritis and for strengthening the stomach. Marjoram is an antidote for narcotic poisons. Marjoram is used for motion sickness and nausea.

Other uses and information:
- Used for convulsions and to stop nightmares.

- Marjoram has been used to lessen the effects of measles.

- This herb can be used in an infusion that can be placed above the nose area to stop hay fever and work with the sinuses.

Caution: Marjoram should not be used by women who are pregnant or during menstruation. Marjoram can irritate the uterus.

MARSHMALLOW (ALTHAEA OFFICINALIS)
Known as moritfication root, sweetweed

Contains:
Vitamins: A, B1 (thiamin), B2 (riboflavin), B3 (niacin), B5 (pantothenic Acid), B6 (pyridoxine), C

Minerals: calcium, iron, magnesium, manganese, phosphorous, potassium, selenium, zinc

Other: asparagin, beta-carotene, betaine, caffeic acid, ferulic acid, iodine, mucilage, pantothenic acid, pectin, quercetin, sodium, sorbitol, tannins, vanillic acid

Plant:
Marshmallow grows in marshy places in Europe and certain areas of the USA. This plant is a perennial that grows to 3-4 ft. tall. The leaves are short and 2-3 inches long. The leaves are soft and velvety on both sides. The plant has small pale flowers. They bloom during August and September.

Parts used: root (most potent part), sometimes leaves and flowers.

Solvent: water

Therapeutic action:
anti-inflammatory, antiseptic, astringent, carminative, cathartic, demulcent, emetic, emollient, expectorant, stomachic.

Uses:
Bladder: Used for bladder infections and urinary bleeding.

Blood: Used in poultice for blood poisoning and gangrene. Used for diabetes.

Bones: Marshmallow has strong anti-inflammatory properties that helps with sore and stiff joints.

Bowels: When the root is boiled in milk, it will treat diarrhea and dysentery. Also used for constipation.

Eyes: Good for sore eyes.

Glands: Used for inflamed glands.

Head: Used to soothe headaches

Intestines: Used for intestinal infection and inflammation. Used when the natural mucus of the intestine has been abraded. Marshmallow, being both mucilaginous and nutritive, is an excellent coating.

Kidneys: Fights kidney infections and relieves irritation.

Liver: Helps to cleanse and support the liver.

Lungs: Helps to soothe the lungs during bronchitis and irritating coughs. Used for the infection and inflammation. The mucilage in marshmallow assists in removing phlegm in the lungs and airways. Used for asthma and emphysema.

Sinuses: Marshmallow relieves sinus problems.

Skin: Marshmallow is used for boils, bruises, burns, carbuncles, softens and soothes the skin, promotes wound healing. The powdered root will extract excess moisture from the skin and has a soothing effect.

Stomach: Used for digestion, gastritis, peptic ulcers.

Throat; Used to soothe sore throats.

Veins: Used for varicose ulcers.

Other uses and information:
- Marshmallow root should be used with a diuretic, to soothe any irritation from the demulcent.

- Used as an eyewash. Used in the following ways: infusion, decoction, tincture and poultice

- When marshmallow root is boiled in milk, it can enrich the milk of the nursing mother and increase the flow (can be combined with blessed thistle)

MEADOWSWEET (SPIRAEA ULMARIA, FILIPENDULA ULMARIA)

Known as meadow queen, meadow-wort, pride of the meadow, queen of the meadow, spirea, sweet meadow

Contains:
coumarin, hyperoside, methyl salicylate, quercetin, rutin, vanillin.

Plant:
Meadowsweet is a small shrub that grows 1 – 4 feet tall. It has small white (sometimes pink) flowers. The leaves are alternate and a dark green. Its native home is Europe with related species in North America.

Parts used: leaves.

Solvent: boiling water, alcohol, oil

Therapeutic action:
anti-inflammatory, astringent, diuretic, stomachic, tonic

Uses:
Bowels: Meadowsweet is used for treating diarrhea.

Muscles: Helps with inflammation of the muscles and reduces aches and cramping.

Prostate: Meadowsweet is used for enlarged prostates.

Skin: Used to help heal skin abrasions and promotes the elimination of excess fluid.

Stomach: Stimulates the parietal cells in the stomach to produce and adjust the HCl acid and pepsinogen. Assist in digestion and helps to regulate it. It is good for gastric ulcers.

Urinary Tract: Used to relieve urogenital irritation

Other uses and information:
- Used to relieve chronic cervicitis and chronic vaginitis with a discharge.

- Used for colds and flus.

Caution: Meadowsweet should not be used by pregnant women or by children with colds, fevers or any childhood diseases. This herb that can cause internal damage to the brain, heart and liver. Used only under the direction of a qualified herbalist.

MELALEUCA (MELALEUCA ALTERNIFOLIA)
Known as tea tree oil.

Contains:
alpha-pinene, alpha-terpinene, aromadendrene, beta pinene, camphor, caryophyllene, cinerol, cymones, limonene, linalool, p-cymene, pinenes, sesqiuterpenes, terpinenes, terpinolene,

Plant:
The melaleuca plant is common to Australia. The plant/oil has over forty-nine different compounds to it that make this a very powerful healer.

Part used: The oil from the leaves is used. The leaves are used in saunas.

Therapeutic action:
antibacterial, anti-inflammatory, antifungal, antimicrobial, anti-parasitic, antiseptic, antiviral, expectorant, fungicide, stimulant

Uses:
Appendicitis: Used to help lessen appendicitis attacks.

Blood: Good for blood circulation.

Bowels: Used to lessen diarrhea.

Ears: Used for earaches and itchy ears.

Diseases: Used for candida, colds, gangrene (diabetic), infections (fungal), infections (genital), infections (viral), infections (yeast).

Head: Used to get rid of lice and good for scalp problems.

Immune system: Support for the immune system.

Intestines: Used to eliminate parasites.

Lungs: Helps with bronchitis, coughs, decongestion, influenza and whooping cough.

Mouth: Used for gingivitis (gum disease), mouth sores and thrush.

Skin: Used for acne, athlete's foot, bed sores, boils, bug bites, burns, cold sores, cuts, eczema, infections, parasites, psoriasis, rash, ringworm, sun burn and warts. Used in sprays as anti-parasitic.

Stomach: Used for digestion and stomach infections.

Teeth: Used to treat tooth abscesses.

Throat: Used in a gargle for sore throat and tonsillitis. (The gargle must be spat out).

Other uses and information:
- Used for hemorrhoids, hysteria, inflammation and vaginitis.

- Good using as a disinfectant for both the body and the home.

- Used as an insect repellant.

Tea tree oil can be mixed with other oils such as citrus oils, eucalyptus, lavender, spice oils.

Bath Water: Can be added to bath water to bring relief to chicken pox or hives.

Disinfectant. Non-toxic disinfectant. This oil can be used with dish soap to clean infected areas of the house or can be used as an aromatherapy to clean the air of bacteria. It can even be used on face cloths to help with skin bacteria.

Douche: Used with water for vaginitis

Face Cleansing: A few drops can be added to the face cloth or wash water.

Gargle: The tea tree oil can be used in a gargle for sore throats and for mouth sores, but you must spit out the gargle.

Hoof sores: For horses and pets use pure oil for a couple of days then use an ointment.

Hygiene: Used in cosmetic and dental products.

Ingrown toe nails: Used for ingrown toe nails applying the oil under the nail

Insect Bites: Add the pure oil to the insect bite. Use the tea tree oil with citronella oil in a spray to prevent bites.

Lice: Using tree oil in shampoo is the best way to use to get rid of lice. For the first application, apply the pure oil to the scalp and hair. Mix in well. Can add tea tree oil to the shampoo and cream rinse. Even use this mixture to deter any potential lice outbreaks.

Radiation wounds: Mix the tea tree oil with oregano oil and thyme oil.

Ringworm: two drops lavender, two drops tea tree oil, two drops thyme. Apply one drop at a time, three times daily for ten days. Then mix two tablespoons carrier oil and thirty drops of tea tree oil and use daily till the ringworm is gone, or wash the area with tea tree oil and water daily.

Shingles: Tea tree oil can mix be mixed with olive or flax oil and applied to the area. One part tea tree ten parts olive/ flax oil.

Skin: Tea tree oil is used in ointments, but the pure oil can be added to the skin.

Venomous insect bites: Apply to the skin right away, two times.

Wood ticks / leeches: Apply the oil to the wood tick/leech right away. Wait a couple of minutes, remove the bug and apply tea tree oil to the puncture wound.

Caution: Should not be used internally.

MILK THISTLE (SILYBUM MARIANUM)

Known as elephant thistle, ivory thistle, Mary thistle, silver milk thistle, wild artichoke

Contains:
Minerals: calcium, iron, magnesium, manganese, phosphorous, potassium, selenium, zinc

Other: beta-carotene, bioflavonoids, carotenoids, fatty acids, flavonoids, fumaric acid, kaempferol, narigenin, quercetin, silandrin, silymarin, taxifolin

Plant:
Milk thistle is native the regions of Europe, North Africa and found in the Middle East. The plant is both an annual or biennial plant. The flower heads are disc-shaped and a pink-to-purple colour, and on the rare occasion can be white in colour.

Parts used: fruit, leaves and seeds.

Therapeutic action:
alterative, anti-cancer, antidepressant, anti-inflammatory, antioxidant, relaxant

Uses:
Arteries: Milk thistle is used to stop plaque build-up, which can cause the arteries to harden.

Blood: For those who have type two diabetes, milk thistle helps to reduce the insulin levels and to lower cholesterol levels. People have used milk thistle to reduce cancer cells that have been found in breast cancer, cervical cancer and prostate cancer. Used as an antioxidant for the blood, it protects the blood from and free radical scavengers. Also known to help break down proteins in the blood. Been used during treatments with chemotherapy.

Bowels: Milk thistle is used for inflamed bowels.

Breast: Milk thistle is used as an anti-cancer formula for the breast.

Gall bladder: Used to help with gall bladder problems and reduce inflammation.

Kidneys: Helps to cleanse and protect the kidneys.

Liver: Cleanses the liver, as it is used as a blood purifier for chronic liver disease and to treat liver cirrhosis and hepatitis. Milk thistle can also be used to block damage that has been done to the liver and help to restore it by stimulating new liver cells. Good to use for alcohol abuse as it helps to regenerate the liver.

Nerves: Milk thistle has been used in the treatment of depression.

Prostate: Milk thistle is used as an anti-cancer formula for the prostate.

Skin: Helps to heal psoriasis which is cause from the liver not working properly. Used for boils.

Spleen: This herb helps to support the spleen.

Stomach: Helps to relief heartburn, gas and stimulates the bile. Used to help increase the appetite.

Other uses and information:
Used to support the adrenals.

- Milk thistle can be found in capsules, extract and tea form. Best used in a capsule format, as milk thistle is not very water soluble as in a tea.

- Used for radiation exposure and helps to protect the body during chemotherapy.

- Been used for depression.

MULLEIN (VERBASCUM THAPSUS)
Known as blanket herb, shepherd's Staff

Contains:

Vitamins: A, B1 (thiamin), B2 (riboflavin), B3 (niacin), B5 (pantothenic Acid), B6 (pyridoxine), B12 (cobalamin), C, D

Minerals: calcium, iron, magnesium, manganese, potassium, selenium, sulfur, zinc

Chemical: fatty acid, malic, phosphoric acid, volatile oil

Plant:

There are 300 species of mullein. This plant is a biannual. It has broad leaves in its first year. The stem grows to 1 – 2 metres tall in second year. There are dense felt like hairs on the stem and leaves.

Parts used: leaves.

Solvent: boiling water, alcohol, apple cider vinegar

Therapeutic action:

anodyne, anti-cancer, anti-inflammatory, antiseptic, antispasmodic, antiviral, astringent, carminative, demulcent, diuretic, nervine, pectoral, stomachic.

Uses:

Bladder: Used to strengthen the bladder tone after childbirth.

Blood: Good for treating tuberculosis and stops hemorrhaging.

Bones: Used for swollen joints and as a pain killer for the pain of the inflammation.

Bowels: Used as a laxative and to stop bleeding in the bowels.

Ears: Mullein flower oil used for earaches.

Diseases: Mullein tea is used for mumps. Used to heal venereal diseases.

Glands: Used to cleanse the glands and reduce swollen glands.

Kidney: Roots are used for a diuretic with an astringent action on urinary tract. Used for dropsy, inflamed kidneys and reducing water retention.

Lungs: Used for lung soothing capabilities for coughs, consumptions, hemorrhage of the lung and pulmonary disease.

Used for asthma, bronchitis, croup, hoarseness, pneumonia and troubles with breathing. Mullein loosens the mucus and moves it out of the body.

Muscles: Mullein is used as a pain killer, and it helps with inflamed muscles.

Sinuses: Used for hay fever and sinusitis.

Skin: The flowers are used fresh and crushed for warts. Used for bruises, diaper rash, sores and wounds.

Stomach: Used for lessening gas.

Testicles: Used for swollen testicles.

Throat: Mullein tea is used for mumps, sore throats and tonsillitis.

Other uses and information:
- Used to help support the lymphatic system.

- Used for soothing hemorrhoids.

- Mullein was used by the Natives as wet smudges for lung problems.

- Used for relaxing and as a sleep aid.

MYRRH (COMMIPHORA MYRRH)
Known as balsmodendron myrrh, gum myrrh

Contains:
Minerals: potassium, sulfur

Chemical: acetic acid, beta-sitosterol, campesterol, dipentene, eugenol, limonene

Plant:
Myrrh is a yellowish-brown to reddish-brown gum resin obtained from a tree found in Arabia and Somalia and grows no more than nine feet tall.

Parts used: Oleo-gun resin from the stem. Used as a fine powder.

Solvent: partially soluble in water, alcohol and ether.

Therapeutic action:
antibacterial, antibiotic, antiseptic, antiviral, astringent, carminative, expectorant, stimulant.

Uses:

Blood: Good for lowering cholesterol. Used as a stimulant and assists the flow of blood to the capillaries.

Immune System: Myrrh supports and strengthens the immune system.

Lungs: Helps with asthma, bronchitis, colds, tuberculosis, and myrrh discharges the mucus in the lungs.

Mouth: Fights off harmful bacteria that can cause gum disease (gingivitis), cankers and is used as a breath freshener.

Menstruation: Used to stimulate menstruation period.Sinus: This herb works with the sinuses.

Skin: Myrrh helps with skin disorders (abscesses), bed sores, boils, cuts, eczema, herpes, nipples (sore), pimples, ulcers, wounds. Disinfectant for washing sores and ulcers.

Stomach: Used for gastric troubles, cleans the stomach and works with the colon. Works with chronic diarrhea.

Throat: Remedy for inflamed throat or as a gargle.

Other uses and information:
-Good fighting off flus and used as a disinfectant.

- Tincture or powder may be applied to the umbilical chord after birth.

- Used for inflammation of hemorrhoids.

NETTLE (URTICA DIOICA)
Known as stinging nettle

Contains:
Vitamins: B1 (thiamin), B2 (riboflavin), B3 (niacin), B5 (pantothenic acid), C, D, E

Minerals: calcium, chromium, copper, folate, rich in iron, magnesium, manganese, phosphorous, rich in potassium, selenium, silicone, sodium, sulfur, zinc

Other: acetic acid, alkaloids, beta-carotene, betaine, caffeic acid, fatty acids, ferulic acid, p-courmaric acid, protein, tannin

Plant:
Nettle grows wild and is known as a common weed in the gardens. The leaves can be eaten when they are young. When the leaves are mature, the plant needs to be boiled first to take out the stinging action of the plant.

Parts used: the flowers, leaves and roots are used.

Therapeutic action:
antihistamine, anti-inflammatory, antispasmodic, astringent, diuretic, expectorant

Uses:
Bladder: Used to help reduce the uric acid and strengthen the bladder.

Blood: As an astringent, nettle is used to stop internal hemorrhaging and external bleeding. Used to replenish the blood with iron when anemic and nettle is a blood purifier. Nettle with also help the blood to absorb the proper nutrients. When the blood has the proper iron, the circulation is better.

Bones: Nettle helps with the bones and lessens the effects or arthritis and rheumatism. Used to reduce hemorrhoids.

Feet: Used in a tonic for goitre (swelling of the big toe.)

Hair: Nettle is used in products for the hair. It helps to regulate the oil on the head and for stimulating the hair follicles.

Heart: Helps to reduce blood pressure.

Intestines: Nettle can be used to reduce diarrhea.

Kidneys: Nettle helps to strengthen the kidneys. It helps to reduce the uric acid. Uric acid is linked to rheumatism. Nettle helps to reduce kidney inflammation. Nettle is used as a diuretic to reduce the water content in the body.

Liver: Cleanses the blood and the liver.

Lungs: Helps with asthma, breathing and hay fever. Also helps to reduce mucous build-up in the lungs and lessen bronchitis.

Menstrual: Nettle tea can help to reduce heavy menstrual flow.

Mouth: Gargling with nettle water will heal mouth sores.

Muscles: Used in a tonic as muscle relaxant and pain reliever.

Nose: Nettle is used to stop nose bleeds.

Prostate: Nettle is used to treat prostates and clear infections.

Skin: Nettle can be used in a salve to heal skin ailments and is used for eczema and hives.

Other uses and information:
- Good as pain reliever and anti-inflammatory.

- Rich in Chromium which assists with appetite regulation.

- Used for vaginitis.

-Body aches: used in a cream or salve for the muscles.

- Sunstroke: Use nettle in a tea or drink and within a couple of hours symptoms should be gone.

OATSTRAW (AVENA SATIVA)
Known as a powerful stimulant and is high in body building properties.

Contains:
Vitamins: A, B1 (thiamin), B2 (riboflavin), B3 (niacin), B5 (pantothenic acid), B6 (pyridoxine), B12 (cobalamin), E

Minerals: calcium, folate, iron, magnesium, manganese, phosphorous, potassium, selenium, silicon, zinc

Other: benzaldehyde, beta-carotene, beta- ionone, beta-sitosterol, betaine, caffeic acid, campesterol, chlorophyll, ferulic acid, campesterol, ferulic acid, lignin, limonene, p-coumaric acid, quercetin, vanillic acid, vanillin

Plant:
Oatstraw is from an oat plant that has been used for cereal for over 3000 years. Oat was a cross between barley and wheat in Europe. The oatstraw and young seed is used for medicinal purposes. The plant has tall stems with long leaves.

When the flower is immature, it expels a white substance known as milky oats and this is used for medicine. The plant itself is known as oatstraw.

Part used: The whole plant is used. Used in capsule or loose-leaf form.

Therapeutic action:
antibacterial, antidepressant, anti-inflammatory, antiseptic, diaphoretic, nervine, stimulant

Uses:
Bladder: Oatstraw is used to stop bed-wetting and to strengthen the bladder.

Blood: Used as a blood cleanser.

Bones: Oatstraw is used for arthritis, bursitis, gout and rheumatism. Helps to strengthen brittle bones.

Bowels: Reduces constipation.

Heart: Helps to strengthen the heart.

Kidney: This herb when heated up will work with reducing pain from kidney stone attacks.

Liver: Oatstraw cleanses the blood and clears liver infections.

Lungs: Strengthens the lungs.

Nerves: Used for its calming effect, as an antidepressant, and it can reduce insomnia.

Pancreas: Used for strengthening the pancreas.

Skin: Oatstraw is used for skin disorders: boils, diseases and wounds.

Stomach: Used to decrease indigestion.

Other uses and information:
- Good for increasing perspiration.

- Used for paralysis.

- Good to use to prevent contagious diseases, supports the immune system.

OLIVE LEAF (OLEA EUROPAEA)

Olive leaf is known for its powerful action against infectious and viral diseases. It is even stronger than antibiotics that are being used, the superbugs that are cropping up in the hospitals. The man made antibiotics cannot stop the super bugs. When using olive leaf extract it attacks the pathogens, and not friendly gut bacteria. This makes it a better antibiotic than the manufactured ones.

Contains:
Minerals: calcium

Other: aglycone, apigenin, beta-sitosterol glucoside, kaempferol, luteolin, mannitol, oleanolic acid, oleuropein quercetin, rutin, tannin

Plant:
Olive trees are thought to have originated by the Mediterranean well over 5,000 years ago. The olive tree was first brought to America in the 15th century.

Therapeutic action:
antibacterial, antibiotic, antifungal, anti-inflammatory, anti-malarial, antimicrobial, anti-parasitic, vermicide

Uses:
Blood: Olive leaf works well with cleaning the blood and killing the bacteria that is caused by AIDS, cholera, Ebola virus, E. Coli, Giardia, hepatitis - A, B, and C, lowers high blood pressure, and inhibits LDL cholesterol from oxidizing and used for malaria.

Bones: Used for inflammatory arthritis.

Diseases: This natural antibiotic has also been used for chlamydia, chronic fatigue, common cold, fever, fibromyalgia, flu, herpes, Lyme Disease, meningitis: both viral and bacterial, pneumonia, Rocky Mountain spotted fever and shingles.

Liver: Olive leaf cleanses the blood and supports the liver.

Lungs: The leaf can assist in clearing up influenza.

Skin: Used to clear psoriasis that is caused by the liver not working properly. Poultices of the olive leaves are used to treat rashes, skin boils and warts.

Other:
Used for vaginitis and yeast infections. (Men can also get yeast infections.)

Used to clear fungus from the body.

Olive leaf can be used as a preventative method against outbreaks or the ongoing battle of infectious disease. The only other herbal remedy that is strong like olive leaf extract is grapefruit seed extract. The olive leaf extract is the chief destroyer or growth inhibitor of many kinds of microorganism such as flatworm, hookworm, roundworm, and tapeworm.

OREGANO & OREGANO OIL
Oregano is high in antioxidant properties. As a herb, it heals and is tasty. As an oil, it is very strong tasting, yet a very strong antioxidant and antimicrobial. Carvacrol, one of oregano's active ingredients, is one of the world's strongest antiseptics

Contains:
Vitamins: A, B1 (thiamin), B2 (riboflavin), B3 (niacin), B5 (pantothenic Acid), B6 (pyridoxine), B12, C, D, E

Minerals: calcium, copper, iron, magnesium, manganese, potassium, zinc

Other: beta-carotene, flavonoids, phenolic acid,

Plant: Oregano is part of the mint family and a perennial. This plant is grown in flower gardens, indoors and outdoors.

Part used: the leaves and the oil extracted from the plant.

Therapeutic action:
antibacterial, antibiotic, anti-emetic, antifungal, anti-inflammatory, anti-malarial, antimicrobial, antioxidant, antiseptic, antispasmodic, antiviral

Uses:
Bladder: Oregano oil can be used for clearing bladder infections

Blood: Oregano oil is excellent for the blood as its properties are antibiotic, antifungal, antioxidant and antiviral. Good for the blood and fighting off hepatitis.

Bones: Works to lessen effects of arthritis.

Diseases: It is an antimicrobial as it works with Lyme disease. As an antiviral, oregano can be used for colds, coughs and the flu.

Ears: Used to reduce ear infections as oregano is an antibacterial.

Head: Used to lessen headaches as it is a muscle relaxant.

Lungs: Oregano can assist in healing asthma, bronchitis, sinusitis, tuberculosis, whooping cough.

Mouth: Used in the mouth for the gums, tooth infection and gum infection.

Muscles: Oregano is an anti-inflammatory- muscular pain. Helps to lessen headaches and back pain.

Skin: Helps with clearing up acne, athlete's foot, bee stings, bites, dandruff, head lice, psoriasis, scabies and warts. Used to heal cold sores, ringworm and good to use on puncture wounds to clean up the bacteria around the wound.

Stomach: Used for indigestion, stimulates appetite and as a purgative.

Throat: Used to soothe sore throats and bring down the inflammation.

Uterus: Used for the prevention of giardia.

Other uses and information:
- The carvacrol in the oil fights off fungi, parasites, yeast and viruses.

- Used for candida, fatigue and fibromyalgia.

- For horses: ringworm – parasites – flies: add to a massage oil to apply to larger areas.

- Oregano does not build up in the body as it dissipates safely.

Caution: Do not use on sensitive or mucus areas of the body.

PARSLEY (PETROSELINUM STAVIUM)
Known as march, persel, persely

Contains:
Vitamins: A, B1 (thiamin), B2 (riboflavin), B3 (niacin), B5 (pantothenic acid), B6 (pyridoxine), C, E, K

Minerals: calcium, folate, iron, magnesium, manganese, phosphorous, potassium, selenium, sodium, sulfur

Other: alpha-pinene, apigenin, benzaldehyde, bergapten, beta-carotene, caffeic acid, carotenoids, chlorogen acid, geraniol, kaempferol, limonene, linalool, myristic acid, myristicin, narigenin, p-coumaric acid, psoralen, quercetin, rosmarinic acid, rutin, xanthotoxin

Plant:
Parsley is a member of the umbelliferea (carrot family). This plant is native to the Mediterranean area. The plant can be grown for two to three years in a row. The leaves, roots and seeds are used. Best grown annually, the plant leaves are not as tough. In the second year of growth, the plant may grow a greenish yellowy flower. After the parsley plant produces flowers, then seeds, the plant will die off. When planted, if it is being used for the root, the plants should be grown further apart. Parsley is good to grow with tomatoes as it helps to attract the moths to them instead of the tomato plant. As the parsley absorbs some of the tomato scent the attraction to the plant gets stronger for the moths, and they stay away from the tomato plants.

Part used: leaves, roots and stems

Therapeutic action:
alterative, antibiotic, anti-cancer, carminative diuretic, tonic

Uses:
Blood: Parsley is used for cleansing the blood and it helps to build up the iron in the blood. The roots and leaves have been used for low blood sugar, where adrenal malfunction is associated.

Diseases: This herb prohibits the growth of cancer cells and venereal diseases.

Gall Bladder: Helps to treat and work with the gall bladder.

Heart: The seeds from the parsley plant can help to reduce blood pressure.

Kidney: Parsley aids in better excretion of water and the sodium in the body, helps to stop bed-wetting and reduces inflammation in the kidneys. Good for children that have weak kidneys.

Liver: Parsley is used to cleanse the liver and clear up jaundice.

Lungs: Has been used to lessen allergies and asthma.

Mouth: Used to refresh the breath.

Prostate: Used for prevention of prostate problems

Stomach: Helps to expel worms. Used for digestion and relieves gas, stimulates the appetite, stimulates gastric secretions and digestive tonic. Can also be used as a laxative.

Other: Works with the thyroid and gout.

Other uses and information:
- Teas: Parsley has a higher vitamin C level than what oranges have. Tea is used for first stage of colds or flu. Drink as much as you can during first day of cold. The roots are stronger than the leaves.

Caution: When pregnant, limit the amount of parsley consumed. Little amounts are usually safe. The plant does affect the uterus if too much is consumed and will also dry up milk during lactation.

PAU D'ARCO (TABEBUIA HEPTAPHYLLA)

Known as lapacho, taheebo

A very powerful antibiotic

Contains:
Vitamins: C

Minerals: iron

Other: beta-carotene, beta-sitosterol, papachol

Plant:
Pau d'arco comes from the inner bark of a tree that grows in the rainforest in South America. The tree grows to 30 metre and 2 – 3 metres wide. The plant has been used by the native people in the rainforests for hundreds of years. The wood is used for bows and arrows (the strength needed for the pressure used) and building products.

Part used: the inner bark

Therapeutic action:
analgesic, anodyne, antibacterial, antibiotic, anti-cancer, antifungal, antiviral, vermicide

Uses:
Blood: Pau d'arco is a blood purifier that is used for cleansing the blood from bacteria, fungus and viruses. Used to stop hemorrhaging. Used to regulate diabetes.

Bones: Used for osteomyelitis and rheumatism.

Bowels: Reduces inflammatory bowel disease and ulcers.

Diseases: Used for Hodgkin's disease that affects the lymphatic system and for lupus. Pau d'arco works with diseases such as AIDS, cancer, gonorrhea, infections (fungal), leukemia, syphilis and other sexually transmitted diseases.

Heart: Used to strengthen the heart and works with the arteries and cardiovascular problems.

Intestines and Colon: Used for colitis and polyps.

Liver: Cleanses the liver and is a powerful blood purifier. Pau d'arco has a high content of iron reduces anemia.

Lungs: Helps to strengthen and protect the respiratory system. Been used for asthma, bronchitis and smoker's cough.

Prostate: Used for prostatitis.

Nerves: Pau d'arco has been used for Parkinson's disease.

Skin: Works on dermatitis, eczema, infections, psoriasis, skin cancer, ulcers and warts.

Spleen: Used to clear spleen infections.

Stomach: Used for gastritis and parasites.

Veins: Used for varicose ulcers.

Other uses and information:
- Works with clearing candida.

- Good working with the immune system to ward off allergies, colds and flu.

- Reduces hernias and tumours.

- Used as a pain reliever.

- Used for Fistulas. This is an abnormal passage that leads from an abscess or hollow organ or part to the body surface or from one hollow organ or part to another. This can be caused by tissue damage during surgery.

PEPPERMINT (MENTHA PIPERITA)
Known as balm mints, brandy mint, common mint, curled mint

Contains:
Vitamins: A, B1 (thiamin), B2 (riboflavin), B3 (niacin), C, E

Minerals: calcium, choline, iron, magnesium, manganese, phosphorous, potassium, selenium, zinc

Other: acetic acid, alpha-carotene, alpha-pinene, azulene, beta-carotene, beta-ionone, betaine, caffeic acid, carotenoids, carvacrol, carvone, chlorogen acid, courmarin, eugenol, flavonoids, hesperidin, limonene, linalool, luteolin, menthol, p-coumaric acid, pectin, phytol, pipmenthol, rosmarinic acid, rutin, tannin, thymol, tocopherols, vanillin.

Plant:
Peppermint originated in the Mediterranean. Peppermint is much stronger than spearmint, and more of a stimulant. Peppermint has a thick spike of purplish flowers and petiole that are dark green. The plant has a square-like stem. The plant should be collected in August to September, just as flowers begin to appear. Every two weeks the plant is cut back when grown for the oil in commercial use.

Parts used: Leaves, stem and oil. The oil is extracted after the flowers have expanded. The fresh and dry leaves can be used in cooking and teas.

Solvent: water. Mint should never be boiled.

Therapeutic action:
antimicrobial, antioxidant, antiviral, carminative, restorative, stimulant, stomachic

Uses:
Bowel: Peppermint helps to cleanse the bowel and is used to slow down diarrhea. Aids in irritable bowel syndrome.

Diseases: Studies show that peppermint oil can help inhibit the Asian flu, cold sores, herpes simplex, mumps, Newcastle disease and sinusitis.

Eyes: Good for strengthening the eyesight.

Head: Been used to treat headaches.

Heart: Used for heart troubles.

Lungs: Used in mixture for influenza.

Menstruation: Peppermint helps to slow down the menstrual flow.

Stomach: Used to stimulate the appetite, used in formulas for colic and in teas for nausea. Stimulating for gastric membrane and helps with indigestion by increasing the stomach acidity. With this it helps to stop the formation of gas in the digestive tract. Activates the secretory organs. Peppermint helps to stimulate the bile flow and relax the sphincter muscles of esophagus.

Throat: Used for sore throats from coughing.

Other uses and information:
- Peppermint provides a stimulation of the vagy's nerve and is used to release tension.

- The leaves and stems are used in teas, vinaigrettes and as a decoration for dishes.

- The oils are used in aromatherapy, lotions, and hand / foot creams.

- Peppermint should never be boiled, it should be seeped and covered to keep in the oils. Peppermint tea and chamomile tea together makes excellent soothing and quenching compound tea.

Caution: Peppermint is not recommended for mothers who are nursing. Overuse can cause nausea.

Peppermint can interfere with the body absorbing iron. It is suggested that pure peppermint oil or leaves not be consumed.

PERUVIAN BARK (CINCHONA SPP.)

Known as Jesuit's bark, countess' powder

Contains:
Mineral: calcium

Other: quinamine, quinine

Plant:
This plant is native to South America. The inner bark is a yellowish colour with the external colour being a light grey or light brown

Parts used: The bark of the tree.

Solvent: alcohol and boiling water.

Therapeutic action:
anti-malaria, antispasmodic, stimulant

Uses:

Bladder: Moderate doses diminish uric and phosphoric acid levels.

Blood: Many strains of malaria are resistant to synthetic quinine, but Peruvian bark is still effective.

Bowels: Peruvian bark is used to assist with the excretion of waste products.

Heart: Small doses aid in flow of heart action, cerebral functions.

Mouth: Powdered bark is used for tooth powder and as a throat astringent. It also helps to strengthen the gums.

Stomach: Small doses aid in flow of saliva and gastric juices. Stimulates taste, smell and improves appetite

Other uses and information:
- Good to use to reduce fevers.

Caution: Large doses over a long time can be poisonous. Peruvian bark's effect goes right through the entire nervous system. Over one gram can cause stomach irritation and vomiting.

Quinine: Quinine used on its own will cause deafness, and should not be used by herbal practitioners. Only the bark should be used.

PLANTAIN (PLANTAGO MAJOR)
Known as broadleaf plantain, white man's foot, greater plantain.

Contains:
Vitamins: A, C, K

Minerals: calcium, iron, potassium, sulfur, zinc

Other: apigenin, benzoic acid, caffeic acid, cinnamic acid, fibre, luteolin, p-coumaric, tannins, trace minerals, vanillic acid

Plant:
This plant is native to Asia and Europe and now is found growing around the world. This is a short plant, known as a weed. The young leaves can be eaten raw and the older leaves cooked in soups and stews.

Part used: leaves and seeds

Therapeutic action:
antibacterial, antibiotic, anti-inflammatory, antiseptic, antispasmodic, astringent, carminative, diuretic, emetic, expectorant, nervine, stimulant, stomachic

Uses:
Bladder: Plantain is used for bladder infections, soothing the urinary tract. Used to stop bed-wetting.

Blood: Used for blood poisoning as plantain neutralizes it. Use for external hemorrhaging and jaundice

Bowels: Plantain is used to stop diarrhea.

Eyes: Good for sore eyes.

Intestines: Used for dysentery.

Kidneys: Used to heal and soothe the kidneys. Used for dropsy.

Liver: Cleanses the liver and stops jaundice.

Lungs: Used for bronchitis, coughing, expelling mucous, respiratory troubles and soothing the lungs. Has assisted in slowing down the growth of tuberculosis. The herb has worked well with young children that have chronic lung problems and can be drunk in a tea.

Menstruation: Used to slow down excessive blood flow.

Nerves: Used for epilepsy.

Skin: Used for the skin: bee stings, bug bites, burns, cuts, infections, sores and to stop the bleeding of wounds.

Stomach: Plantain works with the acids in the stomach and helps to stabilize the stomach secretions. Used to heal stomach ulcers and slow down gas.

Other uses and information:
- Used for hemorrhoids.

- Used in tea to lower high fevers.

- Used as a juice for stomach ulcers.

- Used in a poultice for the skin. The leaves can be applied right to the skin to stop the bleeding of a wound.

- Young leaves can be eaten in salads.

PLEURISY ROOT (ASIEPIAS TUBEROSA)
Known as butterfly weed, celandine, swallow wort, tuber root, white root, wind root,

Contains:
kaempferol, lupeol, mucilage, quercetin, resins, rutin, tannin

Plant:
Pleurisy root is a member of the milkweed genus (does not exude a white latex juice when broken). This plant grows in south-eastern Canada, parts of BC and throughout the USA. Pleurisy root is a perennial with yellowish-brown tubular roots that turn grey with age. Once grey, the plant loses medicinal strength. The flowers are orange/yellow and turn to long narrow pods. The Natives of America consider pleurisy root to be "Great Fathers' best gifts to the children of nature."

Parts used: root

Solvent: boiling water

Therapeutic action:
anodyne, anti-inflammatory, antispasmodic, antiviral, carminative, cathartic, diaphoretic, emetic, expectorant, tonic

Uses:
Blood: Good for treating blood poisoning and tuberculosis.

Bones: Pleurisy root has assisted with treating acute rheumatism.

Diseases: Pleurisy root has been used for treating contagious diseases such as flus, measles, scarlet fever and typhus.

Heart: Has an effect on mucous and serous (visceral membrane) tissue, bringing relief to the heart and arteries of undue tension.

Intestines: Used for dysentery

Kidneys: Assists with the kidneys.

Lungs: Used for the respiratory system and chest pains as the herb helps to stop the inflammation. Helps to expel the mucous from the lungs. Good to use for asthma, bronchitis, coughs, croup, emphysema, influenza, pleurisy and pneumonia. Helps with breathing.

Lymphatic: Used to stimulate the lymphatic system.

Skin: Relaxes the capillaries and has a soothing effect on the skin.

Stomach: Used for gas, indigestion and stomach pain.

Other uses and information:
- Gradually increases skin temperature, promotes a slow steady perspiration and reduces fevers.

- Used for pleurisy.

Caution: Do not use where the pulse is weak and the skin cold.

Not recommended for children.

POKEWEED (PHYTOLACCA AMERICANA)
Known as pokeberry, pokebush, pokeroot

Contains:
Vitamins: A, E

Minerals: calcium, iron, phosphorous

Plant:
This plant has up to thirty-five species: herbs, shrubs and trees. The trees can grow up to 25m tall. The leaves are alternate and evergreen. The stems vary from a green colour to pink and read. The plant has flowers that are from a whitish colour to a pink that turn into berries. The berries go from a green colour to and dark purple/black colour.

Part used: roots and young shoots

Therapeutic action:
anodyne, anti-cancer, anti-inflammatory, antiviral

Uses:
Blood: Pokeweed is a good blood cleanser.

Bones: Good for reducing the inflammation from arthritis and rheumatism.

Bowels: Pokeweed can be used as a laxative.

Glands: Pokeweed is used for enlarged glands: lymphatic, spleen and thyroid. It helps to stimulate the metabolism.

Liver: Cleanses the liver and is a blood purifier.

Lungs: Used for reducing inflammation from respiratory discomforts.

Nose: Used to treat catarrh: helps to reduce the mucus build-up.

Skin: Used for skin abscesses, acne, cancers, infections (fungal), psoriasis and scabies

Stomach: Used for increasing the biliary flow.

Throat: Pokeweed reduces the inflammation from laryngitis, mumps and tonsillitis.

Other uses and information:
- Used for increasing the biliary flow for the liver and gall bladder.

- Pokeweed has been used to nourish someone who has not been eating properly.

- Used in a poultice for the skin.

Caution: This herb should be used sparingly, as it contains steroids and should be recommended by a herbalist.

PRICKLY ASH (XANTHOXYLUM AMERICANUM, XANTHOXYLUM CLAVAHERCULIS, XANTHOXYLUM FRAXINEUM)

Known as prickly ash berry, suterberry, toothache tree, yellow wood

Contains:
acrid resin, alkaloid, gum, xanthoxylin

Plant:
The prickly ash tree grows 8 – 15 feet high. It is native to North America. The flower is greenish-red to a blue black in colour and grows in clusters from April to May.

Parts used: Bark and berries. The bark can be chewed. The bark can be used in power format.

Solvent: Boiling water and dilute alcohol

Therapeutic action:
antibacterial, anti-cancer, anti-inflammatory, antiseptic, astringent, carminative, diaphoretic, rubefacient, stimulant, stomachic, tonic.

Uses:
Blood: Good for purifying the blood and increasing the blood circulation in the whole body. It is a stimulant for paralysis and for cold hands and feet.

Bones: Prickly ash is used as a remedy for arthritis, cold joints and rheumatism.

Bowels: Good for treating diarrhea.

Diseases: Used to treat rheumatic fever and syphilis.

Liver: Cleanses the blood and helps to strengthen the liver.

Mouth: Chewing of bark will reduce toothaches and sores in mouth. The taste of prickly ash is warm and aromatic. It helps to induce the flow of saliva.

Muscles: Used to reduce muscle cramping.

Skin: The powdered bark is used in application for ulcers, new and old wounds, as it cleans the wound and promotes healing of the skin.

Stomach: A tonic made with prickly ash is used for colic, digestive system, reduces gas and is used to treat stomach diseases.

Veins: Induces free capillary circulation.

Other uses and information:
- Removes obstructions in every part of the body.
- Excellent tonic for reducing fevers.
- Promotes perspiration.
- Used to decrease lethargy.

PRIMROSE (OENOTHERA BIENNIS)
Known as evening primrose.

Contains:
Vitamins: E

Minerals: calcium, magnesium, manganese, phosphorous, potassium, zinc

Other: amino acids, beta-sitosterol, caffeic acid, campesterol, essential fatty acids. gallic acid, kaempferol, lignin, p-coumaric acid, quercetin, tannin

Plant:
Primrose plants can be found in many flower gardens. It is a short plant and a perennial. The flowers bloom in the springtime and can be found in many colours.

Therapeutic action:
anti-inflammatory, antispasmodic, astringent, demulcent

Uses:
Bones: Primrose is used for treating arthritis.

Heart: Primrose helps to promote cardiovascular health and reduces high blood pressure.

Menstruation: This herb is used to treat hot flashes, reduces heavy bleeding and menstrual cramping.

Skin: Primrose is good for the skin as it acts like an estrogen and is used to treat skin disorders.

Other uses and information:
- Primrose assists in reducing weight by increasing the metabolism.
- Used to treat alcoholism.
- Primrose has been used for multiple sclerosis.

Caution: Primrose should not be used during pregnancy.

RASPBERRY (RUBUS IDEAUS OR RUBUS STRIGOSUS)
Known as red raspberry, garden raspberry, wild raspberry

Contains:
Vitamins: A, B1 (thiamin), B2 (riboflavin), B3 (niacin), C, D, E, G

Minerals: calcium, chlorine, iron, magnesium, manganese, phosphorous, potassium, selenium, silicon, sulfur, zinc.

Other: alpha-carotene, benzaldehyde, beta-carotene, beta-ionone, caffeic acid, citric acid, ellagic acid, farnesol, ferric citrate, fragerine, gallic acid, geraniol, lutein, tannin,

Plant:
The raspberry plant has a durable root with a biennial stem. The leaves are alternate. The flowers are white and appear in the summer of the second year, producing succulent red fruit that ripens in late July or August. The fruit can be both sweet and sour.

Parts used: bark, leaves and roots

Solvent: water, alcohol

Therapeutic action:
anti-emetic, antifungal, anti-inflammatory, astringent, carminative, emmenagogue, parturient, stimulant, stomachic, tonic.

Uses:
Blood: Raspberry leaves have been used for cleaning cankerous conditions of the mucus membranes throughout the body. High in iron citrate and the leaves are good for a blood builder.

Bones: Promotes healthy bones.

Bowels: Used for dysentery and reducing diarrhea (especially infants).

Childbirth: Helps to ease the discomfort of cramps during childbirth.

Diseases: Aids in controlling herpes, influenza and polio virus 1.

Eyes: Been used as an eyewash.

Menstruation: Raspberry leaves have a mild uterine astringent effect and are used for menstrual problems to reduce excessive flow, cramping and lessens hot flashes.

Mouth: Used to heal canker sores.

Pancreas: Promotes insulin production

Pregnancy: Raspberry is very beneficial during pregnancy. Provides for an easier delivery, easier pregnancy and faster recovery. The nutrients in red raspberry helps to strengthen the uterus wall. Helps to prevent vaginal tearing during delivery along with preventing hemorrhaging after the childbirth. The herb helps to enrich the colostrum in the mother's milk. Been used for morning sickness during the pregnancy.

Stomach: Used for little ones when experiencing colic. Helps to fight nausea and reduces vomiting.

Teeth: Promotes stronger teeth.

Other uses and information:
- Good reducing fevers and kills fungus.

RED CLOVER (TROFOLIUM PRANTENSE)
Known as meadow clover, purple clover, trefoil, wild clover,

Contains:
Vitamins: A, B1 (thiamin), B2 (riboflavin), B3 (niacin), B5 (pantothenic Acid), B6 (pyridoxine), B12, C, E

Minerals: calcium, chromium, iron, magnesium, manganese, phosphorous, potassium, selenium, sodium

Other: beta-carotene, beta-sitosterol, biochanin, caffeic acid, campesterol, chlorogen acid, courmarin, courmestrol, daidzein, eugenol, genistein, methyl salicylate, p-courmaric acid, protein, salicylic acid, sitosteral, trifolianol

Plant:

Red clover is found in meadows and pastures in Europe and North America. The flower head is oval shape and is a purplish brown colour. The plant has a faint aromatic scent, but the taste of the tea is a bit bitter. The roots receive an abundance of nitrogen as they go far into the ground.

Parts used:

The blossoms and sometimes the leaves are used.

Solvent: Boiling water and alcohol.

Therapeutic action:
alterative, antifungal, anti-inflammatory, antispasmodic, stimulant: mild, tonic

Uses:
Blood: Used as a blood purifier and immune stimulation for fighting cancers. Used to treat AIDS, HIV and bacterial infections.

Bowls: Red clover will help to reduce inflamed bowels.

Eyes: Used to help soothe sore eyes.

Gall Bladder: The blossoms are used to activate the gall bladder.

Kidneys: Helps to strengthen the kidneys and has a slight cathartic effect.

Liver: Red clover helps to stimulate and heal the liver, helping to clear up hepatitis.

Lungs: Used for bronchitis, coughing and wheezing. Taken as a warm infusion, red clover will cleanse and soothe the bronchial nerves and is used for asthma.

Menstruation: Red clover has isoflavones, which have estrogenic properties. Used as an alternative to soya products to reduce menopause symptoms.

Nerves: This herb has been used to help lessen nervous tension and has a relaxing effect.

Skin: Used for extreme skin disorders such as eczema and psoriasis along with treating burns.

Other uses and information:
- Used as an appetite depressive.

- Used for rickets (rickets is caused when one does not get enough vitamin D, calcium and phosphorous).

Caution: Red clover should not be used over a long time.

REISHI MUSHROOMS (GANODERMUM LUCIDUM, G. APPLANATUM)
Reishi is known to help support the immune system.

Contains:
adenosine, coumarin, ergosteral, germanium, lanostans, organic acids, polysaccharides, resins, triterpenes

Plant:
The reishi mushroom is a wood composing fungi (mushroom). It has a kidney shaped cap and is divided by growth rings. The colour is a shiny lacquered red to reddish-brown or black. The cap (fruiting body) is woody like the stem and the spores are white to brown. They get darker with age.

Parts used: body and stem

Solvent: water, alcohol

Therapeutic action:
alternative, antibacterial, antifungal, antihistamine, antimicrobial, antioxidant, anti-tumour, antiviral, nervine, relaxant, stimulant

Uses:
Blood: The reishi mushroom is used for circulatory system to lower blood pressure, lower cholesterol level, balance LDL/HDL ratios of cholesterol while reducing other blood lipids. Used to stop blood clots.

Bowels: Good for reducing colitis.

Diseases: The antimicrobial action is effective against bacteria, fungi and viruses. Used as treatment for AIDS and cancer.

Heart: Used for heart and cardiovascular system.

Liver: Reishi helps to cleanse the liver and fight off cancer.

Lungs: Used for allergies, asthma, bronchitis, general upper and lower respiratory problems.

Nerves: Works on central nervous system as a relaxant. Used for chronic fatigue, emotions, insomnia and paranoia.

Pancreas: Used for regulating the blood sugar level (diabetes) and reduces cravings for sugar.

Stomach: Calms down the autonomic nervous system for the digestive tract. Reduces cramping and stomach ulcers.

Other uses and information:
- The reishi mushroom is used to reduce tumours.

ROSE HIP (ROSA CANINA)

Known as rose hip. Rose Hips are known for their high content of vitamin C and natural fruit sugar.

Contains:
Vitamins: A, B1 (thiamin), B2 (riboflavin), B3 (niacin), B5 (pantothenic acid), B6 (pyridoxine), B12 (cobalamin), C, D, E

Minerals: calcium, iron, magnesium, manganese, phosphorous, potassium, selenium, zinc

Other: alpha-pinene, apigenin, beta-carotene, botulin, catechin, flavonoids, isoquercitrin, lycopene, malic acid, pectin, rutin, silica, sulfur, tannin, vanillan

Plant:
Rose hip is the fruit that comes from the flowers of the rose plant. The fruit is from an orange/red colour to a dark purple colour. After the flower has bloomed, it will turn into the rose hip.

Part used: The fruit known as hip.

Therapeutic action:
antibacterial, anti-cancer, anti-inflammatory, antimicrobial, antioxidant, antiseptic, antiviral, astringent, diuretic, expectorant, stomachic, tonic

Uses:
Bladder: Rose Hips are used for treating the bladder.

Blood: Good for to use for blood circulation, as a blood purifier and treating infections.

Bowels: Rose hip is good for bowel cleansing and is used as both a laxative and to reduce diarrhea.

Diseases: Used to prevent contagious diseases such as colds, flus and infections.

Ears: Good for treating earaches and infections

Kidneys: Used to treat water retention. Rose Hips are used to help expel kidney stones.

Liver: Helps to strengthen the liver and prevent cancer.

Mouth: Used for treating mouth sores.

Skin: Used for nourishing the skin and to prevent and treat skin infections. Used for bites, bruises, cuts, psoriasis and stings.

Stomach: Used for sore stomachs and reducing cramping.

Throat: Used to relieve sore throats

Other uses and information:
- Good to use to boost the immunity, high in vitamin C.
- Rose petals are used to shrink inflamed mucous membranes.
- Used to prevent or dispel dizziness.
- Used to reduce fevers.
- Rose Hips are used in infusions, tea, or soup bases.

ROSEMARY (ROSMARINUS OFFICINALIS)

Rosemary is very high in antioxidants.

Contains:
Vitamins: A, B1 (thiamin), B3 (niacin), C

Minerals: calcium, iron, magnesium, manganese, phosphorous, potassium, sodium, zinc

Other: alpha-pinene, apigenin, beta-carotene, beta-sitosterol, betulinic acid, borneol, caffeic acid, camphor, carnosol, carvacrol, carvone, caryophyllene, chlorogenic acid, geraniol, hesperidin, limonene, linalool, luteolin, oleanolic acid, phytosterols, rosmanol, rosmarinic acid, salicylates, tannin, thymol, tocopherols, ursolic acid

Plant:
Rosemary is a perennial plant that is native to the Mediterranean area. This plant can grow up to 1.5m tall. It has evergreen like leaves that are quite fragrant. This plant is also part of the mint family. The plant will get white to purple coloured flowers and can survive in the drier regions.

Parts used: The leaves of the plant are used.

Therapeutic action:
antibacterial, antibiotic, anti-inflammatory, antifungal, anti-inflammatory, antimicrobial, antiseptic, antispasmodic, astringent, decongestant, nervine, stomachic, tonic

Uses:
Blood: Rosemary is high in antioxidants and helps to clean the blood along with fighting cancer causing cells. This herb also will help to increase the circulation of the blood in the body, including the brain. It also helps to regulate the blood pressure.

Head: Used to lessen headaches. This herb can also help to reduce baldness.

Liver: As an excellent antioxidant, rosemary helps to cleanse the blood. This action helps to reduce cancer cells and tumours.

Menstrual: Rosemary had been used to lessen menstrual cramps. It can help to decrease hemorrhaging during the period and is excellent for cleansing the reproductive system.

Muscles: Used to reduce inflammation in the muscles.

Nerves: Rosemary tea has been used to reduce depression and hysteria. The herb works with the nervous system and can reduce stress headaches.

Skin: Rosemary is a great astringent for the skin. It can be used for eczema, bites, rashes and wounds. Its antibacterial properties are very effective.

Stomach: Rosemary helps to soothe the stomach and aids in easing indigestion.

Throat: Rosemary can be used as a gargle to clear any bacterial infections.

Other uses and information:
- Good for increasing memory and helping one to relax.

- Used in cooking and teas.

Caution: Rosemary should not be used during a pregnancy.

SAGE (SALVIA OFFICINALIS)

This herb is found in many dishes and known for its strong taste.

Contains:

Vitamins: A, B1 (thiamin), B2 (riboflavin), B3 (niacin), B5 (pantothenic acid), C

Minerals: calcium, iron, magnesium, manganese, phosphorous, potassium, sodium, sulfur, zinc

Other: alpha-amyrin, alpha-pinene, alpha-terminal, beta-carotene, beta-sitosterol, borneol, boron, caffeic acid, campesterol, camphene, camphor, caryophyllene, chlorogenic acid, cineole, citral, cornsole, cornsolic acid ferulic acid, , flavones, galic acid, genkwanin, hispidulin, limoneme, linalool, lutein, masliinic acid, menthol, mucilage, narigenin, nicotinamide, oleanolic acid, p-coumaric acid, pinene, rosmarinic acid, saponin, silicon, stigmasterol, tannic acid, thujone, thymol, ursonic acid, ursolic acid, vanillic acid

Plant:

Sage is a perennial herb that grows like a small bush. The stems of the plant are woody, and the leaves are greyish-green and thick. The flowers are blue to purple in colour. Sage is a member of the Lamiaceae family (mint) and is native to the Mediterranean area. Sage has a long history of being used for medicinal purposes and culinary uses. Sage was one of the ingredients in the Four Thieves Vinegar that had been used for the plaque. The vinegar was a blend of herbs which was used to ward off the plague.

Parts used: the leaves

Therapeutic action:

antibiotic, antifungal, antimicrobial, antispasmodic, astringent, cathartic, diaphoretic, diuretic, emmenagogue, emollient, pectoral (for the chest), stimulant, tonic

Uses:

Blood: Sage helps clean the blood and works with the liver.

Breast Feeding: Sage is used to stop lactation.

Diseases: Sage is used to treat Alzheimer's, epilepsy, jaundice and the plague.

Gall Bladder: Sage is used to cleanse the gall bladder

Hair: Used to rinse the hair. The tea rinse helps to add shine and will encourage growth of the hair.

Liver: Sage helps to support the liver as it cleanses the blood.

Lungs: Used to treat bronchitis as it works with the chest.

Menstruation: Great for reduce menstrual pains. Used for yeast infections and aids in reducing night sweats and hot flashes due to low levels of estrogen.

Mouth: Used for bleeding gums, toothaches and inflammatory conditions of the mouth and to clean the teeth.

Nerves: Works with the nervous system to provide a calmness.

Skin: Sage is used to treat snake bites,

Stomach: Used for digestion and reduces nausea and works with ulcers.

Other uses and information:
- Used to bring relief for heavy perspiring.

- Used to improve memory.

- Sage that is used in cooking is safer, as it burns off the potent oil called thujone. Too much of this oil can cause convulsions and loss of consciousness. Used in infusions for bathes, rubdowns and for healing sores.

Caution: Too much sage is not good, and it stops the blood from absorbing the minerals that the body needs. Those who are nursing should not consume very much sage, as it will dry up the milk.

Not recommended for those who suffer from seizures.

SASSAFRAS (SASSAFRAS OFFICINALIS, S. ALBIDUM)

Known as saloop, saxafrax, ague tree

Plant:
There are two species that are native to Europe and one from eastern North America. It grows to one hundred feet tall, with a diameter of 6 ft. This tree has a soft dark red to brown brittle bark, deeply furrowed and with a corky texture. All parts of the plant are aromatic and with a spicy taste.

Parts used: bark of the root, sometimes bark of the tree and the oil.

Solvent: boiling water, alcohol, oil.

Therapeutic action:
alterative, anodyne, anti-cancer, anti-inflammatory, diaphoretic, diuretic, tonic

Uses:
Bladder: Sassafras is used for treating and supporting the bladder.

Blood: As a blood purifier, Sassafras is very good at cleansing the blood.

Bones: Used to treat rheumatism.

Bowels: Used to stop diarrhea.

Childbirth: Sassafras helps with lessening the after pains of childbirth.

Diseases: Used to treat syphilis.

Intestines: Used for dysentery.

Kidneys: Sassafras is a diuretic and helps to support the kidneys. Used to treat dropsy.

Liver: Cleanses the liver and fights off cancer.

Lungs: Used to treat bronchitis and to release mucus.

Menstruation: Used to reduce the inflammation of a painful menstruation.

Mouth: Used when a root canal is being done by dentists.

Skin: Used to treat acne, boils, corns, poison ivy, poison oak, psoriasis and skin disease.

Stomach: Used for colic, gas and stomach cramps.

Veins: Used to treat varicose ulcers

Other uses and information:
- Good for treating ulcers

- Used to counteract tobacco poisoning.

- Used for weight loss.

Caution:
Sassafras absorbs slowly into the alimentary canal. Large doses will be thrown off by the kidneys and lungs. Can be poisonous and has caused death.

Should not be taken in early pregnancy.

In the US, the F.D.A. has placed it on the restricted list, as large doses will thin the blood too much.

SENNA (CASSIA SENNA AND SPP.)
Known as purging cassia, ringworm bush

Contains:
alpha-carotene, beta-carotene, beta-sitosterol, chlorophyll, courmarin, crypto-xanthin, daidzein, fumaric acid, genistein, limoneme, lutein, saponin, stigmasterol, zeaxanthin Plantnn

Plant:
Senna grows to .6 – 1 metre tall. The woody stem is usually white. The leaves are 2 – 3.5 cm long and 6 – 10 mm wide. The flowers are large and yellow.

Parts used: Leaves and seed pods.

Solvent: water or alcohol.

Therapeutic action:
alterative, anodyne, antiseptic, astringent, carminative, cathartic, vermicide

Uses:
Bones: Senna is used for rheumatism.

Bowels: Senna is a strong cathartic. It is used as a laxative to decrease constipation.

Gall Bladder: Helps to reduce and remove gull stones.

Intestines: Used for dispelling worms from the intestines.

Liver: Used when the liver has become jaundiced.

Menstruation: Senna assists with the menstruation period.

Mouth: Senna can be used for bad breath and to heal mouth sores.

Skin: Used to treat skin diseases.

Stomach: Used for colic.

Other uses and information:
- Good to use for gout.

- Mix three parts senna to one part ginger (or anise or caraway or fennel).

- Used in parasite cleaning (10 – 20 grains of powder, 1 – 2 tablespoons of tincture, ½ - 1 cup of infusion.)

SKULLCAP (SCUTELLARIA LATERIFLORA AND S. GALERICULATA)
Known as helmet flower, maddog, madweed, pempernel

Contains:
Vitamins: B1 (thiamin), B2 (riboflavin), B3 (niacin), C, E

Minerals: calcium, iron, magnesium, manganese, phosphorous, potassium, selenium, zinc

Other: acetylcholine, beta-carotene, lignin, scullellarin, tannin, volatile oil,

Plant:
Skullcap is a perennial with rhizomes. It has a slender square stem that is 1 – 8 cm. tall. The flowers are blue, rarely pink or white, with helmet like appearance.

Parts used: Entire herb, the leaves and roots, It is best picked and dried in June.

Solvent: diluted alcohol, boiling water.

Therapeutic action:
antihistamine, anti-inflammatory, antispasmodic, astringent, diuretic: mild, nervine, tonic

Uses:
Bladder: Skullcap is used for urinary problems.

Blood: Good for reducing high blood pressure. Used to reduce hypoglycemia caused by low blood sugar.

Bones: Helps reduce the pain from arthritis and rheumatism, along with helping to prevent it.

Diseases: Used for hydrophobia (rabies).

Glandular System: Helps to regulate the thyroid.

Head: Used to reduce headaches.

Heart: Skullcap helps to strengthen the heart muscle and improve circulation. Has helped with cardiovascular disease.

Menstrual: Used to help reducing cramping and PMS symptoms.

Muscles: Helps to reduce muscles cramps and spasms.

Nerves: Skullcap is well known for its nervine properties. Works on the cerebro-spinal centres and sympathetic nervous system to control most nervous irritations. Used for anxiety, chronic fatigue, convulsions, delirium, epilepsy, exhaustion, hyperactivity, hypertension, hysteria, insomnia, Parkinson's disease, neurasthenia (once considered a serious disease), restlessness, rickets, sleeping, spinal meningitis, St. Vitus's Dance (jerking motion) and tremors.

Reproduction: Skullcap has been used to cure infertility.

Skin: Used for poisonous bites (insect and snake).

Other uses and information:
- Good for using when going through drug withdrawals.

- Chinese skullcap (S. baicalensis) root has anti-allergenic and anti-inflammatory properties. Used to reduce fevers.

Caution: An overdose can cause giddiness, stupor, confusion and twitching. Should not be administered to a child under six years old. Don't boil skullcap as this will destroy its properties.

SLIPPERY ELM (ULMAS FULVA, U. RUBRA)

Known as Indian elm, moose elm, red elm.

Known for its ability to heal the whole body.

Contains:
Vitamins: B1 (thiamin), B2 (riboflavin), B3 (niacin), E, K

Minerals: calcium, copper, iron, magnesium, manganese, phosphorous, potassium, selenium, zinc

Other: beta-carotene, iodine, lignin, polysaccharides, tannins

Plant:
This is a small tree that grows in North America. The branches are rough with long leaves that are toothed with rough hairs on both sides. The leaf buds are covered with a dense yellow wool.

Parts used: bark.

Solvent: water

Therapeutic action:
anodyne, antibacterial, anti-inflammatory, antiseptic, antispasmodic, carminative, stomachic

Uses:
Adrenal glands: Slippery elm supports these glands by boosting the output of the cortin hormone that provides the body with blood building substances.

Appendices: Used to reduce the inflammation.

Bladder: Slippery elm helps to soothe the mucous membranes of the urinary tract.

Blood: Helps to clear the blood of impurities.

Bones: Good for reducing the effects of rheumatism.

Bowels: Slippery elm helps to soothe the mucous membranes of the bowels and to reduce both constipation and diarrhea.

Colon: Used to treat Crohn's disease and ulcerated colitis.

Diseases: Used for colds, flus and syphilis.

Head: Used as an anti-inflammatory and pain reliever for headaches.

Heart: Used for cardiovascular disease.

Kidneys: Assists with urinary problems.

Liver: Cleanses impurities from the blood and supports the liver.

Lungs: Used to treat asthma, bronchitis, coughs, croup, reduce mucous, tuberculosis, and other lung problems. Helps the respiratory passages.

Menstruation: Used to reduce pain and cramping.

Skin: Used for boils, burns, diaper rash, herpes, poison ivy, sores, vaginal irritations and wounds.

Stomach: Remedy for weak stomach as it helps to decrease the gas, neutralize stomach acid and soothe the mucous membranes. Helps the stomach digest food and milk.

Throat: Soothes a sore throat.

Other uses and information:
- Used to treat hemorrhoids, tumours and ulcers.
- Used as an anti-inflammatory and to reduce pain.
- Used in poultices and boluses.

SPEARMINT (MENTHA VIRIDIS)
Known as garden mint, Our Lady's Mint, spire mint, lamb mint

Known as the safest plant for even the sickest person to use.

Contains:
Vitamins: A, B1 (thiamin), B2 (riboflavin), B3 (niacin), B5 (pantothenic Acid), B6 (pyridoxine), B12 (cobalamin), C

Minerals: calcium, iodine, iron, magnesium, potassium, sulfur.

Other: acetic acid, alpha-pinene, apigenin, benzaldehyde, beta-carotene, beta-sitosterol, borneol, caprylic acid, carvone, dihydrocarveol acetate, esters of acetic, eugenol, flavonoids, geraniol, limonene, luteolin, menthol, oleanolic acid, phytol, pipmenthol, thymol

Plant:
The spearmint is native to the Mediterranean, Europe, Asia and Northern America. Spearmint is similar to mint but has thinner leaves, and it is a lighter green colour. The flowers grow in spikes and can be pink or white. This plant can be evasive and spreads by its rhizome roots.

Parts used: Entire herb and the oil.

Solvent: water

Therapeutic action:
anodyne, antifungal, anti-inflammatory, antiseptic, antispasmodic, carminative, diaphoretic, diuretic, restorative, stimulant, tonic.

Uses:
Bladder: Used for bladder inflammation and suppressed urine.

Blood: Good as an antioxidant.

Diseases: Used for chills, colds, fevers and flu.

Head: Spearmint is used for reducing inflammation from headaches.

Kidney: Spearmint has a stronger diaphoretic action than peppermint. Used for dropsy, kidney inflammation and kidney stones.

Liver: Spearmints antioxidant properties help to cleanse and support the liver.

Lungs: Used in teas for bronchitis and coughs.

Menstruation: Been used in teas for painful menstruation.

Muscles: Used in lotions on bruises and muscles to lessen the pain and promote better blood flow.

Nerves: Spearmint is used to treat hysteria.

Stomach: Spearmint works with the salivary glands and helps to stimulate the gastric secretion. Used for digestion, gas, nausea (especially during pregnancy) and vomiting. Safe for babies with colic.

Other uses and information:
- Spearmint has been used in teas for women with Hirsutism (excessive hair growth).

- Used to reduce dizziness.

- Used to keep rats and mice away by placing fresh spearmint in a dish in the cupboard or by planting around the house.

- It has been added to milk so that it will not curdle in the stomach or ferment.

- Should always be infused in a closed container, as spearmint has a volatile oil. Spearmint should not be boiled.

- Spearmint leaves can be used whole, chopped, dried and ground.

- Spearmint is used for its oil as a flavouring for toothpaste and candy, along as a fragrance in soups and shampoos.

TEA TREE OIL - SEE MELALEUCA ALTERNIFOLIA

Thyme (Thymus vulgaris)

Thyme is known for its antioxidant properties.

Contains:
Vitamins: B1 (thiamin), B2 (riboflavin), B3 (niacin), B5 (pantothenic acid), B6 (pyridoxine), B12 (cobalamin), C, D

Minerals: iron, silicon, sulfur

Other: alpha-pinene, apigenin, beta-carotene, borneol, caffeic acid, camphor, caprylic acid, carvacrol, carvone, chlorogenic acid, citral, eugenol, iodine, kaempferol, lauric acid, limoneme, linalool, luteolin, myrcene, myristic acid, narigenin, oleanolic acid, p-cymene, phytosterols, rosmarinic acid, salicylates, tannin, thymol, ursolic acid, vanillic acid

Plant:
The whole plant is used. The strong fragrance is from the thymol in the plant. Thyme grows well in hot and sunny spots. The plant is a perennial and can be restarted by seed, clippings or by dividing the plant. The plant can be found in mountain highlands growing wild.

Parts used: the leaves

Therapeutic action:
anodyne, antibacterial, anti-inflammatory, antioxidant, antiseptic, hepatic, vermicide

Uses:
Blood: Thyme is used for anemia, cleansing the blood and lowering the cholesterol level.

Head: Used for headache relief.

Liver: Cleanses and supports the liver.

Lungs: Used for asthma, bronchitis, coughs and croup by infusing the herb in water. Used as a tincture, syrup, salve and steam inhalation.

Menstrual: Used to reduce menstrual discomfort.

Mouth: Good to use as an antiseptic for the mouth and to avoid tooth decay. Can be found in mouthwashes.

Skin: Used for athlete's foot, burns, eczema, psoriasis, sores and warts. The oil has been used on bandages to help heal the wound. Thyme is used in some of the natural hand sanitizers.

Stomach: Soothe the stomach by eliminating gas. You can use the oil to soothe stomach muscles. Used to eliminate worms from the stomach.

Other uses and information:
- Good for reducing fevers.

- Used for crabs and lice.

- Poultice: Mash thyme leaves into a paste and apply to skin, but try a test area first. It may cause irritation.

- Sleeping and dreams: Used to lessen nightmares and induce sleep by placing the thyme under the pillow.

Caution: Do not take the oil internally. It can cause dizziness, nausea, vomiting and sore muscles.

TURKEY RHUBARB (RHEUM PALMATUM)
Known as China rhubarb, East India rhubarb

Contains:
Minerals: calcium

Other: calcium oxalate, cathartic acid, emodin, gallic acid, methyl chrysophanic acid

Plant:
This plant is similar to the garden rhubarb. The root stock is conical, fleshy and has a yellow interior. The large leaves grow to about 12 – 18 inches long.

Parts used: Dried rhizome, root bark mostly used.

Solvent: water and alcohol.

Therapeutic action:
anthelmintic, anti-inflammatory, antimicrobial, anti-tumour, astringent, cathartic, hepatic, purgative, stomachic, tonic.

Uses:

Bowels: Turkey rhubarb is used as a laxative for the bowels and is also used to stop diarrhea.

Intestines: Promotes healthful action of the bile flow.

Liver: Promotes healthful action of the liver.

Muscles: Used to reduce muscle inflammation.

Stomach: In small doses, it is used as stomachic and tonic as it helps to improve digestion. In small doses it is used as stomachic and tonic. Helps to relax the muscles and stop cramping.

Caution: If too much of it is used, urine may turn red (not blood, just by-product).

TURMERIC (CURCUMA LONGA)

Turmeric is known for its antioxidant properties. Possible carcinogenesis inhibitor.

Contains:
Vitamins: B1 (thiamin), B2 (riboflavin), B3 (niacin), C

Minerals: calcium, iron, manganese, phosphorous, potassium, zinc

Other: alpha-pinene, alpha-terpineol, azulene, beta-carotene, beta- caffeic acid, caryophyllene, cinnamic acid, curcumin, eugenol, guaiacol, limonene, linalool, p-courmaric acid, p-cymene, turmerone, vanillic acid

Plant:
Turmeric is a perennial that grows up to 1 metre tall. The leaves are alternate and grow up to 115cm long. This plant is native to Asia and needs the warmer weather and moisture to grow.

Part used: The root of the plant is used.

Therapeutic action:
antibiotic, anti-cancer, anti-inflammatory, antioxidant

Uses:

Blood: Turmeric is good for fighting the free radicals which cause cancer and HIV. A good anti-cancer preventative herb. Turmeric helps to improve the blood circulation and lowers the blood cholesterol levels.

Bones: Turmeric is effective in reducing arthritis.

Heart: Turmeric helps to lower the blood cholesterol levels. It also helps to promote better circulation of the blood for the heart.

Liver: Turmeric is good for fighting the free radicals and helps to cleanse and protect the liver.

Muscles: This herb can help reduce muscle inflammation.

Other uses and information:
- Best used in cooking.

- Turmeric is one of the main ingredients in curry powder.

Caution: If too much of this herb is used, it can cause distress to the stomach.

Not recommended if a person has biliary tract obstruction.

UVA-URSI SEE BEARBERRY

VALERIAN (VALERIANA OFFICINALIS)

Known as all heal, capon's tail, setwell

Contains:
Vitamins: B1 (thiamin), B2 (riboflavin), B3 (niacin), C

Minerals: copper, magnesium, potassium, zinc

Other: azulene, beta-carotene, beta-ionone, beta-sitosterol, bornyl acetate, caffeic acid, chatarine, ellagic acid, quercetin, tannins, valepotriates, valerianine, valeric acid, volatile oils

Plant:
There are many plants in the valerian genus. The conical rootstock or erect rhizome will develop for several years before the plant sends up a flowering stem. It has slender horizontal branches with terminal buds, aerial shoots or stolen which can produce new plant roots. The main stem grows to 3 – 4 feet tall. The flowers are from pink to blue and grow from June to September.

Parts used: The root.

Solvent: water, alcohol

Therapeutic action:
anodyne, anti-inflammatory, antispasmodic, nervine, stomachic, tonic, vermicide

Uses:

Bladder: Valerian is used for removing gravel from the bladder.

Blood: Good for improving the blood circulation.

Bowels: Used for irritable bowel syndrome.

Diseases: Used for measles and scarlet fever.

Head: Used to reduce head congestion.

Heart: Used to slow down the heart rate and for reducing high blood pressure.

Intestines: Used to expel worms and stimulate the intestines.

Lungs: Helps with bronchitis, coughs, for reducing mucous during colds.

Menstruation: Helps to reduce menstrual cramping and to promote the menstruation period. Great for calming nervous conditions during menopause.

Muscles: Valerian reduces muscles spasms and pain.

Nerves: Used for the cerebrospinal system, sedative for afflictions such as convulsions, despondency, epileptic fits, hysteria, insomnia, nervous unrest, neuralgic pain, restlessness, shock and St. Vitus's Dance.

Stomach: Used to stimulate the stomach.

Other uses and information:

- Used for hypochondria.

- Used for inflamed ulcers.

- Used for alcoholism and drug addiction.

Caution:

If taken over a long stretch may cause headache, heaviness and stupor. This herb can be addictive. Only recommended for short-term use.

Never boil the valerian root.

Should not be taken with alcohol.

Keep sealed and away from cats.

WHITE OAK BARK (QUERCUS ALBA)

Known as Tanner's oak

Contains:

Vitamins: B1 (thiamin), B2 (riboflavin), B3 (niacin), B12 (cobalamin), C

Minerals: calcium, iron, magnesium, manganese, phosphorous, potassium, selenium, zinc

Other: beta-carotene, beta-sitosterol, catrechin, cobalt, gallic acid, Iodine, lead, pectin, quercitrin, sodium, sulfur, tannin

Plant:
This plant is found in North America, southward from Canada to the Gulf of Mexico and west to Texas. Grows from 60 – 100 ft. tall. It can grow up to 150 ft. tall with an 8 feet diameter trunk. Bark is pale grey and leaves have rounded or finger shaped lobes.

Parts used: The bark and the acorns.

Solvent: alcohol, water.

Therapeutic action:
anodyne, antibacterial, anti-cancer, anti-inflammatory, antimicrobial, antioxidant, antiseptic, antiviral, astringent, stimulant, stomachic, tonic, vermicide

Uses:
Bladder: White oak bark is used for an ulcerated bladder and bloody urine

Blood: Used for external and internal hemorrhage, helps to cleanse the blood and treat gangrene.

Bowels: White oak bark is often used for chronic diarrhea.

Eyes: Good for inflammatory eye conditions.

Diseases: Used to treat venereal diseases.

Intestines: A decoction of bark is used to expel pinworms and assist in cleansing the entire gastrointestinal tract.

Used for treating damaged tissue in the intestines and reduces diarrhea.

Kidneys: Used to treat and support the kidneys.

Liver: Taken to reduce the deleterious effects of poisonous medicines. Used to strengthen the liver and fight against cancer. Used to counterbalance the effects caused by drug allergies and chemotherapy.

Menstruation: Used to relief menstrual cramping and pain.

Mouth: Used for gum inflammation, mouth sores, strengthening the teeth and to treat pyorrhea.

Prostate: Used for treating prostate cancer.

Skin: Excellent cleansing effect on inflamed surfaces of the skin like eczema. Used for abrasions, bites, bleeding and cleansing for the skin and wounds.

Spleen: Used to support the spleen.

Stomach: Used for treating damaged tissue in the stomach and reduces stomach mucous (excessive stomach mucous can cause nasal drip and sinus congestion.) Used for indigestion, nausea and to stop vomiting.

Throat: Used as a gargle for relief from sore throats and strep throat.

Tonsils: White oak bark is used for inflamed tonsils.

Uterus: A decoction is often used to treat leucorrhea and applied to the vaginal or uterine area, alleviating uterine prolapse or tipped uterus.

Other uses and information:
- White oak bark is often used for chronic mucous discharges and passive hemorrhage.

- An infusion of white oak is well known as a goitre remedy.

- Used as ointment and anal injection to treat hemorrhoids.

- Used internally and externally for varicose veins.

- Helps to improve the metabolism.

- Used to reduce ulcers and glandular swelling.

- Used to reduce fevers.

WHITE POND LILY (NYMPHAEA ODORATA)

Known as American pond lily, water cabbage, water nymph

Named after Theophrastus's water nymphs.

Plant:
Aquatic perennial that is found in ponds in North America. Branched rootstocks produce large orbiculate to oblong orbiculate entire leaves that float on the water surface. Leaves are dark on top and purplish on the bottom. The fragrant white flowers bloom from June to September and open in the forenoon.

Parts used: root

Solvent: water

Therapeutic action:
alterative, anti-inflammatory, astringent

Uses:
Breast: White pond lily is used in a poultice for inflamed breasts and can be taken internally.

Lungs: Used as a chest remedy for asthma and tuberculosis.

Mouth: Used for canker sores.

Skin: Known for its use as a soothing skin astringent, providing youthful look.

Stomach: Used as tea for soothing the digestive tract.

Uterus: Used in a vaginal douche for abrasions of the vagina, leucorrhea and uterine cancer, inflammation and ulceration of the uterus. Used in bolus form to tone up the uterus and remedy vaginal infections.

Other uses and information:
- Used for hemorrhoids.

- Leaves used in soups.

- Both flowers and roots have been eaten extensively.

WHITE POPLAR (APSEN) (POPULAS TREMULOIDES)
Known as American aspen, quaking aspen, trembling aspen

Contains:
Other: Leaves and bark have populin and volatile oil.

Plant:
White popular and grow from small to 30 metres tall. It has a smooth bark, light green of greyish. The bark becomes deeply furrowed with age. The leaves are very slender.

Parts used: Inner bark, sometimes the buds and leaves

Solvent: Boiling water (buds are soaked in alcohol then soaked in water)

Therapeutic action:
antibacterial, diuretic, emmenagogue, stimulant, stomachic, tonic

Uses:
Bladder: White Poplar is used to help stop bed-wetting

Bowels: Good for reducing diarrhea.

Childbirth: The Blackfoot use the inner bark in a tea for women who are about to give birth. Used for, during and after hard labour.

Diseases: White popular has been used to treat gonorrhea and syphilis sores.

Eyes: Good for eye inflammation.

Head: Good for headaches caused by hepatic insufficiency from stomach flatulence and acidity.

Menstruation: Good to use as a female tonic for the menstruation time and the female reproduction system.

Skin: When used as a wash, it helps with treating eczema, infections and skin sores.

Stomach: Used for heartburn, relaxing the stomach and toning the mucous membranes.

Uterus: The tonic is good for supporting the uterus.

Other uses and information:
- Tonic for genitals.

- Used to help reduce fevers.

- Inner bark used as tonic, astringent and diuretic.

WILD INDIGO (BAPTISIA AUSTRALIS)
Known as blue wild indigo, blue false indigo, indigo weed, rattleweed, rattlebush and horsefly weed.

Contains:
alkaloids, baptitoxinebenzin, benzol, cytisine, glycoside indican, rotenone, sophorine, sumatrol, tephorsin, ulexine,

Plant:
The wild indigo is part of the legume family. This plant is found in the north-east and Central America and can be found in the Midwest. This is a plant that can be found at the edge of the woods or in meadows. This plant has a hard time to reproduce as the seed pods of the plant get attacked by weevils. The plant is a perennial and will come back each year. It also spreads by its roots (rhizomes). If the stem of the plant is broken, it will secrete a blue like sap. The pea-like flowers come out in the spring and can be a light purple to a deep violet colour. This plant can also be used as a dye for fabrics. The leaves are soaked to bring out the dye.

Part Used: Both the root and the leaves of the wild indigo plant are medicinal.

Therapeutic action:
alterative, antibacterial, antibiotic, antidepressant, antiseptic, astringent, demulcent

Uses:
Blood: Good for boosting the blood and increasing the immune system. Helps to improve the blood circulation.

Bones: Wild indigo is used for rheumatism.

Bowels: Can help to reduce diarrhea.

Breasts: Used to reduce swelling in female breasts.

Disease: Used to treat thymus and typhoid fever.

Liver: The baptisia in the plant helps to stimulate the liver and helps to increase the biliary secretion.

Lungs: Helps to improve the respiratory movement of the lungs. BUT large doses can harm the lungs and paralyze the respiratory centres. Helps to expel and stop the mucous in the lungs.

Mouth: Wild Indigo can be used in a tea for toothaches. Used to stop foul breath and other septic mouth discharges.

Nerves: Used to treat dementia and melancholia (depression).

Skin: Wild indigo can be used in a salve to heal cuts, infections, gangrene, sores and wounds.

Stomach: Used to help stop nausea. One must be careful not to take large doses. It helps to heal the gastrointestinal tract.

Ulcers: Used to treat ulcers and the foul discharges from the ulcers.

Other uses and information:
- Good for reducing fevers and used at the beginning of a cold.

- Used to treat ulcers and the foul discharges from the ulcers.

- Used to heal cerebral spinal meningitis.

- You can use the roots in teas as a purgative or to treat toothaches and nausea.

WITCH HAZEL (HAMMAMELIS VIRGINIANA)

Contains:
Vitamins: C, E, K

Minerals: copper, manganese, zinc

Other: beta-ionone, gallic acid, iodine, isoquercitrin, kaempferol, myrcetin, phenol, quercitrin, saponin, selenium, tannins

Plant:
Witch Hazel grows from shrub size to a tree of about 7.6m tall and is found in North America. The flowers have four petals that are long and from a dark yellow to a red. The fruit had a shiny black seed. When the seed pods reach maturity, the seeds explode out of the pod. The early settlers in America used the twigs as diving rods to find water.

Part used: leaves, bark and twigs.

Therapeutic action:
anodyne, anti-inflammatory, antiviral, astringent, tonic

Uses:
Blood: Witch hazel contains tannic that helps the varicose veins. Witch hazel will help to stop internal and external bleeding. Used to treat tuberculosis.

Bowels: Good for reducing diarrhea and treating dysentery.

Eyes: Good for treating inflamed eyes and reducing bags under the eyes.

Diseases: Used to treat venereal diseases.

Head: Used to reduce headaches.

Menstruation: Helps to slow down excessive menstruation flow.

Mouth: Used in a mouthwash for bleeding gums and inflammation in the mouth.

Muscles: Witch hazel helps to soothe sore muscles.

Nose: Used to treat nose bleeds and clear the sinuses.

Skin: Use to treat bruises, burns, cuts, insect bites, irritations, scratches, sores, wounds and to clear up yeast infections.

Throat: Used to soothe the throat when inflamed.

Other uses and information:
- Used for sprains to reduce the pain and inflammation.

- Used to reduce hemorrhoids.

- Used to treat tumours.

- Witch hazel can help bring down the swelling in the vaginal area after giving birth.

- Use in a compress for skin irritations, bruises and sprains.

- For yeast infections use infusion from the leaves in a sitz bath.

- Used as an infusion with petroleum jelly and is applied to hemorrhoids. (Witch hazel is found in many hemorrhoid preparations.)

WORMWOOD (ARTEMISIA ABSINTHIUM)
Known as pasture sagewort

Contains:
Vitamins: B1 (thiamin), B2 (riboflavin), B3 (niacin), B5 (pantothenic acid), B6 (pyridoxine), B12 (cobalamin), C

Minerals: calcium, manganese, potassium

Other: beta-carotene, chamazulene, chlorogenic acid, cobalt, isoquercitrin, p-coumaric, rutin, salicylic acid, sodium, tannins, tin, vanillic acid

Plant:
Wormwood is an aromatic dwarf shrub. It grows from 10 – 40 cm tall. The plant is a silvery grey and turns brownish with age. Leaves are alternate and deeply pinnate.

Parts used: plant and leaves.

Solvent: water, alcohol

Therapeutic action:
anodyne, alterative, anthelmintic, anti-inflammatory, astringent, emmenagogue, purgative, stomachic, tonic, vermicide

Uses:

Blood: Wormwood is used for increasing the blood circulation and to stop internal bleeding.

Bones: Used for rheumatism.

Bowels: Good for reducing constipation.

Ear: Good for treating earaches.

Eyes: Used for sore and irritated eyes.

Gall Bladder: Used to treat the gall bladder.

Head: Used to treat headaches, even migraines.

Heart: Works with the vascular system.

Intestines: Used for dispelling worms, and when used with black walnut, will remove parasites.

Kidneys: Used for cleaning and supporting the kidneys and treating dropsy

Liver: Used to cleanse the liver, expel poisons and to support the liver. Treatment for jaundice.

Menstruation: Used to lessen menstrual cramping and to promote the menstrual period.

Mouth: Used for bad breath.

Nerves: Used as a mild sedative.

Skin: Wormwood is used to treat insect bites, blemishes, skin ulcers and wounds. Wormwood can be used to repel insects.

Stomach: Used to increase appetite, digestion, increase stomach acidity, for nausea and to stop morning sickness.

Other uses and information:

- Good for lowering fevers.

- Used to treat gout.

- Used to decrease obesity.

- Oil used as antidote for poisonous mushrooms.

- The tea is used as a hair tonic.

- Oil used as liniment for sprains.

Caution: Do not use during pregnancy. Only for short-term use as it can be addictive.

YARROW (ACHILLEA MILLEFOLIUM)

Contains:
Vitamins: A, C, E, K

Minerals: chromium, copper, iodine, iron, manganese, selenium, sulfur, potassium

Other: achillein, achilleic acid, courmarin, saponin, tannin

Plant:
Yarrow is an aromatic herb that grows to about 3 – 7 cm in height. The flowers are white and sometimes pink. Yarrow can be found growing wild and in flower gardens.

Parts used: whole plant, flowers, leaves and root, especially dried flower heads.

Solvent: water, alcohol

Therapeutic action:
antibiotic, anti-cancer, anti-inflammatory, antiviral, astringent, demulcent, diaphoretic, diuretic: mild, stimulant, tonic

Uses:
Bladder: Yarrow is used for soothing the bladder and to help with urine retention.

Blood: Good for increasing blood circulation, regulating the blood pressure, to help with blood clotting, blood cleanser and reducing jaundice.

Bowels: Used as an enema for piles and hemorrhages of the bowel. Helps to tone the mucous membranes of the bowel, eliminate the waste easier and help stop diarrhea in infants.

Bones: Used to help with rheumatism.

Breast: Good to use in a salve for soar nipples when nursing.

Childbirth: Yarrow is used to hasten the delivery of the unborn child.

Diseases: Used for cancer, chicken pox, colds, fever, flu, measles.

Head: For severe headache, inset a roll of yarrow into the nose to start a nose bleed. This will release the pressure of the headache. Yarrow is used to help promote hair growth.

Heart: Good for regulating the blood pressure.

Glandular System: Yarrow helps to treat and support the glandular system.

Kidneys: Helps the kidneys to function better.

Liver: Yarrow helps to open the skin pores to eliminate toxins. Yarrow is beneficial for the liver and influences the secretion throughout the entire alimentary canal.

Lungs: Helps to reduce bronchitis, lessen congestion, reduce hemorrhaging of the lungs and helps to lessen the effects of pneumonia.

Menstrual: For treating leukorrhea. Leukorrhea is when a white discharge occurs during the menstrual cycle, during pregnancy or during menopause. This can be a sign of infection in the reproductive organs. Yarrow also helps regulate menstrual bleeding.

Mouth: The root is used as a tooth analgesic.

Muscles: Yarrow helps with muscle cramps and pain.

Nerves: Yarrow helps to lessen hysteria and is good for the nerves.

Skin: Yarrow helps to open the skin pores to eliminate toxins. Yarrows green leaves are very effective at stopping bleeding. The dried leaves and flowers may be used. Good to use for skin abrasion, bruises and burns.

Stomach: Used for toning the mucous membranes of the stomach and to help stimulate the appetite.

Ulcers: Yarrow helps to soothe ulcers.

Other uses and information:
- Natives used the dried leaves of yarrow with plantain to stop internal bleeding.
- Used by Natives before going into the sweat lodge.
- Used in an infusion, yarrow increases body temperature. It opens the skin pores and stimulates perspiration.

YELLOW DOCK
Known as curled dock

Contains:
Vitamins: A, B1 (thiamin), B2 (riboflavin), B3 (niacin), C

Minerals: calcium, high in iron, manganese, phosphorus

Other: beta-carotene, hyperoside, quercetin, quercitrin, rutin, tannin

Plant:
Yellow dock is a plant that is native to Asia (western region) and Europe. This plant is a perennial that produces flowers in a stalk. The stalks grow up to 1 metre high. The seeds travel from place to place in the casing that they grow in.

Part used: roots

Therapeutic action:
antibacterial, anti-cancer, anti-inflammatory, antioxidant, antiscorbutic, antiviral, astringent, cathartic, demulcent, hepatic, stomachic, tonic

Uses:
Bladder: Used for cleansing the bladder.

Blood: Yellow dock is an excellent blood builder, cleanses the blood and treats leukemia.

Bones: Used for rheumatism.

Bowels: Good to stop bowel bleeding, stimulating elimination and helps to improve the bile flow.

Colon: Used to cleanse the colon.

Eyes: Good for treating ulcerated eyelids.

Diseases: Used to assist in treating cancer, leprosy and scurvy.

Liver: Yellow dock is used for anemia, as a blood purifier, to cleanse the liver and treat jaundice. An excellent blood builder.

Lungs: Used to treat bronchitis and stop bleeding in the lungs. Helps to reduce inflammation in the airways.

Lymphatic: Used to strengthen the lymphatic system. Used to support the thyroid glands.

Skin: Used for dyspepsia, eczema, hives, itching, psoriasis and rashes. Used with sarsaparilla in a tea to treat skin disorders.

Spleen: Used to strengthen the spleen.

Stomach: Helps to produce the bile needed to digest the food.

Other uses and information: - Used to treat tumours and ulcers.

Caution: Do not use yellow dock in soups or salads.

CHAPTER 10

Legumes

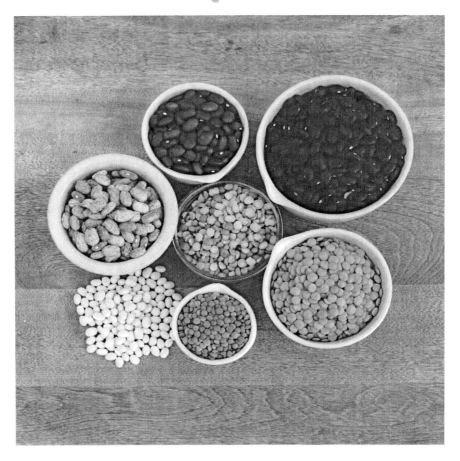

LEGUMES ARE ANOTHER ONE OF OUR SUPER FOODS. THIS FOOD GROUP PROVIDES SO many benefits and is used in so many dishes. As I was doing research for the book, it was fun to learn how we need to be combining our food to maximize the benefits of the food groups to receive the fullest potential of the nutrients.

When a person eats little meat, we need to supplement the proteins that meat provides. To have complete protein we have two options that we use, and this provides a lot of ideas and ways of creating healthy meals.

1. Beans with brown rice, corn, nuts, seeds or wheat.

2. Brown rice with beans, nuts, seeds or wheat.

Beans are an amazing food group. They help to regulate the blood sugar level, lower cholesterol and they help to reduce the risk of cancer. They are an excellent source of fibre, which is good for the bowels. Beans have two types of fibre: insoluble and soluble. Both work differently for our body. As we eat the beans, the soluble fibre is part that gathers up the cholesterol and removes it from the body. Beans are also high in antioxidants. The darker the bean, the higher the antioxidant properties of the beans.

THE FOLLOWING VITAMINS AND MINERALS WERE COMMON IN MOST OF THE BEANS:

B2, B3, and B6 appeared in most of the beans but in very low amounts.

B5: Can be found in all the beans. For our adrenal hormones, anti-stress, immune system, metabolism of carbs, fats and proteins and for our neurotransmitters.

B6: Can be found in all the beans. Amino acids for better absorption, arthritis: relieves pain, brain support, burning sensations, convulsions, immune system, leg cramps, liver support and nerves.

Choline: Can be found in all the beans. Choline helps the other vitamins to work properly, works with our memory and muscles. It is also used to help treat Alzheimer's, dementia, Friedreich's Ataxia, Gilles de la Tourette's disease, Huntington's disease, manic depression and Tardive dyskinesia.

Folate: Can be found in all the beans. For our arteries, bone marrow, brain, DNA, energy production, fingernails, hair, immune system, metabolism, red blood cells, RNA and white blood cells.

Inositol: Can be found in all the beans. For our arteries, bowels, heart muscles, nerves, skeletal muscles and skin.

E: This is good for cardiovascular disorders, endocrine glands, fatty acid protection, healthy heart, immune system, nervous system, PMS and healing of the skin.

Calcium: Can be found in almost of the beans. Anti-cancer, blood clotting, blood pressure (lower), bones (growth), cholesterol (lowers it), DNA, gums, heart, heartbeat, muscle growth, RNA, and teeth.

Chromium: Can be found in all the beans. Regulates sugar levels, reduces body fat and helps the fetus develops properly.

Copper: Can be found in all the beans. Formation of the blood cells, energy, hair, immune support, joints, skin and nerves.

Iron: Can be found in all the beans. Good for blood (red cells), energy and our immune system.

Magnesium: Can be found in all the beans. Good for bowels, energy production, heart, insomnia (better sleep), kidneys, muscles and nerves.

Manganese: Can be found in most beans. For blood sugar regulation, bone growth, cartilage, joints, immune system, metabolism (protein and fats) and for our nerves (calming).

Phosphorus: Can be found in most of the beans. For blood clotting, bone formation, heart, kidneys, teeth formation. Helps our body process food so that we utilize the vitamins.

Potassium: Can be found in all the beans. For our heart, muscles and nervous system.

Sulfur: Can be found in all the beans. Antioxidant, disinfect our blood, bacteria resistant, proper bile secretion.

Zinc: Can be found in most beans. For the immune system, prostate glands, reproductive organs and skin.

WE WILL BE COVERING THE FOLLOWING:

Bean (black, red and white), black-eyed peas, carob, garbanzo bean, kidney bean, lentil, lima, navy bean, peanut, pinto and soybean.

BEAN (BLACK)

Black beans are high in antioxidant properties, molybdenum, folate, fibre, copper, manganese, B1, phosphorus, magnesium and iron.

Benefits:
- anti-cancer, anti-inflammatory

- Other benefits: blood cholesterol (lower), blood sugar (regulate), colitis prevention, colon support, digestive tract, heart (cardiovascular support), heart disease (prevention), intestine support, liver support, muscle support, pancreas support, tumour prevention.

Contains:
Vitamins: B1 (thiamin), B2 (riboflavin), B3 (niacin), B5 (pantothenic acid), B6 (pyridoxine), choline, folate, inositol, E

Minerals: calcium, chromium, copper, iron, magnesium, manganese, phosphorus, potassium, sulfur, zinc

Other: omega-3, omega-6, fibre, protein

BEAN (RED)

Red beans are the highest in antioxidant properties. Red beans contain no fat or cholesterol and are high in protein and fibre.

Benefits:
- antioxidant

- Other benefits: blood (support), bone support, depression, digestive tract, eyes, heart (support), liver support, muscle support, skin care

Contains:
Vitamins: B1 (thiamin), B2 (riboflavin), B3 (niacin), B5 (pantothenic acid), B6 (pyridoxine), C, E, choline, folate, inositol, K

Minerals: calcium, chromium, copper, iron, magnesium, manganese, molybdenum, potassium, selenium, sodium, sulfur, zinc

Other: omega-3, omega-6

BEAN (WHITE)

White beans contain no fat or cholesterol and are high in protein and fibre.

Benefits:
- Other benefits: blood sugar (regulate), bowel support, cholesterol (lower), heart disease prevention

Contains:
Vitamins: B1 (thiamin), B2 (riboflavin), B3 (niacin), B5 (pantothenic acid), B6 (pyridoxine), C, choline, E, folate, inositol, K

Minerals: calcium, chromium, copper, iron, magnesium, manganese, phosphorous, potassium, sodium, sulfur, zinc

Other: omega-3, omega-6, fibre, protein

BLACK-EYED PEA

Black-Eyed Peas are a bean.

Benefits:
- anti-inflammatory

- Other benefits: anemia, blood pressure: too high, bowel support, constipation prevention, digestion, eyes, heart: support, inflammation (chronic), skin: care.

Contains:
Vitamins: A, B1 (thiamin), B2 (riboflavin), B3 (niacin), B5 (pantothenic acid), B6 (pyridoxine), folate C, E, K

Minerals: calcium, copper, iron, magnesium, manganese, phosphorous, potassium, selenium, zinc

Other: fibre, protein

CAROB

Carob is a part of the pea/legume family. The carob trees grow to 49' tall. The carob is loaded with antioxidants and has no caffeine or gluten.

Benefits:
- antidepressant, anti-inflammatory, antioxidant.

- Other benefits: blood cleanse, cancer prevention, depression, eyes, heart: support, liver: support, muscles: inflammation, muscles: support, nerves: calming, organ: support, skin care.

Contains:
Vitamins: A, B1 (thiamin), B2 (riboflavin), B3 (niacin), B6 (pyridoxine), choline, folate, inositol, E

Minerals: calcium, copper, iron, magnesium, manganese, potassium, selenium, sodium, zinc

Other: omega-3, omega-6, fibre, protein

GARBANZO BEAN

Garbanzo beans are also known as chick peas. They contain no fat or cholesterol and are high in fibre and protein. Garbanzo beans have a large amount of folate and manganese.

Benefits:
- anti-inflammatory, antioxidant.

- Other benefits: anemia, blood cleanser, blood sugar: regulate, bone growth, bowel support, cancer prevention, cholesterol: to lower, colon support, depression, heart: cardiovascular, heart: support, immune system, liver, muscle support, pregnancy: folate (development of unborn baby).

Contains:
Vitamins: A, B1 (thiamin), B2 (riboflavin), B3 (niacin), B5 (pantothenic acid), B6 (pyridoxine), C, E, choline, folate, inositol, K

Minerals: boron, calcium, chromium, copper, iron, magnesium, manganese, molybdenum, phosphorous, potassium, selenium, sodium, sulfur, zinc

Other: omega-3, omega-6, fibre, protein

KIDNEY BEAN

Kidney Beans are in the top ten of antioxidants. They contain no fat or cholesterol and high in protein and fibre. Kidney beans are excellent for women who are pregnant and need their iron.

The red beans are the highest in antioxidant properties that work to ward off cancers. Red beans contain no fat or cholesterol and are high in protein and fibre.

Benefits:
- anti-inflammatory, antioxidant.

- Other benefits: anemia, arteries, blood cleanser, blood pressure (regulate), blood sugar (regulate), bowel support, brain support, cholesterol (lower), diabetes, digestive tract, energy, heart (cardiovascular support), heart support, IBS prevention, muscle support, veins.

Contains:
Vitamins: B1 (thiamin), B2 (riboflavin), B3 (niacin), B5 (pantothenic acid), B6 (pyridoxine), C, D, E, choline, folate, inositol, K

Minerals: calcium, chromium, copper, iron, magnesium, manganese, molybdenum, phosphorous, potassium, sodium, sulfur, zinc

Other: omega-3, omega-6, fibre, protein

Served as:
Before eating, kidney beans should be soaked in water for at least five hours. The water needs to be drained, and then the beans should be boiled in clean water at 212°F (100°C) for at least 10 minutes. Kidney beans should not be eaten raw.

LENTIL

Brown lentils are known for their ability to lessen hot flashes in females. Lentils can be black, brown, green and red.

They are high in folate, iron, manganese, phosphorus and B1 (Thiamin).

Benefits:
- anti-inflammation, antioxidant

- Other benefits: anemia, appetite: to reduce, blood pressure (too high), brain support, cancer prevention, constipation, diabetes prevention, digestion, energy, exhaustion, heart support, immune system, tumours, weight: reduction.

Contains:
Vitamins: B1 (thiamin), B2 (riboflavin), B3 (niacin), B5 (pantothenic acid), B6 (pyridoxine), C, choline, folate, inositol, E, K

Minerals: calcium, chromium, copper, iron, magnesium, manganese, molybdenum, phosphorous, potassium, selenium, sulfur, zinc

Other: omega-3, omega-6, fibre, protein

LIMA BEAN

Lima beans are known as "butter beans." The bean has a buttery texture. Lima beans can be brown, black, green, purple, red or white.

Benefits:
- anti-cancer, antioxidant

- Other benefits: blood cholesterol (to lower), blood cleanser, blood sugar (regulate), breast cancer prevention, cancer prevention, colon support, diabetes, heart support, muscle support.

Contains:
Vitamins: B1 (thiamin), B5 (pantothenic acid), B6 (pyridoxine), choline, folate, inositol, E

Minerals: chromium, copper, iodine, iron, magnesium, molybdenum, phosphorous, potassium, sulfur, zinc

Other: L-lysine, fibre, protein

NAVY BEAN

Navy beans contain no fat or cholesterol and are high in fibre, folate, manganese, copper, phosphorus and B1.

Benefits:
- anti-inflammatory, antioxidant

- Other benefits: arteries, blood circulation, blood pressure (regulate), blood support, blood sugar (regulate), bones (support), bowels, cholesterol (lowering), constipation prevention, diabetes, DNA, energy, heart support, hypoglycemia, memory, muscle inflammation, muscle support, veins.

Contains:
Vitamins: B1 (thiamin), B2 (riboflavin), B3 (niacin), B5 (pantothenic acid), B6 (pyridoxine), C, choline, folate, inositol, K

Minerals: boron, calcium, chromium, copper, iron, magnesium, manganese, phosphorous, potassium, sulfur, zinc

Other: omega-3, omega-6, fibre, protein

PEANUT

The peanut really is a legume and is also known as a groundnut. The peanut is high in copper, manganese and B3. The roasted peanuts increase the antioxidant properties of the peanut by about 20%.

Benefits:
- anti-cancer, antioxidant.

- Other benefits: Alzheimer's disease, colon cancer, colon: support, gall stone prevention, heart: cardiovascular support, heart support, liver support, stroke prevention, weight reduction.

Contains:
Vitamins: B1 (thiamin), B2 (riboflavin), B3 (niacin), B5 (pantothenic acid), B6 (pyridoxine), biotin, folate, C, E, Coenzyme Q10

Minerals: boron, calcium, copper, iron, magnesium, manganese, phosphorous, potassium, selenium, sodium, zinc

Other: omega-6, fibre, protein

PINTO BEAN

Pinto beans are high antioxidant properties. Pinto beans are low in fat and contain no saturated fat, trans fats, or cholesterol. They are high in molybdenum, folate, fibre, copper, manganese, phosphorus, protein, B1 and B6.

Benefits:
- anti-cancer, antioxidant

- Other benefits: blood pressure (regulate), blood sugar regulator, bowel support, cancer prevention, cholesterol (lower), diabetes, digestive tract, energy, heart (cardiovascular support), heart disease prevention, heart (support), hypoglycemia, muscle support, stroke prevention.

Contains:
Vitamins: B1 (thiamin), B5 (pantothenic acid), B6 (pyridoxine), choline, folate, inositol, E

Minerals: calcium, chromium, copper, iron, magnesium, manganese, molybdenum, phosphorous, potassium, sulfur, zinc

Other: fibre, protein

SOYBEAN

This product may be high in many vitamins and minerals, but the product itself can deplete the land of the nutrients. This plant is also used as a milk or in a cheese as an alternative to having to milk for those who are lactose intolerant.

Benefits:
- antioxidant

- Other benefits: blood circulation, bone support, cancer prevention, diabetes prevention, digestion, fetus development, heart support, menopause, metabolism.

Contains:

Vitamins: B2 (riboflavin), B5 (pantothenic acid), B6 (pyridoxine), B12, biotin, choline, folate, inositol, E, K, P

Minerals: calcium, chromium, copper, iron, magnesium, manganese, molybdenum, phosphorous, potassium, silicon, sulfur, zinc

Other: omega-3, fibre, protein

Caution: Studies are showing that soy beans can create an imbalance in the estrogen levels and for men it may bring about infertility by lowering the sperm count. Too much soy products can disrupt the function of the thyroid gland and hormones.

It is interesting that research done shows the benefits of using soy is higher than eating meat and dairy. Yet the impact of the land can also be at stake by the soy bean production.

CHAPTER 11

Meats

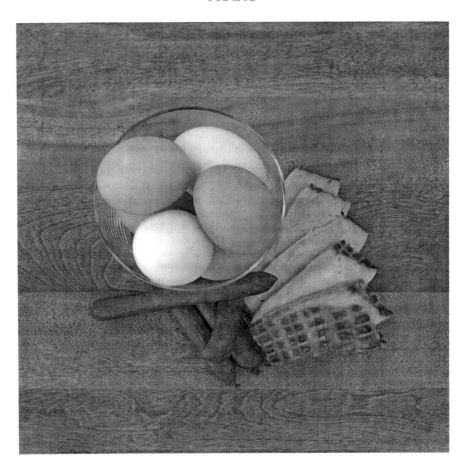

MEAT HAS BEEN A STAPLE IN MANY REGIONS AROUND THE WORLD. COWS, GOATS, SHEEP, poultry are raised on the farms. Fish in now being farmed in large pools. Wildlife is still being hunted for food. At one time, this staple was cherished, and people were not allowed to hunt for sport only. Every part of the animal was used, and there was no waste.

Now the livestock is loaded with hormones and antibiotics. Human beings are having difficulty digesting the meat, and some of us can smell and even taste these manmade chemicals. This becomes hard for those who don't know how to replace their enzymes, iron and proteins properly as vegetarians. If your body cannot digest today's meat, look for the nearest organic farmer in your area. The meat may cost more, but your body is worth it.

Today there are so many different lifestyles and ways that people feel comfortable with what they eat. When we listen to our bodies, we will notice when food products are slowing us down or increasing our energy. For myself, I know when my body is craving beef or poultry. This will happen about once a month or so. Eggs are a part of my daily diet for the nutrition and protein. As for the meat, I can do without it until I get that craving. I do make sure that the proper food is consumed for all the requirements that I need, which might be more legumes or vegetables that are high in iron and proteins. Over the last few years I have met a few people who are vegan. Their complexion is pale. They lack energy and seem to be sporting colds all the time. I want to say and ask: "You look sick. What are you really eating?"

If you choose to be vegan or vegetarian, take a good look at Chapter 4 and read up on all the nutrients that our bodies need to be healthy and make sure you can replace the nutrients that meat has to offer. If you are an avid meat eater, research into how the meat is being raised to see if you are really consuming healthy food.

Another huge concern today is the processed meats: hot dogs, package sandwich meat and some of the smoked meats. The smell of sandwich meats with the effects of smoked meat in my digestive tract and the ill feeling I get after eating hot dogs lets me know that these products are toxic for my body. I can smell the chemicals in the turkey meat. I have learned to pay attention to the processed meats and know better what not to buy.

It was interesting going through the meats and seeing that some of the beef and more so the fish has enzymes that we need for better digestion. If a person is unable to eat a lot of meat, we do have the option of finding digestive enzymes on the shelf in the health food stores and some of the prescription stores. As we age, our bodies sometimes require more enzymes, and we could benefit from having them in our diet daily. Some of the fish has the omega-3 oils that are essential for our brain and our heart. It is interesting to really see what we are consuming and how it can heal the body when eaten in moderation, not fried and cooked properly.

IN THE BEEF, THE MAIN NUTRIENTS ARE:

B1: abdomen, antibodies, appetite, blood circulation, brain, chest pain, depression, eye health, fatigue, memory, nerve impulses.

B2: adrenal glands, birth defects (preventative), blood, eyes, detox, growth, metabolism, nerves, respiratory, skin, thyroid, weight loss

B3: anxiety, arthritis, blood, blood circulation, cholesterol (lower), depression, diarrhea, fatigue, headaches, heart disease, insomnia, liver, mental illness, nerves, respiration

B5: For our adrenal hormones, anti-stress, immune system, metabolism of carbs, fats and proteins and for our neurotransmitters.

B6: amino acids (better absorption), arthritis (reliefs pain), brain support, burning sensations, convulsions, immune system, leg cramps, liver support, nerves.

B12: anemia, mental health, nervous system, small intestine, red blood cells.

D: Better absorption of calcium, kidneys, osteoporosis, rickets, teeth

E: This is good for cardiovascular disorders, endocrine glands, fatty acid protection, healthy heart, immune system, nervous system, PMS and healing the skin.

Iron: Good for blood (red cells), energy and our immune system.

L-Lysine: bone development, cold sores, concentration, building block for proteins, hair loss, herpes.

L-Tyrosine: anxiety, dehydration, digestion (fats and vitamins), epilepsy, hyperactive, hypertension, nervous system, seizers,

L-Tyrosine: depression, metabolism, nervous system, thyroid gland, pituitary gland, restless legs, weight control.

It is interesting that B12 is needed to activate the folate in our food, and the lack of this vitamin is also what creates the pallor look in vegetarians who are not eating properly. B12 is also needed for our mental health, and a lack of it can cause severe depression.

The iron in the meats is essential for the blood. When the iron level is low, a person can become anemic and lethargic. I remember how I needed to take an iron supplement when I was pregnant. The tablets were bad and made a person constipated. Now we have liquid iron supplements that are easier on the body, and a lot of foods with iron in them.

L-lysine, L-taurine and L-tyrosine are amino acids and protein that our body requires. These are not found in a lot of food groups and are found more in the beef and seafood.

THE MAIN NUTRIENTS FOUND IN LAKE, OCEAN, RIVER, SEA:

B2, B3, B5, B6, iodine, sulfur, zinc, L-lysine, L-taurine and L-tyrosine are more present. The B5 is good for reducing stress, converting the food properly and providing the body with more energy. The iodine is good for thyroid health.

B2: adrenal glands, birth defects (preventative), blood, eyes, detox, growth, metabolism, nerves, respiratory, skin, thyroid, weight loss

B3: anxiety, arthritis, blood, blood circulation, cholesterol (lower), depression, diarrhea, fatigue, headaches, heart disease, insomnia, liver, mental illness, nerves, respiration.

B5: For our adrenals, hormones, anti-stress, immune system, metabolism of carbs, fats and proteins and for our neurotransmitters.

B6: amino acids (better absorption), arthritis: relieves pain, brain support, burning sensations, convulsions, immune system, leg cramps, liver support, nerves.

Iodine: diarrhea, fatigue, metabolism, mouth sores, thyroid gland, weight gain.

Sulfur: antioxidant, disinfect our blood, bacteria resistant, proper bile secretion.

Zinc: For the immune system, prostate glands, reproductive organs and skin.

L-Lysine: bone development, cold sores, concentration, building block for proteins, hair loss and herpes.

L-Tyrosine: anxiety, dehydration, digestion: fats and vitamins, epilepsy, hyperactive, hypertension, nervous system, seizers,

L-Tyrosine: depression, metabolism, nervous system, thyroid gland, pituitary gland, restless legs, weight control.

Beef

BEEF

Vitamins: B5 (pantothenic acid), B6 (Pyridoxine), Folate

Minerals: iron, phosphorous, selenium, zinc

Other: L-lysine, L-taurine, L-tyrosine

Benefits:
- antibacterial, anti-inflammatory, antioxidant.
- Other benefits: adrenal glands, anxiety, arthritis, bone growth, brain support, exhaustion, immune system, liver, metabolism, nerves (support), immune system.

BEEF: CALF LIVER

Vitamins: A, Biotin, E

Minerals: calcium, chromium, iron, zinc

Benefits:
- antibacterial, anti-cancer.

- Adrenal glands, blood cleanse, blood clotting, bone support, endocrine system, energy, eyes (night vision), infections (bacterial), heart (cardiovascular), immune system, kidney, liver, menstruation (depression) and hormone, skin care, teeth.

BEEF: KIDNEY

Vitamins: B1 (thiamin), B5 (pantothenic acid), B12, biotin, PABA, E

Minerals: iron, selenium

Benefits:
- anti-inflammatory

- Other benefits: adrenals, anemia, arthritis, blood circulation, brain support, eyes, exhaustion, hair, memory, menstruation (depression) and hormones, mental well-being, metabolism.

A note of interest or something to think about

The liver is what helps to cleanse our body of all the toxins. What if the cattle had been fed hormones or other chemicals? Would not the liver be full of this? Even though there are many nutrients in the liver, how much of it would be effective if it loaded with toxins. My gut instinct would tell me, if I needed to eat the liver for the iron, I would only eat the liver from organically raised cattle.

BEEF: LIVER

Vitamins: A, B1 (thiamin), B3 (niacin), B5 (pantothenic acid), B12, biotin, choline, folate, D, E, K, P

Minerals: calcium, chromium, iron, molybdenum, phosphorous, zinc

Benefits:
- anti-aging, relaxant

- Other benefits: adrenal glands, anemia, anxiety, appetite: to stimulate, blood: circulation, blood: support, bone: growth, bone: support, brain: support, depression, eye, fetus growth, heart: cardiovascular, memory, nerves: support, skin: care, teeth, thyroid.

Lake, Ocean, River, Sea

CLAMS

Vitamins: B3 (niacin), B12, E

Minerals: iron, magnesium, selenium, zinc

Other: protein

Benefits:
- Anti-inflammatory.

- Other benefits: anemia, anxiety, arthritis, blood circulation, blood (red blood cells), heart (cardiovascular), heart support, nerves, skin care.

FISH: FRESH WATER

Vitamins: A, B1 (thiamin), B2 (riboflavin), B3 (niacin), B5 (pantothenic acid), B6 (pyridoxine), B12, choline, E,

Minerals: potassium, sulfur, zinc

Other: L-lysine, L-taurine, L-tyrosine, omega-3

Benefits:
- antioxidant.

- Other benefits: adrenal glands, anemia, brain support, depression, heart (cardiovascular system), immune system, memory, nerves (support), skin care.

FISH: OILS

Vitamins: A, B2 (riboflavin), D

Other: omega-3, omega-6

Benefits:
- antioxidant.

- Other benefits: adrenal glands, blood circulation, bone support, brain, eyes, heart (cardiovascular), metabolism, nerves (support), teeth: growth.

FISH: SALTWATER

Vitamins: B1 (thiamin), B2 (riboflavin), B3 (niacin), B5 (pantothenic acid), B6 (pyridoxine), B12, biotin, E

Minerals: iodine, potassium, sulfur, zinc

Other: L-lysine, L-taurine, L-tyrosine

Benefits:
- antidepressant, anti-inflammatory

- Other benefits: anxiety, blood support, brain, depression, immune system, memory, mental health, nerves (support).

HALIBUT

Vitamins: B1 (thiamin), B2 (riboflavin), B3 (niacin), B5 (pantothenic acid), B6 (pyridoxine), B12, biotin, D

Minerals: iodine, potassium, sulfur, zinc

Other: L-lysine, L-taurine, L-tyrosine

Benefits:
- antidepressant, anti-inflammatory

- Other benefits: anxiety, blood support, brain, depression, heart (cardiovascular support), immune system, memory, mental health, muscle inflammation, nerves: support, pituitary gland, skin care.

HERRING

Vitamins: B1 (thiamin), B2 (riboflavin), B3 (niacin), B5 (pantothenic Acid), B6 (pyridoxine), B12, biotin, D

Minerals: iodine, potassium, sulfur, zinc

Other: L-lysine, L-taurine, L-tyrosine, omega-3

Benefits:
- antidepressant, anti-inflammatory

- Other benefits: anxiety, blood support, bone support, brain, depression, heart (cardiovascular support), eyes, immune system, memory, mental health, muscle inflammation, muscle support, nerves, pituitary gland, skin: care, thyroid support.

MACKEREL

Vitamins: B1 (thiamin), B2 (riboflavin), B3 (niacin), B5 (pantothenic acid), B6 (pyridoxine), B12, biotin, D, CoQ10

Minerals: iodine, potassium, sulfur, zinc

Other: L-lysine, L-taurine, L-tyrosine

Benefits:
- antidepressant, anti-inflammatory

- Other benefits: anxiety, blood support, brain, depression, heart (cardiovascular support), immune system, memory, mental health, muscle support, nerves (calming), pituitary gland, skin care.

SALMON

Vitamins: A, B1 (thiamin), B2 (riboflavin), B3 (niacin), B5 (pantothenic acid), B6 (pyridoxine), B12, folate, D, CoQ10

Minerals: calcium, copper, magnesium, phosphorous, selenium, sulfur, zinc

Other: L-lysine, L-taurine, L-tyrosine, omega-3

Benefits:
- antidepressant, anti-inflammatory, antioxidant

- Other benefits: anxiety, blood support, brain, depression, heart (cardiovascular support), immune system, liver, memory, mental health, muscle support, nerves, pituitary gland, skin care.

SARDINES

Vitamins: B1 (thiamin), B2 (riboflavin), B3 (niacin), B5 (pantothenic Acid), B6 (pyridoxine), B12, biotin, D, CoQ10

Minerals: calcium, iodine, sulfur, zinc

Other: L-lysine, L-taurine, L-tyrosine, omega-3

Benefits:
- antidepressant, anti-inflammatory

- Other benefits: anxiety, blood support, brain, depression, heart (cardiovascular support), immune system, memory, mental health, muscle support, nerves (support), pituitary gland, skin care.

TUNA

Vitamins: A, B1 (thiamin), B2 (riboflavin), B3 (niacin), B5 (pantothenic Acid), B6 (pyridoxine), B12, folate, D

Minerals: iodine, potassium, selenium, sulfur, zinc

Other: L-lysine, L-taurine, L-tyrosine, omega-3

Benefits:
- antidepressant, anti-inflammatory, antioxidant

- Other benefits: anxiety, blood support, brain, depression, heart: cardiovascular support, immune system, liver: support, memory, mental health, muscle: support, nerves: support, pituitary gland, skin: care.

Lamb

LAMB

Vitamins: B3 (niacin), B12, folate

Minerals: phosphorous, selenium, zinc

Other: omega-3, protein

Benefits:
- antioxidant

- Other benefits: anemia, anxiety, arthritis, asthma, blood clotting, blood support, cholesterol, depression, fetus development, heart support, kidney support, lung, mental health, prostate cancer prevention, skin care, teeth.

Pork

PORK

Vitamins: B1 (thiamin), B3 (niacin), B5 (pantothenic acid), B6 (pyridoxine), B12, folate

Minerals: iron, phosphorus, selenium, zinc

Other: omega-3, omega-6, protein, L-taurine

Benefits:
- antioxidant

- Other Benefits: adrenal glands, anemia, anxiety, blood circulation, blood cleanser, bone development, brain, depression, eye, fetus development, heart (cardiovascular), hypertension, hypoglycemia, immune system, insomnia, kidney support, liver, memory, metabolism - stimulate (fat and protein), nerves, teeth, thyroid.

Poultry

CHICKEN

Vitamins: B1 (thiamin), B2 (riboflavin), B6 (pyridoxine)

Minerals: iron, magnesium, potassium, selenium

Benefits:
- anti-inflammatory, antioxidant

- Other benefits: adrenal glands, arthritis, blood circulation, depression, eye, metabolism, muscle inflammation, nerves (support), thyroid.

EGG

Vitamins: A, B1 (thiamin), B2 (riboflavin), B3 (niacin), B5 (pantothenic acid), B6 (pyridoxine), B12, D, E

Minerals: calcium, chromium, iron, magnesium, phosphorous, sulfur

Other: L-lysine, L-taurine, L-tyrosine

Benefits:
- antibacterial, antidepressant, anti-inflammatory, antioxidant

- Other benefits: adrenal glands, arthritis, blood circulation, blood support, brain, depression, eyes, heart (cardiovascular), heart support, infections (bacterial), kidney support, memory, metabolism, muscles (inflammation), muscle support, nerves (support), skin care, teeth, thyroid.

EGG YOLK

Vitamins: B1 (thiamin), B2 (riboflavin), biotin, choline, K, P

Minerals: manganese, zinc

Other: L-lysine, L-taurine, L-tyrosine

Benefits:
- antidepressant

- Other benefits: blood circulation, brain support, depression, eyes, fatigue, metabolism, skin care, thyroid.

TURKEY

Vitamins: B1 (thiamin), B2 (riboflavin), B5 (pantothenic acid), B6 (pyridoxine), choline

Minerals: calcium, iron, magnesium, phosphorous, potassium, selenium, sodium, zinc

Other: omega-3, omega-6, protein

Benefits:
- antidepressant, relaxant

- Other benefits: blood support, bone support, brain, depression, eye, heart (cardiovascular), memory, muscle cramp, nerves, relaxant, skin.

CHAPTER 12

Nuts, Oils & Seeds

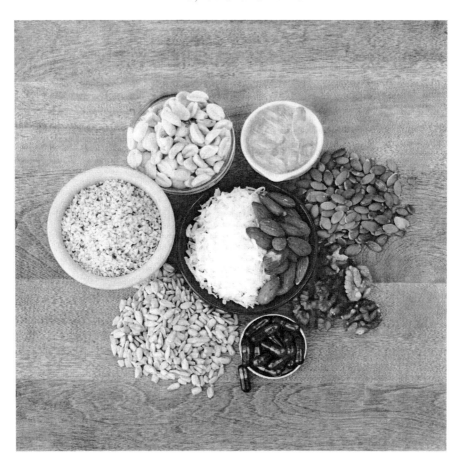

I AM LOVING BEING ABLE TO PUT THIS INFORMATION TOGETHER AND SEE WHERE I HAVE gone wrong with the combination of my foods as I learn how to maximize the nutrients. As I reviewed the nutrients of nuts and seeds, previous information was coming back to me from my data bank within, and I knew I had to reread the information on proteins.

As I had started with almonds, I noticed that the protein for the nuts and seeds was missing. I eat both of them almost on a daily basis, as I am not a big meat eater and require the additional protein. With the way that the meats are being filled with hormones and antibiotics, the meat is not as healthy, and many are finding alternatives for the proteins that we can find in our plant-based foods.

With more research, I found that we have complete protein when we combine the following:

Beans with brown rice, corn, nuts, seeds or wheat.

Brown rice with beans, nuts, seeds or wheat.

With this, we can put together amazing salads and dishes that can cover many of our daily requirements.

It is suggested that we consume nuts and seeds raw as they hold more of the nutrients, especially with boron and omega-6 oil.

THE NUTS HAVE A LOT OF FOLATE AND C:

Folate: For our arteries, bone marrow, brain, DNA, energy production, fingernails, hair, immune system, metabolism, red blood cells, RNA and white blood cells.

C: allergies, enzyme activation, heart, fatigue, immune system, iron absorption, mental illness, stress, skin (wounds).

NUTS AND THE SEEDS HAVE A LOT OF THE FOLLOWING NUTRIENTS:

B1: abdomen, antibodies, appetite, blood circulation, brain, chest pain, depression, eye health, fatigue, memory, nerve impulses.

B2: adrenal glands, birth defects (preventative), blood, eyes, detox, growth, metabolism, nerves, respiratory, skin, thyroid, weight loss

B3: anxiety, arthritis, blood, blood circulation, cholesterol (lower), depression, diarrhea, fatigue, headaches, heart disease, insomnia, liver, mental illness, nerves, respiration

B5: For our adrenal hormones, anti-stress, immune system, metabolism of carbs, fats and proteins and for our neurotransmitters.

B6: amino acids (better absorption), arthritis (reliefs pain), brain support, burning sensations, convulsions, immune system, leg cramps, liver support, nerves.

Boron: Used for our bones, brain function and mental alertness. Boron helps the body to metabolize calcium, phosphorus and magnesium. It also helps to derive energy from the fats and sugar.

Calcium: Anti-cancer, blood clotting, blood pressure (lower), bones (growth), cholesterol (lowers it), DNA, gums, heart, heartbeat, muscle growth, RNA, and teeth.

Copper: formation of the blood cells, energy, hair, immune support, joints, skin and nerves.

Iron: Good for blood (red cells), energy and our immune system.

Magnesium: Good for bowels, energy production, heart, insomnia (better sleep), kidneys, muscles and nerves.

Manganese: For blood sugar regulation, bone growth, cartilage, joints, immune system, metabolism (protein and fats) and for our nerves (calming).

Phosphorus: For the blood (to help clot), bone formation, heart, kidneys, teeth formation. Helps our body process food so that we utilize the vitamins.

Potassium: For our heart, muscles and nervous system.

Selenium: antioxidant, cancer prevention, fetus development

NUT, OILS AND SEEDS HAVE:

E: This is good for cardiovascular disorders, endocrine glands, fatty acid protection, healthy heart, immune system, nervous system, PMS and healing the skin.

Omega-3: This oil is essential for our brain function. Omega-3 lso plays a huge role in fighting cardiovascular diseases.

Omega-6: Fatty Acid (Linoleic acid) is best combined with the omega-3 fatty acid.

Protein: Proteins contain the following: amino acids, carbon, hydrogen, nitrogen, oxygen, and sometimes phosphorus and sulfur. Proteins help to form the structure of most of our organs. These proteins contribute to making the enzymes and hormones that our body needs to function.

Nuts

WE WILL BE COVERING THE FOLLOWING:

almond, Brazil nut, cashew, coconut, hazelnut, macadamia, pecan, pine nut, pistachio and walnut.

ALMOND

Almonds are known for their high content of vitamin E, calcium and magnesium. Almond milk is used as a substitute for dairy milk. This nut is gluten free.

Benefits:
- antioxidant

- Other benefits: blood (circulation), blood cholesterol (lower), blood (support), cancer prevention, celiac disease, colon support, heart support, liver.

Contains:
Vitamins: B1 (thiamin), B2 (riboflavin), B3 (niacin), B5 (pantothenic acid), folate, E

Minerals: boron, calcium, copper, iron, magnesium, phosphorous, potassium, zinc

Other: L-tyrosine, omega-6, omega-9, protein

BRAZIL NUT

The Brazil nut is high in B1, E, copper, magnesium, manganese, phosphorus and selenium. This nut is gluten free.

Benefits:
- antioxidants

- Other benefits: anemia, arteries, blood cholesterol (lower), blood support, cancer prevention, celiac disease, liver, osteoporosis, skin (dry).

Contains:
Vitamins: B1 (thiamin), B2 (riboflavin), B3 (niacin), B5 (pantothenic acid), B6 (pyridoxine), olate, C, E

Minerals: boron, calcium, copper, iron, magnesium, manganese, phosphorous, potassium, selenium, zinc

Other: L-tyrosine, omega-3, omega-6, protein

CASHEW

Cashews are known for their low fat content and high level of protein. This nut is great for good heart health and the cardiovascular system. The cashew is high in copper, phosphorus, magnesium, manganese and zinc.

Benefits:
- anti-inflammatory, antioxidant

- Other benefits: asthma, bone and tendon support, diabetes, energy, gall stone prevention, heart (cardiovascular system), heart support, insomnia, migraines, muscle cramps, muscle spasms, nerve support, skin care.

Contains:
Vitamins: B1 (thiamin), B2 (riboflavin), B3 (niacin), B5 (pantothenic acid), B6 (pyridoxine), B12 (cobalamin), E

Minerals: boron, calcium, copper, iron, magnesium, manganese, phosphorous, potassium, selenium, zinc

Other: omega-6, omega-9, protein

COCONUT

Coconut is high in fibre and magnesium. Coconut is also high in a health fat that helps and supports our body and organs. This fat helps the body to lose the unhealthy fat that has caused weight gain.

Benefits:
- antibacterial, antifungal, antimicrobial, antioxidant, antiviral

- Other benefits: AIDS, blood cholesterol (lower), bone support, candida, digestion, giardia, hair support, heart support, herpes, immune system, influenza, kidney support, liver, pancreas, skin care, skin (dermatitis), skin (eczema), skin (dry), skin (infections), skin (psoriasis), stress, teeth infections, thyroid support, weight reduction, yeast infections.

Contains:
Vitamins: B1 (thiamin), B2 (riboflavin), B3 (niacin), B5 (pantothenic acid), B6 (pyridoxine), folate, E, K

Minerals: boron, calcium, copper, iron, magnesium, manganese, phosphorous, potassium, selenium, sodium, zinc

Other: L-tyrosine, omega-3, omega-6, protein

Filbert See: Hazelnut.

This nut is related to the hazelnut. When looking for information, the web took me to the hazelnut each time.

HAZELNUT

Hazelnut is very like the filbert nut. The hazelnut is high in B1, B6, E, fibre and magnesium. This nut is gluten free.

Benefits:
- antioxidant

- Other benefits: anemia, arteries, blood support, bone support, bowel support, cancer prevention, constipation, fetus development, liver support, skin care.

Contains:
Vitamins: B1 (thiamin), B2 (riboflavin), B3 (Niacin), B5 (pantothenic acid), B6 (pyridoxine), folate, C, E, K

Minerals: boron, calcium, copper, iron, magnesium, manganese, phosphorous, potassium, selenium, zinc

Other: omega-3, omega-6, omega-9, protein

MACADAMIA NUT

The macadamia nut is high in B1, fibre and magnesium. This nut also contains a healthy fat that is good for our heart and blood. This nut has no gluten.

Benefits:
- antioxidant

- Other benefits: blood support, bowel, coronary support, heart support, liver support, stroke prevention.

Contains:
Vitamins: B1 (thiamin), B5 (pantothenic acid), B6 (pyridoxine), C, E

Minerals: boron, calcium, iron, magnesium, manganese, potassium

Other: omega-3, omega-6, protein

PECAN

Pecans are known for their antioxidant properties. Pecans are high in B1, copper, iron, magnesium, manganese, phosphorus and zinc.

Benefits:
- antibacterial, anti-cancer, anti-inflammatory, antioxidant

- Other benefits: arteries, arthritis, blood (cleanser), blood (red blood cell), blood pressure (too high), brain support, cholesterol (lower), diabetes, heart (cardiovascular support), heart support, infections (bacterial), metabolism, osteoporosis, skin care, stress, weight reduction.

Contains:
Vitamins: A, B1 (thiamin), B2 (riboflavin), B3 (niacin), B5 (pantothenic acid), B6 (pyridoxine), folate, C, E

Minerals: boron, calcium, copper, iron, magnesium, manganese, phosphorous, potassium, selenium, zinc

Other: fibre, omega-3, omega-9, protein

PINE NUTS

This nut is gluten free. Pine nuts are high in B1, E, K, copper, magnesium, manganese and phosphorus.

Benefits:
- antioxidant

- Other benefits: appetite (reduce), arteries, blood support, celiac disease, cholesterol (lower), immune system, liver support, skin care, stroke prevention, weight reduction.

Contains:
Vitamins: B1 (thiamin), B2 (riboflavin), B3 (niacin), B5 (pantothenic acid), B6 (pyridoxine), folate, C, E, K

Minerals: calcium, copper, iron, magnesium, manganese, phosphorous, potassium, selenium, zinc

Other: fibre, protein

PISTACHIO

The pistachio is high in B1, B6, copper, magnesium, manganese, phosphorus and potassium.

Benefits:
- anti-cancer, antioxidant

- Other benefits: cancer prevention, cataract prevention, cholesterol (lower), diabetes, energy, eye, heart support, metabolism, sexual stimulant, skin care, weight control, weight reduction.

Contains:
Vitamins: A, B1 (thiamin), B2 (riboflavin), B3 (niacin), B5 (pantothenic acid), B6 (pyridoxine), folate, C, E, K

Minerals: boron, calcium, copper, iron, magnesium, manganese, phosphorous, potassium, selenium, zinc

Other: omega-3, omega-6, fibre, protein

WALNUTS

Walnuts are high in omega-3, copper and manganese. Walnuts also have melatonin that helps with relaxing and better sleep. Walnuts are high in copper, magnesium, manganese and phosphorus.

Benefits:
- anti-cancer, anti-inflammatory, antioxidant

- Other benefits: blood pressure (regulate), blood sugar (regulate), bone support, breast support, cancer prevention, diabetes (type 2), heart (cardiovascular support), insomnia, liver support, memory, nerves, prostate support, sleep, tumour (reduce).

Contains:
Vitamins: B1 (thiamin), B2 (riboflavin), B3 (niacin), B5 (pantothenic acid), B6 (pyridoxine), biotin, folate, C, E, K

Minerals: boron, calcium, copper, iron, magnesium, manganese, molybdenum, selenium, zinc

Other: omega-3, omega-6, protein

Oils

Saturated Fat: It has a solid consistence at room temperature. The American Heart Association suggests 5 – 6% saturated fat daily. Too much saturated fats increase the LDL, which is unhealthy for your heart.

Types of saturated fat: beef, butter, margarine.

Unsaturated fat: This is a liquid at room temperature. This is a much healthier fat than saturated fats. Helps to lower heart disease.

Types of unsaturated fats: avocado, fish (omega-3), nuts, olive oil, plant oil.

Monounsaturated fat is healthy dietary fat. Helps to lower heart disease.

Type of monounsaturated fat: olive oil

Polyunsaturated fat is at a liquid state at room temperature. Another form of unsaturated fat.

Cholesterol has a complex structure and is bound to protein. This is a low density lipoprotein (LDL).

LDL is a low density cholesterol and can create health risks.

HDL is a high density cholesterol that is a good cholesterol.

FATTY ACIDS:

Fatty acids: Helps every cell in our body to build a protective outer layer.

Omega-3 Fatty Acids: Reduces diseases that are causing inflammation.

When we add the healthy oils to our diet, especially with salad, the oil increases our absorption of carotenoid antioxidants.

Note: Cold pressed oils are better to use. There are more nutrients left in the oil with this process. Cooking the oils deletes the benefits of the oils.

Disclaimer: With the following information, the amounts of fats per oil is an estimate. When doing research in books and on the internet the amounts varied, and I tried to find an average rating to provide an idea of what is in each oil for the saturated, monounsaturated and polyunsaturated oils.

WE WILL BE COVERING THE FOLLOWING OILS:

almond oil, coconut oil, cotton seed oil, grapeseed oil, hazelnut oil, hemp seed oil, olive oil, sesame seed oil, Siberian pine nut oil and walnut oil.

ALMOND OIL

Almond oil has the highest vitamin E content. This oil is an unsaturated fatty acid and also a monounsaturated fatty acid that helps with the heart.

Per 1 cup:

Saturated Fat	17.9 g
Monounsaturated Fat	152 g
Polyunsaturated Fat	37.9 g

Benefits:
- antioxidant

- Other benefits: blood: cholesterol (to lower), cancer prevention, cardiovascular disease, colon support, coronary heart disease, diabetes (type 2), digestion, ear infections, heart support, laxative, pancreas support, rectal, rectal prolapse (children), skin care, skin (dry), skin (eczema), weight loss.

Contains:
Vitamins: choline, E, K

Other: omega-3, omega-6, protein

AVOCADO OIL

Even though avocado is a fruit, the oil needs to be mentioned here. About 70% of the avocado is a monounsaturated omega-9 fatty acid. Avocado is also high in lutein that is good for the eyes.

Per 1 cup:

Saturated Fat	25.2 g
Monounsaturated Fat	154 g
Polyunsaturated Fat	29.4 g

Benefits:
- anti-inflammatory, antioxidants

- Other benefits: arthritis, blood cholesterol (lower), bone and cartilage support, cataracts, cholesterol (lower), cataracts, diabetes (type 2), eye, gum disease, hair, heart support, macular degeneration, osteoarthritis, psoriasis, skin care, skin (psoriasis), skin (wound)

Contains:
Vitamins: E

Other: omega-3, omega-6, omega-9

COCONUT OIL

Coconut oil is an amazing additive to your food and has many health benefits. Again, make sure the oil is cold pressed and a virgin oil (no chemicals or high heat used).

Per 1 cup:

Saturated Fat	189 g
Monounsaturated Fat	12.6 g
Polyunsaturated Fat	3.9 g

Benefits:
- antibacterial, antioxidant

- Other benefits: Alzheimer's, blood (lower LDL), cholesterol (lower), candida, cardiovascular diseases, colon support, diabetes 2, heart (cardiovascular support), hair, immune system, skin care, skin (dry), weight reduction.

Contains:
Vitamins: E, K

Minerals: iron

Other: omega-6

COTTON SEED OIL

This oil is low in monounsaturated fats. If used in smaller quantities the oil can have a bit of a benefit. The cottonseed oil does have a good polyunsaturated fat.

Per 1 cup:

Saturated Fat	56.5 g
Monounsaturated Fat	38.8 g
Polyunsaturated Fat	113 g

Benefits:
- Other benefits: blood: HDL, LDL Regulate

Contains:
Vitamins: E

Minerals: magnesium

Other: omega-3, omega-6, protein

GRAPESEED OIL

If too much grapeseed oil is used, it can cause health problems like weight gain and inflammation. Grapeseed oil is safer to bring to the higher temperatures compared to olive oil.

Per 1 cup:

Saturated Fat	20.9 g
Monounsaturated Fat	35.1 g
Polyunsaturated Fat	152 g

Benefits:
- anti-inflammatory, antioxidant

- Other benefits: arthritis, blood cholesterol (lower), brain, cancer prevention, hair, heart (cardiovascular), heart support, inflammation, menstruation (hormones), skin care

Contains:
Vitamins: E

Other: omega-3, omega-6

HAZELNUT OIL

Higher concentration of monounsaturated fats.

Per 1 cup:

Saturated Fat	16.1 g
Monounsaturated Fat	170 g
Polyunsaturated Fat	22.2 g

Benefits:
- antibacterial, antioxidants, astringent

- Other benefits: cancer prevention, digestion, earaches, gall stones, hair (all hair on the body), skin (acne), skin care, skin (wounds), skin (wounds infected), snoring (sip before bed helps the throat muscles), UV protection.

Contains:
Vitamins: E

Other: omega-6

HEMP SEED OIL

Hemp oil has the right balance of the omega-3 and -6 fatty acids, which is great for vegetarians.

Per 1 cup:
Saturated Fat	10%
Polyunsaturated Fat	75%

Benefits:
- anti-inflammatory, antioxidant

- Other benefits: aging, arteries, blood clots (reduce), blood sugar (regulate), cholesterol (lower), hair (good in a conditioner), heart (cardiovascular), immune system, intestines (support), menstruation (hormone), metabolism, nerve support, skin care, skin (dry), skin (psoriasis), varicose veins.

Contains:
Vitamins: E

Other: omega-3, omega-6

OLIVE OIL

Olive oil is high in calories but very rich with the monounsaturated fatty acids. Extra virgin olive oil has the highest grade of olive oil, and it is cold pressed with very little heat used to extract the oils.

Per 1 cup:
Saturated Fat	30 g
Monounsaturated Fat	158 g
Polyunsaturated Fat	23 g

Benefits:
- anti-inflammatory, antioxidant

- Other benefits: blood (HDL, LDL), breast support, depression, DNA protection, heart (cardiovascular support), heart support, hypertension, inflammation, metabolism, stroke prevention, tumour (reduce)

Contains:
Vitamins: choline, E, K

Minerals: iron

Other: omega-3, omega-6

SESAME SEED OIL

Per 1 cup:
Saturated Fat	31 g
Monounsaturated Fat	86 g
Polyunsaturated Fat	90 g

Benefits:
- anti-inflammatory, antioxidants

- Other benefits: Alzheimer's disease, arteries, blood (decrease LDL), blood (increase HDL), bone support, brain, cancer prevention, coronary artery disease, coronary support, diabetes, heart (cardiovascular support), heart support, inflammation, nerve support, skin care

Contains:
Vitamins: E, K

Minerals: calcium, iron, magnesium, potassium

Other: omega-3, omega-6, protein

SIBERIAN PINE NUT OIL

The Siberian pine nut oil is a powerful healer and is used for so many ailments.

Per 1 cup:
Saturated Fat	30 g
Monounsaturated Fat	158 g
Polyunsaturated Fa	23 g

Benefits:
- antibacterial, antioxidant

- Other benefits: appetite suppressant, artery support, blood cholesterol (lower LDL), dandruff, gastritis, hair loss, hemorrhoids, immune system, influenza, lactation, liver, nervous system, pancreas support, respiratory system, skin (scars), skin (wounds), stomach (gas), tonsillitis, ulcer, weight reduction,

Contains:
Vitamins: A, E, K, P

WALNUT OIL

Walnut oil should be stored in the fridge and used within the year to maintain the benefits.

Per 1 cup

Saturated Fat	19 g
Monounsaturated Fat	49 g
Polyunsaturated Fat	138 g

Benefits:
- anti-cancer, anti-inflammatory, antioxidant

- Other benefits: blood clots (reduce), brain (memory), brain support, cancer fighting, heart (cardiovascular support), heart support, inflammation, nerves.

Contains:
Vitamins: B1 (thiamin), B2 (riboflavin), B3 (niacin), E

Minerals: magnesium, phosphorous, selenium, zinc

Other: omega-3

Seeds

WE WILL BE COVERING THE FOLLOWING:

Seeds: chia seed, cacao, flaxseed, hemp seed, mustard seed, pumpkin seed, sesame seed and sunflower seed.

CHIA SEED

Chia seeds are native to South America and have been a staple in Mayan and Aztec diets for centuries. Chia seeds are high in antioxidants, omega-3, -6, -9 fatty acids and fibre. Chia seeds are gluten free and assist with lowering the cholesterol level and regulating the blood sugar levels.

Benefits:
- antioxidant

- Other benefits: adrenal glands, appetite suppressant, blood support, blood sugar (regulate), bowel, cholesterol (lower), energy, glandular support, heart support, intestine support, metabolism, muscle support, skin care, thyroid, weight loss

Contains:
Vitamins: B1 (thiamin), B2 (riboflavin), B3 (niacin), D, E

Minerals: boron, calcium, copper, iron, magnesium, manganese, phosphorous, potassium, zinc

Other: omega-3, omega-6, omega-9, protein

CACAO

Cacao is known for its powerful antioxidant actions. Raw cacao has four times the antioxidants than that of regular dark chocolate. Cacao is not only healthy, but it brings a nice flavour to our food.

Benefits:
- anti-cancer, anti-inflammatory, antioxidant

- Other benefits: blood cleanser, blood pressure (lower), brain (to stay alert and focused), cancer fighting, cholesterol (lower LDL levels), depression, heart (cardiovascular support), heart support, immune system, liver support, organ support.

Contains:
Vitamins: B1 (thiamin), B2 (riboflavin), B6 (pyridoxine), E

Minerals: calcium, iron, magnesium, potassium, sodium, sulfur

Other: omega-6, protein

FLAX SEED

Flaxseeds are high in fibre and the magnesium in the oil from the flaxseed is good for the bowels. This seed is gluten free.

Benefits:
- anti-cancer, anti-inflammatory

- Other benefits: blood sugar (regulate), bowel, cancer prevention, candida, cholesterol (lower), constipation, Crohn's Disease, digestion, cancer prevention, colon cleanser, colon support, estrogen, hair, menstruation (hormones), osteoporosis, rosacea, skin (acne), skin care (estrogen), skin (dry), skin (eczema), weight loss.

Contains:
Vitamins: B1 (thiamin), B6 (pyridoxine), C, E

Minerals: boron, calcium, copper, iron, magnesium, manganese, phosphorous, potassium, selenium, sodium, zinc

Other: fibre, omega-3, omega-6, protein

HEMP SEED

Hemp has been around for a long time. Years ago, when the province of Alberta was just starting up, hemp was grown for its oil and seeds.

Benefits:
- anti-cancer, anti-inflammatory, antioxidant

- Other benefits: ADHD, arthritis, asthma, blood pressure (lower), breast support, cancer fighting, diabetes (blood sugar regulator), digestion, heart (disease), heart (support), menstruation (hormones), MS, muscle support, rheumatoid arthritis, skin care, skin diseases, skin inflammation, weight loss.

Contains:
Vitamins: A, B1 (thiamin), B2 (riboflavin), B6 (pyridoxine), C, D, E

Minerals: iron, magnesium, phosphorous, zinc

Other: fibre, omega-3, omega-6, omega-9, protein

MUSTARD SEED

There are four types of mustard seeds: black, brown, yellow and white. The black seeds have a stronger taste. The yellow seed is mild.

Benefits:
- anti-cancer, anti-inflammatory

- Other benefits: arthritis, asthma, blood pressure (lower), gastrointestinal tract, heart disease, menopause, migraine, rheumatoid arthritis, sleep.

Contains:
Vitamins: B1 (thiamin), B3 (niacin), B6 (pyridoxine), folate, C, E, K

Minerals: calcium, copper, iron, magnesium, manganese, phosphorous, potassium, selenium, zinc

Other: fibre, omega-3, omega-6, protein

PUMPKIN SEED

Pumpkin seeds are known for their ability to paralyze worms and parasites in the intestine. This seed is found in some of the colon cleanse products. Pumpkin seeds are high in manganese, phosphorus, magnesium and copper. The unshelled pumpkin seeds contain more zinc.

Benefits:
- antifungal, antimicrobial, antioxidant, anti-parasitic, antiviral

- Other benefits: blood cleanser, cancer prevention, colon, diabetes, infections (viral), intestine (cleanse), liver: cleanse and support, parasites, prostate support, skin care, worms

Contains:
Vitamins: A

Minerals: calcium, copper, iron, magnesium, manganese, phosphorous, potassium, zinc

Other: L-tyrosine, omega-3, omega-6, protein

SESAME SEED

Sesame seeds are high in copper, manganese, calcium, magnesium and phosphorus. Sesame seeds have more calcium in them when they are not hulled.

Benefits:
- anti-inflammatory, antioxidant

- Other benefits: arthritis, asthma, blood (cholesterol), blood support, blood pressure (too high), bone support, cholesterol (lower), colon support, diabetes, liver, lungs, menopause, menstruation (cramping), migraines, osteoporosis, rheumatoid arthritis, sleep, stroke prevention

Contains:
Vitamins: B1 (thiamin), B6 (pyridoxine)

Minerals: boron, calcium, copper, iodine, iron, magnesium, manganese, molybdenum, phosphorous, selenium, zinc

Other: L-tyrosine, fibre, omega-6, protein

SUNFLOWER SEED

Sunflower seeds are high in E, copper, B1, manganese, selenium, and phosphorus. They are known as an polyunsaturated oil.

Benefits:
- anti-inflammatory, antioxidant

- Other benefits: arteries, asthma, blood cholesterol (lower), blood support, brain, cardiovascular disease, cholesterol (lower), colon support, depression, diabetes prevention, heart (cardiovascular support), hot flashes, immune system, menopause, muscle support, nerves (calming), osteoarthritis, rheumatoid arthritis.

Contains:
Vitamins: A, B1 (thiamin), B2 (riboflavin), B3 (niacin), B5 (pantothenic acid), B6 (pyridoxine), folate, C, E

Minerals: boron, calcium, copper, iron, magnesium, manganese, phosphorous, potassium, selenium, silicon, zinc

Other: omega-3, omega-6, protein

CHAPTER 13

Vegetables

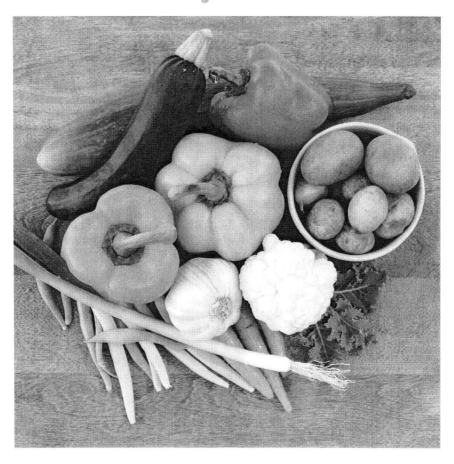

OF ALL THE FOOD GROUPS, VEGETABLES ARE MY FAVOURITE. THEY HAVE SO MANY DIFferent tastes and sensations, and there are so many ways of preparing vegetables for the platter. The energy from the veggies along with the herbs that I add provides a meal that feels good in the belly, does not leave one feeling lethargic and provides the body with the nourishment that can last for hours.

While doing research for on vegetables, I noticed that they also have good proteins with the vitamins and minerals that we need for our bones. The folate in the vegetables is essential for pregnant mothers to provide proper development for the unborn child. What was even more surprising was finding out that there is vitamin c in vegetables, especially when you grow up only thinking of it being in the fruit.

FOLLOWING ARE THE MOST COMMON MINERALS AND VITAMINS IN THE VEGETABLES:

A: Adrenal glands, anemia, infections, bone growth, eyes (night vision), teeth growth.

B1: Abdomen, antibodies, appetite, blood circulation, brain, chest pain, depression, eye health, fatigue, memory, nerve impulses.

B2: Adrenal glands, birth defects (preventative), blood, eyes, detox, growth, metabolism, nerves, respiratory, skin, thyroid, weight loss.

B3: Anxiety, arthritis, blood, blood circulation, cholesterol (lower), depression, diarrhea, fatigue, headaches, heart disease, insomnia, liver, mental illness, nerves, respiration.

B5: For our adrenal hormones, anti-stress, immune system, metabolism of carbs, fats and proteins and for our neurotransmitters.

B6: Amino acids (better absorption), arthritis (relieves pain), brain support, burning sensations, convulsions, immune system, leg cramps, liver support, nerves.

Folate: For our arteries, bone marrow, brain, DNA, energy production, fingernails, hair, immune system, metabolism, red blood cells, RNA and white blood cells.

C: Allergies, enzyme activation, heart, fatigue, immune system, iron absorption, mental illness, stress, skin (wounds).

E: This is good for cardiovascular disorders, endocrine glands, fatty acid protection, healthy heart, immune system, nervous system, PMS and healing the skin.

K: Blood clotting.

Calcium: Anti-cancer, blood clotting, blood pressure (lower), bones (growth), cholesterol (lowers it), DNA, gums, heart, heartbeat, muscle growth, RNA, and teeth.

Iron: Good for blood (red cells), energy and our immune system.

Magnesium: Good for bowels, energy production, heart, insomnia (better sleep), kidneys, muscles and nerves.

Phosphorus: For the blood (to help clot), bone formation, heart, kidneys, teeth formation. Helps our body process food so that we utilize the vitamins.

Potassium: For our heart, muscles and nervous system.

Sodium: Blood pressure, kidney, liver, muscle contraction, nerve transmission, PH levels.

Zinc: For the immune system, prostate glands, reproductive organs and skin.

FOLLOWING ARE THE VEGETABLES THAT WE ARE COVERING IN THIS CHAPTER:

Artichoke - Asparagus

Bean (Lima) - Bean (Snap) - Beet - Beet Green – Broccoli - Brussel sprout

Cabbage – Carrot – Cauliflower – Celery – Collard – Corn -Cucumber

Dulse

Garlic

Kale – Kelp - Kohlrabi

Lettuce (iceberg and romaine)

Mushroom - Mustard Green

Onion (Green and Red)

Parsnip – Peas - Pepper (bell) – Potato - Pumpkin

Radish - Rutabaga

Spinach – Squash - Sweet Potato - Swiss chard

Turnip and Turnip Greens

ARTICHOKE

- Artichoke has more antioxidant properties than cranberries and is low in calories.

Benefits:
- anti-cancer, antioxidants

- Other benefits: blood cholesterol (lowers), bone health, brain support (cognitive), digestive support, fetus growth (needed by pregnant mothers), liver support.

Contains:
Vitamins: B1 (thiamin), B2 (riboflavin), B3 (niacin), B6 (pyridoxine), folate, C, K

Minerals: calcium, copper, iron, magnesium, manganese, phosphorous, potassium, sodium, zinc

Other: fibre, protein

ASPARAGUS

- Asparagus is known for its antioxidant properties.

Benefits:
- anti-inflammatory, antioxidant

- Other benefits: blood pressure (regulate), blood sugar (to regulate), pancreas support, tumours (prevention)

Contains:
Vitamins: A, B1 (thiamin), B2 (riboflavin), B3 (niacin), B5 (pantothenic acid), B6 (pyridoxine), choline, folate, C, E, K

Minerals: calcium, copper, iron, magnesium, manganese, phosphorous, potassium, selenium, zinc

Other: fibre, omega-3, protein

BEAN (LIMA)

- The molybdenum in the lima bean helps to detox the sulfites in our body.

Benefits:
- anti-cancer, antidepressant

- Other benefits: blood sugar (stabilize), bowel support, energy from the iron, heart support (reduces risk of heart attack), pancreas health.

Contains:
Vitamins: B1 (thiamin), B2 (riboflavin), B3 (niacin), B5 (pantothenic acid), B6 (pyridoxine), B12, folate, C, E, K

Minerals: calcium, copper, iron, magnesium, molybdenum, phosphorous, potassium, sodium, zinc

Other: fibre, protein

BEAN (SNAP)

- Green or yellow snap beans are low in calories and contain healthy amounts of calcium, vitamin C, beta-carotene, vitamin K and Lutein.

Benefits:
- antidepressant, anti-diabetic

- Blood: lowers blood pressure, blood sugar (regulates), bone and tissue support (silicon), diabetes (decreases the risk), heart support.

Contains:
Vitamins: B1 (thiamin), B2 (riboflavin), B3 (niacin), B5 (pantothenic acid), B6 (pyridoxine), B12, choline, folate, C, E, K

Minerals: calcium, chromium, copper, iron, magnesium, manganese, molybdenum, phosphorous, potassium, zinc

Other: fibre, omega-3, protein

BEET

- Beets are used for their detoxifying properties and for cleansing of the liver. Beets are a source of folate, which is necessary for proper development of the unborn fetus.

Benefits:
- anti-inflammatory, antioxidant, hepatic

- Other benefits: anemia, blood cleanser, fetus development, heart (cardiovascular support), liver cleanser.

Contains:
Vitamins: A, B2 (riboflavin), B3 (niacin), B5 (pantothenic acid), B6 (pyridoxine), folate, C

Minerals: calcium, copper, iron, magnesium, phosphorous, potassium, silicon, sodium, zinc

Other: fibre, protein

Served as:
- Best to cook beets as little as you can.

- Served cooked, steamed, raw and processed.

BEET GREEN

- Beets greens contain a large amount of vitamins K and A, along with a large amount of antioxidants beta-carotene and lutein.

Benefits:
- antioxidant, hepatic, nervine

Other benefits: anemia, blood, eyes, liver, nervous system.

Contains:
Vitamins: A, B1 (thiamin), B2 (riboflavin), B3 (niacin), B5 (pantothenic acid), B6 (pyridoxine, folate, C, E, K

Minerals: calcium, copper, iron, magnesium, manganese, phosphorous, potassium, zinc

Other: fibre, protein

Served as:

Steamed or sautéed, can be blanched then frozen for the winter

BROCCOLI

- Broccoli is known for its calcium and vitamin K.

Benefits:
- anti-cancer, anti-inflammatory, antioxidant

- Other benefits: bladder cancer, blood, breast cancer, colon cancer, eye support, heart support, liver support, nerves, ovarian cancer, prostate cancer prevention, stomach (digestion).

Contains:
Vitamins: A, B1 (thiamin), B2 (riboflavin), B3 (niacin), B5 (pantothenic acid), B6 (pyridoxine), choline, folate, C, E, K

Minerals: calcium, chromium, copper, germanium, iron, magnesium, manganese, phosphorous, potassium, selenium, sodium, zinc

Other: fibre, omega-3, protein

Served as:
Can be eaten raw, baked, boiled and stir fried.

Broccoli is best steamed than boiled.

BRUSSEL SPROUT

- Brussel sprouts are high in antioxidant properties, vitamin K and C.

Benefits:
- anti-cancer, anti-inflammatory, antioxidant

- Other benefits arthritis: blood cleanser, blood sugar (to regulate), bowel support, Crohn's disease, heart support, irritable bowel, liver support, prostate cancer, rheumatoid arthritis, stomach (digestion), weight reduction

Contains:
Vitamins: A, B1 (thiamin), B2 (riboflavin), B3 (niacin), B5 (pantothenic acid), B6 (pyridoxine), choline, folate, C, K

Minerals: calcium, copper, iron, magnesium, manganese, phosphorous, potassium, sulfur, zinc

Other: fibre, omega-3, protein

CABBAGE (RED)

- Cabbage is known as a prevention to type 2 diabetes. Red cabbage has more benefits than the green cabbage.

Benefits:
- anti-inflammatory, antioxidant

- Other benefits: blood sugar (to regulate), cancer prevention, heart (cardiovascular support), stomach cleanser, stomach (digestion), stomach (support).

Contains:
Vitamins: A, B1 (thiamin), B2 (riboflavin), B3 (niacin), B5 (pantothenic acid), B6 (pyridoxine), choline, folate, C, E, K

Minerals: calcium, copper, iron, magnesium, phosphorous, potassium, selenium, sodium, sulfur, zinc

Other: fibre, protein

Served as:
Cabbage can be eaten raw in salads, cooked in dishes or soups and pickled.

Cabbage is the main ingredient in sauerkraut. Sauerkraut is known to help support the stomach flora.

CARROT
- Carrots are high in antioxidant properties and beta-carotene. Carrots contain a very large amount of vitamin A, and they also contain falcarinol, which helps to prevent cancer.

Benefits:
- anti-cancer, antioxidant

- Other benefits: cataract reduction and prevention, colon support, eye health, heart (cardiovascular support), optic nerve support, stomach (digestion).

Contains:
Vitamins: A, B1 (thiamin), B2 (riboflavin), B3 (niacin), B5 (pantothenic acid), B6 (pyridoxine), biotin, folate, C, E, K

Minerals: boron, calcium, copper, iron, magnesium, manganese, molybdenum, phosphorus, potassium

Other: fibre, protein

Served as:
Carrots can be eaten raw alone, in salads, used as a garnish, cooked alone or in soups and stews, pickled, added to baking and can be blanched then frozen for the winter. Good keepers in a cold room.

CAULIFLOWER
- Cauliflower forms into a head shape and is white to a yellowish colour.

Benefits:
- anti-inflammatory, antioxidant

- Other benefits: blood cholesterol, heart (cardiovascular), immune system, liver cleanser, organ support, prostate cancer, stomach (digestion), weight regulation.

Contains:
Vitamins: B1 (thiamin), B2 (riboflavin), B3 (niacin), B5 (pantothenic acid), B6 (pyridoxine), choline, folate, C, K

Minerals: iron, magnesium, manganese, phosphorous, potassium, sodium

Other: fibre, protein, omega-3

Served as:
Cauliflower is eaten raw and cooked.

CELERY

- Celery grows upright in stalks.

Benefits:
- anti-inflammatory, antioxidant

Other benefits: blood pressure regulation, blood support, digestive tract support, heart (cardiovascular), muscle relaxant, stomach support, stomach ulcer preventative.

Contains:
Vitamins: A, B2 (riboflavin), B5 (pantothenic acid), B6 (pyridoxine), folate, C, K

Minerals: calcium, copper, germanium, iron, magnesium, manganese, molybdenum, phosphorous, potassium, sodium

Other: fibre

Served as:
Celery is eaten both raw and cooked. This is a good additive to smoothies.

COLLARD

- Collards are long dark leaves. They grow upward like Swiss chard.

Benefits:
- anti-inflammatory, antioxidant

- Other benefits: blood cleanser, blood (cholesterol), cancer preventative, colitis, Crohn's disease, diabetes (type 2), digestive support, heart (cardiovascular support), liver cleanser, muscle (inflammation), rheumatoid arthritis.

Contains:
Vitamins: A, B1 (thiamin), B2 (riboflavin), B5 (pantothenic acid), B6 (pyridoxine), choline, folate, C, E, K

Minerals: calcium, copper, iron, magnesium, manganese, phosphorous, potassium

Other: fibre, protein, omega-3

Served as:
Collards are steamed and used in stews.

CORN
- Eating corn with legumes provides a better absorption of vitamins and minerals.

Benefits:
- antioxidant, hepatic
- Other benefits: blood cleanser, blood sugar stabilizer, colon cancer preventative, heart, immune system, liver support.

Contains:
Vitamins: A, B1 (thiamin), B2 (riboflavin), B3 (niacin), B5 (pantothenic acid), B6 (pyridoxine), folate, E

Minerals: calcium, chromium, copper, iron, magnesium, manganese, phosphorous, potassium, selenium, sodium, zinc

Other: fibre, protein

Served as:
Corn is cooked on the cob and eaten with butter. The corn can be cut off the cob to go into several different dishes, cold, hot and warm.

CUCUMBER
- Cucumber is part of the gourd family. The cucumber appears to be lower in vitamins and minerals compared to the other vegetables, yet still has amazing healing properties.

Benefits:
- anti-cancer, anti-inflammatory, antioxidant
- Benefits: digestion, estrogen balancing, intestinal tract, muscle inflammation, skin care, skin regeneration.

Contains:
Vitamins: A, B1 (thiamin), B5 (pantothenic acid), biotin, choline, C, K

Minerals: calcium, copper, iron, magnesium, manganese, phosphorous

Other: fibre, protein

Served as:
Cucumber is usually served cold. Some varieties of cucumbers are wonderful to pickle as a garnish for meals.

Cucumbers are used in face masks. The estrogen helps to replenish the skin.

DULSE

- Dulse is a red seaweed vegetable. It is high in iron, potassium and protein. Dulse grows in the Northern Hemisphere.

Benefits:
- antioxidant

- Benefits: anemia, blood pressure (lower), blood (circulation), blood support, bone support, brain, digestion, eye (improve vision), heart support, immune system, liver, nervous system, thyroid support.

Contains:
Vitamins: A, B1 (thiamin), B2 (riboflavin), B12, C, E

Minerals: calcium, chromium, iodine, iron, magnesium, potassium, selenium, sodium, zinc

Other: fibre, omega-3

Served as:
Dulse is used as a medicine for the thyroid.

Used as a flavouring for salads and soups.

Caution: Dulse is good if used moderately. If overused the iodine can harm the thyroid.

GARLIC

- Garlic is high in antioxidant properties. It is known as one of the best viral preventative foods.

Benefits:
- antibacterial, anti-cancer, antifungal, anti-inflammatory, antioxidant

- Benefits: blood cleanser, blood sugar regulator, candida, cancer fighting, digestion, endocrine system, heart (cardiovascular), heart (support), immune system, liver support.

Contains:
Vitamins: A, B1 (thiamin), B6 (pyridoxine), Folate, C, K

Minerals: calcium, copper, germanium, iodine, iron, magnesium, manganese, phosphorous, potassium, selenium, sulfur

Other: fibre, omega-3, protein

Served as:
Garlic can be sautéed with olive oil and garlic, added to soups, stews or stir-fries and can be blanched then frozen for the winter.

The young tender leaves of the garlic can be used in a salad.

Garlic is used fresh, dried and in oils.

KALE
- Kale is high in antioxidant properties: vitamin A, C and K. It is also known for its lutein content.

Benefits:
- anti-cancer, anti-inflammatory, antioxidant

- Other benefits: arteries: cleanses of plaque, blood cleanser, cancer fighting, cataract prevention, cholesterol (lower), digestion, heart (cardiovascular support), liver support, pulmonary disease,

Contains:
Vitamins: A, B1 (thiamin), B2 (riboflavin), B3 (niacin), B6 (pyridoxine), folate, C, E, K

Minerals: calcium, copper, iron, magnesium, manganese, phosphorous, potassium, sulfur

Other: fibre, omega-3, protein

Served as:
The young kale leaves are good in salads. Kale can be steamed and used in soups and stews.

KELP
- Kelp is different from dulse, being that they grow in different regions. Kelp is a sea vegetable, brown algae, known for its high content of iodine. Japan harvests a lot of the sea vegetables.

Benefits:
- anti-cancer, anti-coagulant, anti-inflammatory, antioxidant, antiviral

- Other benefits: blood (support), cholesterol (lower), colon cancer prevention, heart (cardiovascular support), herpes simplex (virus 1 and 2), liver support, osteoarthritis, thyroid support

Contains:
Vitamins: A, B1 (thiamin), B2 (riboflavin), B3 (niacin), B5 (pantothenic acid), B6 (pyridoxine), B12, C, E, K, P

Minerals: calcium, copper, iodine, iron, magnesium, manganese, phosphorous, potassium, selenium, sodium, zinc

Other: omega-3, omega-6, protein

Served as:
Kelp is used in a powder form or in its natural form.

KOHLRABI

- Kohlrabi is a wonderful source of vitamins and minerals, especially vitamin C.

Benefits:
- antioxidant

- Other benefits: anemia, blood circulation, blood pressure (regulate), bones (strengthen), cancer prevention, constipation, digestive health, heart, eye health, immune system (to boost), metabolism (regulate), muscle support, nerve function, stomach (bloating), stomach (cramp), weight loss.

Contains:
Vitamins: B1 (thiamin), B2 (riboflavin), B3 (niacin), B5 (pantothenic acid), B6 (pyridoxine), C, E

Minerals: calcium, copper, iron, magnesium, phosphorous, potassium, sodium

Other: fibre, protein

Served as:
Raw with a dip, cooked in soups or stews or blanched then frozen for the winter.

LETTUCE (ICEBERG)

- Green leaf lettuce contains a large amount of vitamins A and K, plus the antioxidants beta-carotene and lutein.

Benefits:
- antioxidant

- Other benefits: blood cleanser, liver support

Contains:
Vitamins: A, B5 (pantothenic acid), B6 (pyridoxine), folate, C, E, K

Minerals: calcium, iron, magnesium, manganese, potassium

Other: fibre, protein

Served as:
Served raw in salads, as a garnish, on sandwiches and in wraps.

LETTUCE (ROMAINE)
- Low in calories and is an excellent source of vitamin A and Lutein.

Benefits:
- anti-inflammatory, antioxidant

- Other benefits: arteries, blood pressure (lower), bone support, cancer preventative, cholesterol (lower), colon support, digestion, eye support, heart support, immune support, pregnancy (folate), skin (acne), skin health, weight loss.

Contains:
Vitamins: A, B1 (thiamin), B2 (riboflavin), B5 (pantothenic acid), B6 (pyridoxine), biotin, folate, C, E, K

Minerals: calcium, chromium, copper, iron, manganese, molybdenum, phosphorous, potassium

Other: fibre, omega-3, omega-6

Served as:
Served raw and in salads, as a garnish and in sandwiches or wraps.

MUSHROOMS (WHITE)
- There are so many varieties of mushrooms, and we could easily do a whole book on them. The common mushroom sold in the grocery stores is the white mushroom.

Benefits:
- anti-inflammatory, antioxidant

- Other benefits: arthritis prevention, blood support, bone support, breast cancer prevention, diabetes prevention, DNA protection, heart (cardiovascular protection), heart support, immune system, prostate cancer prevention.

Contains:
Vitamins: A, B1 (thiamin), B2 (riboflavin), B3 (niacin), B5 (pantothenic acid), B6 (pyridoxine), B12, choline, folate, PABA, C, D

Minerals: chromium, copper, magnesium, manganese, phosphorus, potassium, selenium, zinc

Other: omega-6, protein

Served as:
Mushrooms can be used raw, sauted and using in dishes and sauces.

MUSTARD GREEN

- Mustard greens are known for having a high content of fat soluble antioxidant vitamins and vitamin E and K.

Benefits:
- antioxidant

- Other benefits: atherosclerosis prevention, blood cleanser, blood cell (support), cancer prevention, digestive support, heart (cardiovascular support), intestinal support, liver protection, stomach health.

Contains:
Vitamins: A, B1 (thiamin), B2 (riboflavin), B3 (niacin), B5 (pantothenic acid), B6 (pyridoxine), B12, folate, C, E, K

Minerals: calcium, copper, iron, magnesium, manganese, phosphorous, potassium

Other: fibre, protein

Served as:
Mustard greens can be eaten raw, sauted and stewed.

ONION: GREEN

- Green onions are a tasty onion. The only drawback is that the green onion does not have a long shelf life. The eastern doctors use the white part of the green onion for medicinal purposes.

Benefits:
- antibacterial, antifungal, anti-inflammatory, antiviral, expectorant

- Other benefits: allergies, appetite (increase), arthritis prevention, asthma, blood circulation, blood sugar control, bone health, chills, cholesterol (lower), colds, colon cancer prevention, diarrhea, DNA protection, eyes, hay fever, headaches, heart, hives, immune system, indigestion, insomnia, respiratory (infection), respiratory tract, sweat glands, throat (sore - used in a compress and/or eaten).

Contains:
Vitamins: A, B1 (thiamin), B2 (riboflavin), B3 (niacin), B5 (pantothenic acid), B6 (pyridoxine), folate, C, E, K

Minerals: calcium, copper, iron, germanium, magnesium, manganese, phosphorous, potassium, selenium, sodium, sulfur, zinc

Other: fibre, protein

Served as:
Green onions are usually eaten raw and in salads.

ONION: RED

- Red onions are source of fibre, vitamin C and vitamin B6, which helps to level the blood pressure. Red onions have a lot of quercetin.

- If you are sick with a cold or flu, a red onion can be cut in half and placed cut side up in the room that you are in. The onion will absorb the virus and clean the air.

Benefits:
- antibiotic, anti-inflammatory, antioxidant

- Other benefits: athlete's feet, bee stings, blood pressure (to regulate), cancer preventative, cholesterol (lowers), constipation, digestion, endocrine system, heart, immune support, infections (bacterial), liver, organ support, red blood support, skin burns.

Contains:
Vitamins: B1 (thiamin), B3 (niacin), B5 (pantothenic acid), B6 (pyridoxine), folate, C, E, K

Minerals: calcium, copper, iron, magnesium, manganese, phosphorous, potassium, selenium, sulfur, zinc

Served as:
Raw in salads, sandwiches, as a garnish, cooked in soups and stews.

PARSNIP

- Parsnips have a high content of vitamins, minerals and fibre. The folate in the parsnips is necessary for the unborn baby to develop properly.

Benefits:
- anti-depression, anti-diabetic

- Other benefits: blood pressure (lowers), cholesterol (lowers), constipation, depression, diabetes, digestive tract, heart support, immune system, metabolism, weight reduction.

Contains:
Vitamins: B1 (thiamin), B3 (niacin), B5 (pantothenic acid), B6 (pyridoxine), folate, C, E, K

Minerals: calcium, copper, iron, magnesium, manganese, phosphorous, potassium, selenium, sodium**,** zincOther: fibre, protein

Served as:
Eaten raw with a dip, shredded and added to salads, cooked in soups and stews.

PEA

- Peas are an excellent source for vitamin A, B complex vitamins, C and lutein.

Benefits:
- anti-inflammatory, antioxidant

- Other benefits: arthritis, blood sugar regulator, diabetes 2, digestive tract, heart (cardiovascular health), heart disease, muscle inflammation, stomach cancer, stomach support.

Contains:
Vitamins: A, B1 (thiamin), B2 (riboflavin), B3 (niacin), B6 (pyridoxine), choline, folate, C, E, K

Minerals: calcium, copper, iron, magnesium, manganese, molybdenum, phosphorous, potassium, zinc

Other: fibre, protein, omega-3

Served as:
Eaten raw in salads or added raw as a last addition to a dish, in stews, soups and can be blanched then frozen for the winter.

PEPPER (BELL)

- Bell peppers can be green, red and yellow in colour. The red and yellow ones are a bit sweeter.

- The green pepper has more of the carotenoids that are good for the eyes.

- The red peppers have more vitamin C, antioxidant and anti-inflammatory benefits.

Benefits:
- anti-cancer, anti-inflammatory, antioxidant

- Other benefits: blood cholesterol (lowers), blood support, cataract prevention, diabetes (regulate), eyes, heart, immune system, liver, muscle cramps, muscle spasm.

Contains:
Vitamins: A, B1 (thiamin), B3 (niacin), B5 (pantothenic acid), B6 (pyridoxine), folate, inositol, PABA, C, E, K,

Minerals: calcium, copper, iron, magnesium, manganese, molybdenum, phosphorous, potassium, zinc

Other: fibre, protein

Served as:
Peppers can be eaten raw or cooked.

POTATO

- When potatoes are cooked and eaten without the unhealthy oils (butter, cheese, sour cream and cooking oils) they can be a very healthy vegetable.

- The russet potatoes have the highest antioxidant properties.

- White potatoes have a higher source of sulfur and can bother sensitive stomachs. The red potato has a lower sulfur content.

Benefits:
- Antioxidants

- Other benefits: athletic endurance, blood pressure (regulate), brain cells, cancer prevention (free radicals), heart health, muscle support, nerve support.

Contains:
Vitamins: A, B1 (thiamin), B3 (niacin), B5 (pantothenic acid), B6 (pyridoxine), folate, C, E, K

Minerals: calcium, copper, iron, magnesium, manganese, phosphorous, potassium, selenium, sodium, zinc

Other: Fibre, L-glutamine, L-lysine, L-tyrosine, protein

Served as:
- Potatoes are best served baked as most of the nutrients are retained. They can be fried, cooked, and used in soups and stews. Keeps well in a cold storage room over the winter months.

- When eating your potato, don't forget to eat the skin, this part has the highest content of potassium. Potatoes are gluten free.

PUMPKIN

- Pumpkins are a large source of beta-carotene, vitamin A and other carotenoids. Carotenoids are powerful antioxidants. - Pumpkin seeds are a source of good polyunsaturated oils and recommended to help avoid prostate cancer.

Benefits:
- antioxidant

- Other benefits: brain (support), cancer prevention, eye vision, immune support, lungs, mouth support (cancer prevention), nerves (calming), nerve support, prostate health.

Contains:
Vitamins: A, B1 (thiamin), B2 (riboflavin), B3 (niacin), B5 (pantothenic acid), B6 (pyridoxine), folate, C, E, K

Minerals: calcium, copper, iron, magnesium, manganese, phosphorous, potassium, selenium, zinc

Other: fibre, protein

Served as:
Seeds: shelled, raw, roasted and used in salads and alone.

The fruit of the pumpkin: baked, roasted, in stews and of course used for jack o' lanterns.

RADISH
- Radishes have a high source of foliate, calcium, potassium and fibre.

Benefits:
- antifungal, antioxidant, diuretic

- Uses: asthma, blood cleanser (free radicals), blood pressure (regulate), bones, bowel, cancer prevention, congestion, heart support, kidney stones, liver support, skin care, skin infections, urinary (support), worms.

Contains:
Vitamins: B2 (riboflavin), B6 (pyridoxine), folate, C

Minerals: calcium, copper, iron, magnesium, manganese, potassium, sodium, vanadium

Other: fibre

Served as:
Radishes are usually served raw in salads.

RUTABAGA
- Rutabagas are an excellent source of vitamin C, folate, fibre and minerals.

Benefits:
- anti-aging, anti-cancer, antioxidant

- Helps with: aging (slows down), blood cleanser (free radicals), blood pressure (too high), bowel support, cholesterol (lower), constipation prevention, digestion, eyesight, heart support, immune system, metabolism, muscle support, skin care, weight control.

Contains:
Vitamins: A, B1 (thiamin), B2 (riboflavin), B3 (niacin), B5 (pantothenic acid), B6 (pyridoxine), B12, folate, C, E, K

Minerals: calcium, copper, iron, magnesium, manganese, phosphorous, potassium, selenium, sodium, zinc

Other: fibre

Served as:
-Raw with a dip, cooked in soups and stews. Can be blanched then frozen for the winter.

SPINACH

Spinach has twice the iron of other greens. It has lots of calcium, folate, manganese, vitamins A and K.

Benefits:
- anti-cancer, anti-inflammatory, antioxidant

- Helps with: anemia, appetite (regulate), blood sugar (regulate), cataract prevention, cholesterol levels (lower), diabetes (type 2), digestion, memory loss prevention.

Contains:
Vitamins: A, B1 (thiamin), B2 (riboflavin), B3 (niacin), B5 (pantothenic acid), B6 (pyridoxine), B12, choline, folate, PABA, C, E, K, CoQ10

Minerals: calcium, copper, iodine, iron, magnesium, manganese, molybdenum, phosphorous, potassium, selenium, sodium, zinc

Other: fibre, L-glutamine, omega-3, protein

Served as:
-Served raw in salads and sandwiches, steamed and can be blanched then frozen for the winter.

SQUASH

- Summer squash, zucchini, crookneck, straight neck and scallop squash. A high source of lutein.

Benefits:
- anti-inflammatory, antioxidant

- Other benefits: asthma prevention, blood: cholesterol (lower), blood pressure (lower), blood protection (free radicals), bone tissue development, diabetes prevention, energy, eyes (sore/ inflamed), eyes (vision), heart health, muscle support, nerves, prostate gland, skin (wounds), teeth.

Contains:
Vitamins: A, B1 (thiamin), B3 (niacin), B5 (pantothenic Acid), B6 (pyridoxine), folate, C, E, K

Minerals: calcium, copper, iodine, iron, magnesium, manganese, phosphorous, potassium, selenium, zinc

Other: omega-3

Served as:
- Raw in salads (zucchini), baked on the Bar-B-Que, baked in the oven, stewed, sautéed and some can be shredded and frozen for the winter. Can be used in baking.
- Summer squash and zucchini have a very thin skin, which can be eaten.
- The flowers of this plant are eaten raw and deep-fried.

SWEET POTATO

- Sweet potatoes are high in A, C, manganese, copper and B6.
- Known as an antioxidant and have a higher source of vitamin A than the other vegetables.

Contains:
- antibacterial, antifungal, anti-inflammatory, antioxidant
- Other benefits: arthritis, asthma, blood cleanser, blood (to regulate clotting), blood sugar (regulate), brain (support), diabetes 2, digestive tract, gout, heavy metal, liver, muscle cramps, muscle spasm, nerve tissue, skin (wounds).

Vitamins: A, B1 (thiamin), B2 (riboflavin), B3 (niacin), B5 (pantothenic acid), B6 (pyridoxine), folate, C, D, E

Minerals: calcium, copper, iron, magnesium, manganese, phosphorous, potassium, selenium, sodium, zinc

Other: fibre, protein

Served as:
- Yams can be eaten raw in a dip, cooked, stewed and steamed.

Note: Make sure it is sweet potato that you are buying. They have a lot more nourishment than yams.

SWISS CHARD

- Swiss chard grows in an upward leaf. This plant can be in a variety of bright colours.

Benefits:
- anti-inflammatory, antioxidant
- Helps with: arthritis, blood cleanser, blood pressure (to lower), blood sugar (regulate), bone health, diabetes (type 2), eyes, muscle inflammation, nervous system, stress, weight.

Contains:
Vitamins: A, B1 (thiamin), B2 (riboflavin), B3 (niacin), B5 (pantothenic acid), B6 (pyridoxine), choline, folate, C, E, K

Minerals: boron, calcium, copper, iodine, iron, magnesium, manganese, molybdenum, phosphorous, potassium, selenium, sodium, zinc

Other: fibre, omega-3, protein

Served as:
Raw in salads (younger leaves), steamed and served with raw toppings. They can be blanched then frozen for the winter. You can pickle the stalks and leaves and use it in relish.

TOMATO: SEE CHAPTER 7: FRUIT

TURNIP & TURNIP GREENS

- Turnips have a high content of vitamin K, A, C, folate and copper.

Benefits:
- anti-inflammatory, antioxidant

- Other benefits: anemia, arthritis, blood cholesterol (lower), blood circulation, blood cleanser, bone health, bone support, cancer prevention, chronic pain, constipation, cramping, diarrhea, digestion, gout, heart, liver support, metabolism, osteoporosis, rheumatoid arthritis, stomach support

Contains:
Vitamins: A, B1 (thiamin), B2 (riboflavin), B3 (niacin), B5 (pantothenic acid), B6 (pyridoxine), B12, choline, folate, C, E, K

Minerals: calcium, copper, iodine (turnip greens), iron (turnip), magnesium (turnip), manganese (turnip), phosphorous, potassium, sodium, sulfur (turnip), zinc

Other: fibre, omega-3, protein

Served as:
Turnip can be served raw with a dip, cooked in soups and stews, deep-fried as chips and can be blanched and frozen.

Caution: For those who have problems with their thyroid, you need to consult a doctor before turnips become a large part of your diet.

ZUCCHINI: SEE SQUASH

Enjoy your vegetables!

Don't like them on their own?

Add herbs, legumes, nuts and seeds.

~~~ So many ways to enjoy one of Mother Earth's amazing food groups. ~~~

CHAPTER 14

Essential Oils

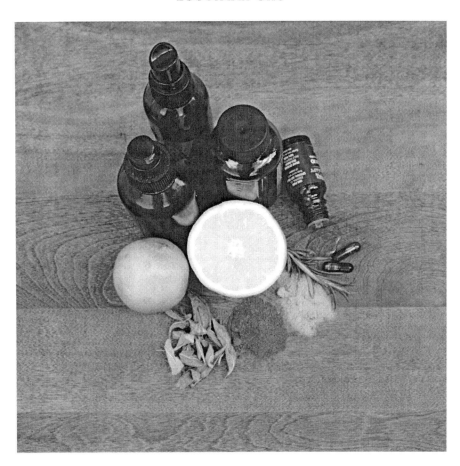

OILS ARE DERIVED FROM THE PLANTS FROM MOTHER EARTH. OILS PROVIDE US WITH many fresh and relaxing scents along with providing several and powerful healing properties. There are now about 100 oils that are known that have antibacterial, antifungal and antiviral components with several more healing properties.

Essential oils have been used since the beginning of time. One of the original uses of the rose oil or rose water was to cover the scent of sweat and dirt. Our grandmothers and great-grandmothers used lavender perfume or soaps and eucalyptus oils for the chest. Oregano oils were used to ward off colds and flus, and calendula oils and balms were for healing wounds. We have many more oils to work with now and many different combinations that we can use on a daily basis.

Essential Oils are extracted from bushes, flowers, plants, roots, shrubs, seeds and the barks of trees. The oil is the resin of the plant, and the resin is considered as the life force of the plant. The resin contains all of the healing properties of the plant, whether it is revitalizing, healing of organs or used as muscle relaxants.

Clean oils should have no toxic chemicals and should not be cut or diluted. The oil should have been extracted from the plant and not mechanically reproduced. Essential oils are known as ethereal oils or volatile oils, and they are the essence of the plant that they came from.

Extraction of oils

Most oils are either extracted by the process of distillation or solvent extraction. Citrus oils are either cold pressed or mechanically expressed. When the oils are cold pressed, the oil does not lose any of its potency. Oils, such as many of the flower oils are usually extracted by using ethyl alcohol. When you use the ethyl alcohol, another step is needed to leave behind only the pure oil.

Steam distillation is done by placing the plant in a still, and the steam is then forced over the plant. The steam causes the plant to sweat so that the oils are forced out of the plant and evaporates into the steam. The temperature of the steam needs to be carefully regulated so that the oil does not get too hot or burn. When the steam with the essential oil in it goes through the cooling system, the oil and water separate.

The steam method is good for lavender oil as it is heat sensitive. The heat will decompose the acetic acid and the linalool acid, which are essential healing properties.

Water distillation is done by placing the plant into the still covered in water. The still needs to come to a boil. The water and plant is cooled down, the oil is separated and then used as essential oil. Since water distillation can be done with reduced pressure, it helps to preserve the original plant and essence of the oils that have been extracted.

The water that has been separated from the oil can then be used as floral water such as orange water, lavender water and rosewater. Oils extracted this way include neroli oil. Neroli oil is made from thousands of citrus fruits. It is highly concentrated and very pricey.

The plants that are high with esters are not recommended for the water distillation process.

Cold pressing: When oil is extracted from plants, the plant is placed into a container over water. The heated water causes the plant material to vapourize and the oil vapours will flow through a coil where they are cooled off. This vapour becomes a liquid that is collected. This kind of process produces water products such as rose water or orange blossom water.

Oils such as citrus oils are cold pressed or mechanically expressed. When the oils are cold pressed, the oil does not lose any of its potency. When extracting oil from seeds, the cold pressing method is preferred. This process is used for most carrier oils and many of the essential oils.

Jojoba oil cannot exceed 45 degrees and extra virgin oil olive cannot exceed 25 degrees for cooking, or both oils will diminish.

WHEN OIL IS EXTRACTED FROM SEEDS:

- This begins with the filtering stage, in which the seeds will be passed through a series of spaces with an air system. This process removes any impurities.

- Milling: The fruits, nuts and seeds are placed in the granite bowl and ground to a paste. In the factories they would have larger stainless steel presses that are used.

- Pressing: The pulp of the fruit, nuts and seeds is stirred and pressure is applied to slowly draw out the oils. Again, very little heat is used so that the oils are not harmed.

- The oil is then filtered to keep out any of the impurities.

PROPERTIES OF OILS

Other interesting properties of essential oils:

- they contain oxygenating molecules

- have a bio-electrical frequency

- help to ward off bacteria, diseases, viruses and fungus

- oils have a higher frequency than food

Essential oils have the same healing properties as herbs, but oils have a higher concentration than the dry herb or fruit. With the oil the healing effect can be much quicker, and the body heals a lot faster.

Essential oils have small molecules that are easy for the skin to absorb. The effect is this is quicker than if we were to eat a food or herb or to drink a tea. The oil absorbs into the skin and into the body on a cellular level faster than the dry herb.

Like our liver, the skin of our body is our personal armour, and it provides the function of detoxing the chemicals in our environment. The products with chemicals and heavy metals cause skin irritations and problems as the chemical sits on top of the skin and will irritate it. The essential oils can penetrate through the skin faster and bring the required oxygen and nutrients to the nervous system, blood and organs.

Other interesting properties of essential oils:

- contains oxygenating molecules

- have a bio-electrical frequency

- help to ward off bacteria, diseases, viruses and fungus

- oils have a higher frequency than food

NOTE: Essential oils have the same healing properties herbs, but due to the concentration of the oils they are more powerful. The oils are absorbed faster into the body and don't need to be broken down in the intestine to extract the healing properties. Most of the oils listed in the essential oils will be also in the lists for fruit, herbs and vegetables.

Applications of Oils

Oils can be used in the following ways as applications for the environment and self-healing:

Bathwater: Add four to five drops of the oil to your bath water. Wait till you get into the water so that your body can absorb the oils through the skin and airways.

Diffusers for the home: Helps to release oxygen, ions and ozone in the house. Oils can have an aromatic scent as well as being a disinfectant for the air. Oils can also be used as a perfume

Internally: Some of the oils can be used internally but proceed with caution. Oils are very potent and only certain ones can be ingested.

Massage Therapy and Reflexology: Essential oils can be added to a carrier such as olive oil, almond oil and used in the treatments.

Skin: The oils again can be applied to the skin, but you need to do a small test area first to make sure you don't react to the oil. One or two drops should do then gently rub it into the skin. The oils can be added to carriers, even coconut oil, and then applied to the skin.

As a cleanser in the home or office: Your citrus oils are excellent antibacterial oils and are wonderful to use to use for cleaning the house. They leave a nice scent in the home without leaving chemicals in the air (like air fresheners that can cause neurological damage to the body). Oregano oil and melaleuca both are both excellent disinfectants for the home and can be added to your cleaning water.

DISCLAIMER - PLEASE NOTE that we cannot claim that any of the essentials oils are cures for any diseases. They are however a very beneficial support to have for our health and well-being, along with providing many healing effects for our bodies, organs and mental and spiritual growth.

Essentials Oils and Their Properties

BASIL (OCIMUM BASILICUM)

It is known best for its calming effect and is an enhancer.

Therapeutic Action: antibacterial, antidepressant, anti-infectious, antiseptic, antispasmodic, restorative (stimulant for nerves)

Uses: anxiety, bronchitis, colds, concentration, depression, digestion, earaches, energizing, epilepsy, fainting, fevers, gout, headaches, hiccups, insomnia, mental fatigue, menstruation (scanty periods), migraine, stomach and intestinal cleanser, vomiting, whooping cough

BERGAMOT (CITRUS BERGAMIA)

Known best for calming, enhancer and modifier.

Therapeutic Action: antidepressant, antiseptic, antispasmodic, anti-parasitic

Uses: anxiety, appetite stimulation, bronchitis, candida, colic, depression, digestion, gonorrhea, infections, intestinal parasites, lungs, respiratory infection, sedative, skin (psoriasis), tonsillitis (acute)

BIRCH (BETULA ALLEGHANIANSIS)

Known best for being an enhancer and personifier.

Therapeutic Action: anti-inflammatory, pain relief, stimulant

Uses: arthritis, bone spurs, cramps, gout, hypertension, muscular pain, osteoporosis, rheumatism, tendinitis, ulcers.

CEDARWOOD (CEDRUS ATLANTICA)

Known best for its calming effect.

Therapeutic Action: antiseptic, astringent, diuretic, insect repellant, sedative

Uses: anger, anxiety, asthma, bronchitis, calming, cellulite, constipation, cystitis, dandruff, hair loss, lungs, nerves, respiratory, sedative, skin (acne), skin diseases, skin (eczema), urinary infections

CHAMOMILE

Known best for being a relaxant.

Therapeutic Action: anti-convulsive, antiseptic, anti-suppressant

Uses: depression, digestion, gingivitis, insomnia, menstruation, skin (eczema), throat (sore), toothache

CHAMOMILE: BLUE (MATRICARIA RECUTITA)

Known best for being a relaxant.

Therapeutic Action: anti-inflammatory, anti-infectious, antispasmodic, gastritis (chronic), pain reliever

Uses: colic, convulsions, cystitis, decongestant, digestion tonic, emotion stabilizer, gall bladder, hypersensitivity, liver, menstruation (hormone stabilizer), menstruation (irregular period), muscle spasms, neuralgic aches, skin (acne), skin (eczema), skin (wounds), ulcers.

CHAMOMILE: ROMAN (CHAMAEMELUM NOBILE)

Known best for its calming effect.

Therapeutic Action: anti-inflammatory, anti-parasitic, anti-spasm, nervine

Uses: asthma, balancing of the body, calming for the nerves, muscles (reduces inflammation), muscles (reduces spasm), parasites

CINNAMON (CINNAMOMUN VERUM)

Known best for its antibacterial, anti-infection properties and being a blood sugar stabilizer.

Therapeutic Action: antibacterial, antibiotic, anti-diuretic, antifungal, anti-infectious, anti-parasite, antiseptic, anti-viral, astringent, immune stimulant

Uses: blood sugar stabilizer, circulation, colds, coughs, decongestant, digestion, exhaustion, infections, rheumatism, throat (sore), toothache, tropical infections, typhoid fever, vaginitis

CITRONELLA

Known best for warding off mosquitoes.

Therapeutic Action: insect repellant

Uses: insect repellant

CLARY SAGE (SALVIA SCLAREA)

Known best for being used in the bath for relaxation.

Therapeutic Action: anti-convulsive, anti-infectious, antiseptic, antispasmodic, antiviral, astringent, nerve tonic, sedative

Uses: bronchitis, cholesterol, depression, digestion - tonic, exhaustion, frigidity, genitals, hemorrhoids, impotence, infections, insect bites, insomnia, intestinal cramps, kidney disorders, menopause, menstrual cramps, menstrual (hormones), relaxation, skin (dry), throat infection, ulcers, whooping cough

CLOVES (EUGENIA CARYOPHYLLATA)

Known best for its antibiotic and antiviral properties.

Therapeutic Action: antibacterial, anti-cancerous, antifungal, anti-tumour, antiviral, insect repellant, pain reliever

Uses: arthritis, bad breath, bronchitis, diarrhea, headaches, hypertension, impotence, intestinal cramps, intestinal parasites, kidney disorders, leg ulcers, lupus, memory, menopause (pre), mouth sores, nausea, pain, plaque, rheumatism, skin diseases, skin infections, skin wounds infected, spleen, stomach cleanser, toothache, tuberculosis, vomiting

Caution: Avoid use when pregnant.

CYPRESS (CUPRESSUS SEMPERVIRENS)

Known best for its antibacterial and anti-infectious properties.

Therapeutic Action: antibacterial, anti-infectious, anti-mucus, antiseptic, astringent, decongestant, diuretic, refreshing, relaxing,

Uses: Arthritis, asthma, blood circulation, bronchitis, coughs, cramps, fluid retention, hemorrhoids, influenza, insomnia, intestinal parasites, laryngitis, liver, lymphatic, decongestant, menstrual pain, muscle cramps, nervous tension, pancreas discomforts, pleurisy, rheumatism, skin (dry0, spasms, throat, tuberculosis, veins (varicose), warts, whooping cough

Caution: Not recommended for use after menopause.

EUCALYPTUS (EUCALYPTUS GLOBULUS)

Eucalyptus oil and leaves have been used in saunas and hot tubs for years. The oil from the leaves and young twigs helps to clear out the sinuses and ward off virus and infections in the lungs.

Therapeutic Action: analgesic, antiseptic, anti- viral, diuretic, insect repellant, stimulant

Uses: asthma, bronchitis, burns, candida, colds, coughs, cystitis, diabetes, diarrhea, fevers, gall stones, gonorrhea, herpes, influenza, malaria, measles, migraine, muscular pain, respiratory infection, sinusitis, skin (infections), skin (wounds infected), tuberculosis, viruses

This oil can be used on its own or blended with cedar wood, lemon oil, peppermint and tea tree oil.

Caution: I found a note in one book that warned against using this oil on infants and young children.

FENNEL (FOENICULUM VULGARE)

Known best for its liquorice taste and soothing properties for the stomach.

Therapeutic Action: antiseptic, antispasmodic, antitoxin, diuretic, expectorant

Uses: cellulite, colic, constipation, cystitis, digestion tonic, flatulence, gout, intestinal, kidney stones, lactation (increase), menopause, nausea, obesity, parasites, skin (oily), urinary stones

FIR (ABES ALBA)

Known best for bringing relief for the throat and lungs.

Therapeutic Action: antiseptic, expectorant, refreshing, sedative,

Uses: asthma, bronchitis, chest congestion, colds, energy, influenza, lungs: mucus

FRANKINCENSE (BOSWELLIA CARTERII)

Known best for its antiseptic properties.

Therapeutic Action: anti-catarrhal, antidepressant, anti-inflammatory, antiseptic, anti-tumour, astringent, digestive, diuretic, expectorant, immuno-stimulant, sedative

Uses: asthma, bad breath, bites (insect), bites (snake), blood pressure (high), bronchitis, cancer, carbuncles, coughs, diarrhea, diphtheria, gonorrhea, headaches, hemorrhoids, herpes, inflammation (aging), jaundice, laryngitis, meningitis, pneumonia, skin (wounds infected), staph, syphilis, tonsillitis (acute), tuberculosis, typhoid, ulcers, warts

GERANIUM (PELARGONIUM GRAVEOLENS)

Known best for getting rid of the toxins in the blood and organs.

Therapeutic Action: antidepressant, anti-infectious, antiseptic, astringent, diuretic, insect repellant, sedative

Uses: diabetes, diarrhea, digestion - tonic, gall bladder, insomnia, jaundice, kidney disorders, liver, menstruation, nervous tension, rheumatism, ringworm, shingles, skin diseases, skin (dry), skin (oily), skin (psoriasis), sterility, throat (sore), ulcer: gastric, urinary stones, wounds.

GINGER (ZINGIBER OFFICINALE)

Known best for the soothing effect for the stomach and prevention of contagious diseases.

Therapeutic Action: anti-inflammatory, antiseptic, expectorant, laxative, stimulant

Uses: alcoholism, angina, aphrodisiac, appetite (loss of), bones (broken), colds, constipation, contagious diseases, diarrhea, digestion, expectorant, flatulence, heartburn, impotence, laxative, muscles: sore, nausea, rheumatism, scurvy, sprains, stimulant, throat (sore), tonsillitis

GRAPEFRUIT (CITRIS PARADISI)

Known best for its enhancing properties and helping the body with digestion and cleansing.

Therapeutic Action: antibacterial, antidepressant, antiseptic, diuretic, stimulant

Uses: appetite stimulant, cellulite, depression, digestion, disinfectant, dyspepsia, eating disorders, fluid retention, gall stones, headaches, heart (vascular system), jet lag, kidney cleansing, liver, lymphatic, menstruation-pre (relief tension), migraines, skin tightening, stress, weight reduction

Caution: If on heart medication, it is not recommended to consume grapefruit or use the oils.

HELICHRYSIUM/STRAWFLOWER (HELICHRYSUM ITALICUM)

Known best for its blood cleansing properties for the organs.

Therapeutic Action: anti-catarrhal, anti-coagulant, anti-inflammatory, astringent

Uses: Blood cleansing, cholesterol, circulation, colitis, dermatitis, detoxifying, gall bladder, hematoma, liver, lymph drainage, pancreas stimulant, pain, psoriasis, sinus infections, skin, skin (eczema), stomach cramps,

JUNIPER BERRY (JUNIPERUS COMMUNIS)

Known best for its stimulant properties and for helping with depression.

Therapeutic Action: anti-infectious, antioxidant, antiseptic, antispasmodic, astringent, diuretic, stimulant, tonic

Uses: depression, dermatitis, detoxifier, digestive, kidney stones, MS, muscles (sore), nerves, rheumatism, skin (acne), skin (eczema), skin (wounds), urinary infections

LAVENDER (LAVANULA ANGUSTIFOLIA)

Known best for being used to lessen anxiety, calm the nerves, increase clairvoyance and aid with sleep.

Therapeutic Action: anti-convulsive, antidepressant, anti-infectious, anti-inflammatory, antiseptic, antispasmodic, antitoxin, anodyne, sedative

Uses: acne, allergies, anxiety, arthritis, asthma, blood pressure (lowers it), bronchitis, burns, carbuncles, convulsions, cramps, dandruff, depression, diaper rash, fainting, flatulence, fluid retention, gall stones, hair loss, headaches, herpes, hysteria, indigestion, influenza, insomnia, laryngitis, lymphatic system, menstruation (cramping), depression and pain, migraines, mouth abscesses, nausea, muscles (inflammation), nervous tension, phlebitis, rheumatism, skin (burns), skin (eczema), skin (psoriasis), skin (scars), skin (stretchmarks), skin (wounds), sleep, sunstroke, throat infection, thrush, tuberculosis, typhoid, whooping cough

LEMON (CITRIS LIMONUM)

Known best for its fresh smell and antiviral actions.

Therapeutic Action: antibacterial. anti-infectious, antiseptic, antiviral, astringent, restorative.

Uses: air disinfectant, anemia, anxiety, asthma, bleeding (stops the bleeding), blood (cleanses and stimulates the formation of the red and white blood cells), circulation, colds, digestion, disinfectant, fevers, gall stones, germicide, gout, heart burn, immune system, infections (viral), insomnia, intestinal parasites, respiratory, rheumatism, throat (sore), ureter infections, varicose veins, water purifier

LEMONGRASS (CYMBOPOGON CITRATUS)

Known best for being used as an insect repellant.

Therapeutic Action: anodyne, anti-inflammatory, antiseptic, insect repellant, pain reliever, relaxant, restorative, sedative

Uses: arteries, bladder infection, cellulite, digestion, edema, eyes, fevers, fluid retention, headaches, heart: vascular system, infections (viral), kidney, lymphatic system, muscles (inflammation parasympathetic system - regulates), relaxant, respiratory, skin regeneration, throat, varicose veins, vascular walls (strengthens the walls)

MARJORAM (ORIGANUM MARJORANA)

Known best as an antispasmodic and muscle relaxant.

Therapeutic Action: antiseptic, antispasmodic, digestive stimulant, expectorant, sedative, tonic

Uses: anxiety, arteries, arthritis, asthma, blood circulation, blood pressure (lowers it), bronchitis, colds, colic, constipation, headaches, insomnia, intestinal: spasms, menstruation, migraines, muscles cramps, muscles (pain), parasympathetic nerves (increases the tone), relaxant, rheumatism, sprains

MELALEUCA/TEA TREE OIL (MELALEUCA ALTERNIFOLIA)

Known best for its disinfectant properties.

Therapeutic Action: antibacterial, antifungal, anti-infectious, anti-inflammatory, antioxidant, anti-parasitic, antiseptic, antiviral, expectorant, insect repellant, stimulant

Uses: appendicitis, athletes foot, bacteria, blood circulation, burns, bronchitis, candida, colds, cold sores, coughs, decongestion, depression, diarrhea, digestive, disinfectant, gingivitis, gum disease, hemorrhoids, herpes, hysteria, infections (fungal), infections (viral), inflammation, influenza, lice, parasites, psoriasis, rash, respiratory (infection), ringworm, shock, skin (acne), skin (burns), skin (eczema), skin (infections), skin (wounds), throat (infections), throat (sore), tonsillitis, toothaches and abscess, vaginitis, warts, whooping cough, yeast infections

MYRRH (COMMINPHORA MYRRHA)

Known best for its antiviral actions.

Therapeutic Action: anti-infectious, anti-inflammatory, antiseptic, antiviral, astringent, tonic

Uses: appetite (stimulant), bronchitis, catarrh, candida, diarrhea, digestion, dysentery, hepatitis, infections (fungal), inflammation, mouth sores, skin (infections), skin (stretch marks), thyroid (hyper), ulcers

MYRTLE (MYRTUS COMMUNIS)

Known best for its respiratory repair.

Therapeutic Action: anti-infectious, anti-parasitic, antiseptic, antispasmodic, astringent, expectorant

Uses: anger (soothing), bronchitis, candida, cystitis, decongestant, diarrhea, dysentery, hemorrhoids, infections, inflammatory, insomnia, menstruation: hormones, muscle relaxant, psoriasis, pulmonary disorders, sinusitis, skin (acne), skin (bruises), sleep (promotes), thyroid (hyper), urethritis

NUTMEG (MYRISTICA FRAGRANS)

Known best for its aromatic scent and as a digestive aid.

Therapeutic Action: anti-parasitic, antiseptic, carminative, laxative,

Uses: appetite stimulant, blood circulation, cerebral stimulant, diarrhea, digestion for starchy foods and fat, fainting, gall stones, hair tonic, infections, intestinal (cleanser), intestinal (parasites), menstruation (cramps), menstruation (scanty), nausea, rheumatism, vomiting

Avoid in pregnancy: Nutmeg can cause discomfort, heart problems and delirium.

ORANGE (CITRUS AURANTIUM)

Known best for its citrusy fresh aroma.

Therapeutic Action: antidepressant, anti-inflammatory, antiseptic, antispasmodic, decongestant, relaxant

Uses: angina, appetite (stimulant), blood circulation, bronchitis, calming, cardiac spasm, cholesterol, colds, constipation, diarrhea, digestion, dyspepsia, flatulence's, heart (cardiac spasm), heart palpitation, insomnia, menopause, muscles (sore), relaxant, skin (diseases), skin (dry), skin (regeneration), stomach (spasms)

OREGANO OIL (ORIGANUM COMPACTUM)

Known best for natural antibiotic properties.

Therapeutic Action: antibacterial, antibiotic, antifungal, anti-infectious, antiparasitic, antioxidant, antiseptic, anti-viral

Uses: asthma, bronchitis, colds, cysts, digestion, dysentery, hypotension, infections (bacterial), infections (fungal), immune system stimulant, parasites, pneumonia, respiratory infection, rheumatism, throat infection, tuberculosis, viruses, whooping cough

PATCHOULI (POGOSTEMON CABLIN)

Known best for its anti-inflammatory properties.

Therapeutic Action: antidepressant, anti-infectious, anti-inflammatory, antiseptic, astringent, digestive stimulant, diuretic, insect repellant, sedative

Uses: allergies, anxiety, appetite (curb), cellulite, dandruff, decongestant, depression, dermatitis, diarrhea, digestive, hemorrhoids, infections (fungal), inflammation, insect bites, inflammation, insecticide, parasites, skin (acne), skin (eczema), skin (infections), skin (regeneration), skin (tightening), snake bites, water retention, weight reduction

PEPPERMINT (MENTHA PIPERITA)

Known best for soothing of the stomach and assists in digestion.

Therapeutic Action: anodyne, antibacterial, anti-infectious, anti-inflammatory, antiseptic, antispasmodic, expectorant, pain reliever, refreshing, stimulant

Uses: arthritis, asthma, bronchitis, colds, colitis, cysts, decongestant, diarrhea, digestion stimulant, exhaustion, eyes (vision), fevers, flu, fungicide, headaches, heartburn, hemorrhoids, hepatitis, hot flashes, hypertension, hypotension, indigestion, infections (bacterial), infections (viral), inflammation, intestinal tract (gas), laryngitis, liver, menstrual (regulator), migraines, muscles (spasms), nausea, prostate, shock, sinusitis, skin care, skin (eczema), skin (itchy), throat infection, toothache, travel sickness, tuberculosis, ulcers, varicose veins, vomiting

PINA (PINUS SYLVESTRIS)

Known best for its decongestant properties.

Therapeutic Action: anti-diabetic, anti-infectious, antiseptic, decongestant

Uses: allergies, arthritis, asthma, bronchitis, decongestant, diabetes, digestion, hypertension, infections, menstrual: hormone regulation, rheumatism, sinusitis

RAVENSARA (RAVENSARA AROMATICA)

Known best for its viral action.

Therapeutic Action: antibacterial, antiviral, expectorant

Uses: bronchitis, herpes, infections: viruses, muscle (inflammatory), muscle (spasms), sinusitis, stimulant

ROSEMARY (ROSMARINUS OFFICINALIS)

Known best for its strong herbal flavour in cooking and antibacterial properties.

Therapeutic Action: antibacterial, anti-catarrhal, anti-infectious, anti-inflammatory, antispasmodic

Uses: arthritis, blood pressure (low), bronchitis, cellulite, cholera, colds, dandruff, diabetes, fluid retention, hair loss, headaches, hepatitis, infections: viral, memory, menstrual (irregular periods), mental fatigue, muscle (inflammatory), reproductive organ regulator, sinusitis, vaginitis

ROSEWOOD (ANIBA ROSAEODORA)

Known best for its bacterial and infection fighting properties.

Therapeutic Action: antibacterial, antifungal, anti-infectious, antiviral

Uses: candida, depression, fungus, infections (bacterial), infections (viruses), mouth infections, skin: acne, skin (dry), skin (eczema), vaginitis

SAGE (SALVIA OFFICINALIS)

Known best for its detoxing properties.

Therapeutic Action: antibacterial, anti-cancer, antifungal, anti-infectious, antiseptic, antispasmodic, antiviral, diuretic, expectorant, relaxant

Uses: adrenal, arthritis, asthma, blood circulation, blood pressure (too low), bronchitis, catarrh, cellulite, digestive system, disinfectant, fibrosis, glandular support, gripe, hot flashes, infections (bacterial), infections (viral), liver, lymphatics, meningitis, menopause, Menstrual (depression and hormone balancer), menstrual: (irregular), nervous system, night sweats, plague, pulmonary, respiratory problems, rheumatism, sinusitis, skin infections, skin (tighten), sprains, stimulant, urinary

SANDALWOOD

Known best for its relaxing properties.

Therapeutic Action: antibacterial, antidepressant, antifungal, antiseptic, astringent, relaxant, sedative

Uses: aphrodisiac, bronchitis, nerves, candida, catarrh, decongestant, depression, diarrhea, hemorrhoids, hypertension, impotence, menstruation (hormone balancer), nerves, pulmonary, respiratory, skin (acne), skin (infections), urinary

SPEARMINT (MENTHA SPICATA)

Known best for its digestive and calming properties.

Therapeutic Action: anti-inflammatory, antispasmodic, digestion, insect repellant including spiders, relaxant, restorative, stimulant

Uses: appetite: stimulant, bad breath, candida, constipation, cysts, depression, diarrhea, digestion, fevers, flatulence, headaches, hiccups, kidney stones, kidney support, menstruation (heavy), menstruation (irregular period), mouth (sore gums), nausea, nerves, skin (acne), skin (dry), skin (eczema), throat infections, vaginitis, vomiting

Caution: Careful when using it on children. Pregnant mothers should not drink the tea or absorb the oil. It may cause an abortion.

SPRUCE (PICEA MARIANA)

Known best for its anti-inflammatory actions.

Therapeutic Action: antibacterial, antidepressant, anti-infectious, anti-inflammatory, anti-parasitic, antiseptic, antispasmodic, disinfectant

Uses: adrenal, arthritis, bones, bronchitis, candida, cortisone, depression, joints (sore), menstrual (hormones), muscle (spasms), prostate, relaxing, rheumatism, thymus gland, thyroid (hyper)

TANGERINE

Known best for its fresh citric aroma.

Therapeutic Action: antiseptic, antispasmodic, relaxant

Uses: cellulite, constipation, depression, diarrhea, digestion, fluid retention, gall bladder, insomnia, intestinal (spasms), irritability, limbs: tired and aching, liver, lymphatic, parasites, stress.

TARRAGON (ARTEMISIA DRACUNCULUS)

Known best for its anti-inflammatory relief.

Therapeutic Action: antibacterial, anti-cancer, anti-infectious, anti-inflammatory, antiseptic, antispasmodic, antiviral, laxative, stimulant

Uses: anorexia, appetite stimulant, arthritis, belching, colitis, digestion, diuretic, flatulence (gastric complaint), hiccups, intestinal (spasms), kidney support, laxative, menstrual, nausea, nerves, parasites, rheumatism, sciatica, skin (wounds infected)

Tea Tree Oil see Melaleuca

THYME (THYMUS VULGARIS)

Known best for its viral fighting properties.

Therapeutic Action: antibacterial, antifungal, anti-infectious, antiseptic, antispasmodic, antiviral, nervine, stimulant

Uses: anthrax, aphrodisiac, asthma, bronchitis, candida, circulation, colitis, cysts, depression, digestion, fatigue, flus, headaches, immune system, infections (bacterial), infections (viral), intestinal tract (gas), nerves (stimulates nerve endings), parasites, prostate, psoriasis, rheumatism, skin infections, staph infections, tuberculosis, urinary infections, urinary, vaginitis

YLANG YLANG (CANANGA ODORATA)

Known best for its calming effect.

Therapeutic Action: antidepressant, antiseptic, antispasmodic, relaxant.

Uses: anxiety, arterial hypertension, blood pressure (high), depression, diabetes, frustration, hair growth, heart palpitation, hypertension, impotence, insomnia, intestinal – infections, mental fatigue, shock, skin care

Have fun learning about your oils. They have amazing healing properties both externally and internally. The oils can heal our bodies on a cellular level, and it takes very little oil to have an amazing effect.

Another medicine and blessing from Mother Earth.

CHAPTER 15

Ailments and Alternative Options

WE HAVE JOURNEYED THROUGH THIS BOOK, GONE ON ADVENTURES LEARNING ABOUT how we can heal the body energetically with the foods that are healthy and how we can live in a non-toxic home. Everything takes time to shift and change within. While we work on these changes, our body gets stronger each day. As the body starts to flourish, life becomes a new journey of hope and happiness.

When we achieve that status of good health, we still need to feed and nourish our bodies daily. Yes, we can cheat here and there and have those foods that are not on the health list. You will find it interesting, though, once you choose that good living state, how your body will react to certain foods. These reactions can lead again to distress if we don't return to the healthier eating. I do grab that odd bag of potato chips, four times a year maybe or that package of liquorice of the kind that is almost pure sugar. I try not to beat myself up over it and enjoy for the moment. Then I go right back to the foods that nourish my body, heart, spirit and soul all at once. Look at what is in your grocery cart or basket and see what you are taking home. Is it good for you? Is it just comfort food? Is it healthy for you, and is it comfort food like black bean dip and veggies or hummus and veggies?

We can observe and watch others, and know where they are stuck in life situations and how it affects their bodies. We can also see how we can overcome illnesses and maintain a state of well-being by bringing in the products that we require to healing from within.

This chapter will first focus on the therapeutic actions that can be provided by the foods and essential oils that we covered. Then we will see some of the diseases/illness that are in the write-ups for the food groups. The aim is to show the description of the ailment and offer some of the foods that can assist with the healing process.

Disclaimer: The following information is for reading and exploring. I do not or will not prescribe any of the following to the reader.

PLEASE use this following section to add all your notes along with other options that you have heard about. Let this be the book that you write in, update and use as your personal healing go to book. There are a lot more options that can go under the sections in this chapter, like the vitamins and minerals. When you find what you are looking for in chapter 4, bring the information forth to this chapter too as a reminder.

Therapeutic Actions and Natural Alternatives

ALTERATIVE

Herbs: bayberry, bistort, black cohosh, blessed thistle, burdock, chaparral, chickweed, cleaver, eyebright, garlic, goldenseal, kelp, mandrake, milk thistle, parsley, red clover, reishi mushroom, sassafras, senna, white pond lily, wild indigo, wormwood

ANALGESIC

Essential Oils: eucalyptus

Herbs: balm of Gilead, echinacea, Pau d'arco

ANODYNE

Amino Acids, Minerals, Omega Oils, Vitamins:

Vitamin: P

Essential Oils: birch, chamomile (blue), cloves, lavender, lemongrass, peppermint

Herbs: cannabis, dandelion, Lady's slipper root, lavender, Pau d'arco, pleurisy root, pokeweed, sassafras, senna, slippery elm, spearmint, thyme, valerian, white oak bark, witch hazel, wormwood

ANTHELMINTIC

Herbs: bistort, garlic, gentian, hops, turkey rhubarb, wormwood

ANTI-AGING

Amino Acids, Minerals, Omega Oils, Vitamins:

Mineral: silicon

Vitamin: coenzyme Q10

Fruit: cranberry, peach, plum / prune, Saskatoon berry, tangerine

Herb: Ashwagandha

Meat: beef liver

Vegetable: rutabaga

ANTIBACTERIAL

Amino Acids, Minerals, Omega Oils, Vitamins:

Amino Acids: l-glutamine, l-lysine

Minerals: germanium, sulfur, zinc

Vitamins: A, paba, C

Dairy: cheese (cow), cheese (goat)

Fruits: cranberry, lemon, pineapple

Essential Oils: cinnamon, cloves, cypress, grapefruit, lemon, melaleuca/tea tree oil, oregano oil, peppermint, ravensara, rosemary, rosewood, sage, sandalwood, spruce, tarragon, thyme, rose hips, slippery elm

Grains: barley, oat

Herbs: aloe vera, anise seed, Ashwagandha, astragalus, balm of Gilead, basil, bayberry, bearberry, blue cohosh, borage, burdock, chlorella, cinnamon, cloves, dandelion, echinacea, fennel, ginger, horseradish, Lady's slipper root, lemon balm, lemongrass, licorice root, melaleuca, myrrh, oatstraw, olive leaf, oregano, Pau d'arco, plantain, prickly ash, reishi mushroom, rosemary, thyme, white oak bark, white popular, wild indigo, yellow dock

Meat:

Beef: beef, beef: calf liver

Lake, ocean, river, sea: fish oils

Poultry: egg

Nuts, Oils, Seeds:

Nut: coconut, pecan

Oil: coconut oil, hazelnut oil, Siberian pine nut oil

Vegetables: garlic, onion (green), sweet potato

ANTIBIOTIC

Amino Acids, Minerals, Omega Oils, Vitamins:

Vitamins: paba

Essential Oils: cinnamon, oregano oil

Herbs: cinnamon, eucalyptus, gentian, goldenseal, juniper, myrrh, olive leaf, oregano, parsley, plantain, rosemary, sage, turmeric, wild indigo, yarrow

Vegetable: onion (red)

ANTI-CANCER

Amino Acids, Minerals, Omega Oils, Vitamins:

Mineral: calcium

Dairy: buttermilk, whey

Essential Oils: cloves, sage, tarragon

Fruit: apple, blueberry, cherry, date, fig, goji berry, gooseberry, grape/raisin, grapefruit, guava, kiwi, lemon, lime, mango, orange, peach, pear, pineapple, rhubarb, tomato

Grains: barley, rye

Herbs: cannabis, comfrey, dandelion, fennel, ginseng, Irish moss, lemongrass, licorice root, milk thistle, mullein, parsley, Pau d'arco, pokeweed, prickly ash, rose hips, turmeric, white oak bark, yarrow, yellow dock

Legumes: bean (black), lima bean, peanut, pinto bean

Meat:

Beef: calf liver

Nuts, Oils, Seeds:

Nut: pecan, pistachio, walnut

Oil: walnut oil

Seed: Cacao, flaxseed, hemp seed, mustard seed

Vegetables: artichoke, bean (lima), broccoli, Brussel sprouts, carrots, cucumber, garlic, kale, kelp, pepper (bell), rutabaga, spinach

ANTI-CATARRHAL

Essential Oils: frankincense, helichrysium/strawflower, rosemary

ANTI-COAGULANT

Vegetables: kelp

ANTI-CONVULSION

Essential Oils: chamomile, clary sage, lavender

Herbs: anise seed, lavender

ANTIDEPRESSANT

Amino Acids, Minerals, Omega Oils, Vitamins: Amino Acid: l-tyrosine

Dairy: milk (goat), whey

Essential Oils: bergamot, frankincense, geranium, grapefruit, lavender, orange, patchouli, sandalwood, spruce, ylang ylang

Herbs: Ashwagandha, lavender, milk thistle, oatstraw, wild indigo

Legumes: carob

Meat:

Lake, ocean, river, sea: fish: saltwater, halibut, herring, mackerel, salmon, sardines, tuna

Poultry: egg, egg yolk, turkey

Vegetables: bean (lima and snap), parsnip

ANTI-DIABETIC

Fruits: cranberry

Essential Oils: cinnamon, pina

Herbs: cinnamon

Vegetables: bean (snap), parsnip

ANTI-EMETIC

Herbs: cannabis, cloves, ginseng, Irish moss, lemongrass, oregano, raspberry

ANTI-FLATULENT

Herbs: fennel, kelp

ANTIFUNGAL

Essential Oils: cinnamon, cloves, melaleuca/tea tree oil, oregano oil, rosewood, sage, sandalwood, thyme

Fruit: grape / raisin.

Herbs: black walnut, burdock, cilantro, cinnamon, juniper, lemongrass, olive leaf, Pau d'arco, raspberry, red clover, reishi mushroom, rosemary, sage, spearmint

Nuts, Oils, Seeds:

Nut: coconut

Seed: pumpkin seed

Vegetable: garlic, onion (green), radish, sweet potato

ANTIHISTAMINE

Herbs: caraway seed, green tea, nettle, reishi mushroom, skullcap

ANTI-INFECTIOUS

Essential Oils: chamomile (blue), cinnamon, clary sage, cypress, geranium, juniper berry, lavender, lemon, melaleuca/tea tree oil, myrrh, myrtle, oregano oil, patchouli, peppermint, pina, ravensara, rosemary, rosewood, sage, spruce, tarragon, thyme

Herbs: anise seed, bilberry, buchu, lavender

ANTI-INFLAMMATORY

Amino Acids, Minerals, Omega Oils, Vitamins: Amino Acids: l-glutamine, l-taurine

Minerals: germanium, magnesium, manganese

Vitamins: paba, C, D, P

Diary: whey

Essential Oils: birch, chamomile (blue), chamomile (roman), cypress, frankincense, ginger, helichrysium/strawflower, lavender, lemongrass, melaleuca/tea tree oil, myrrh, orange, patchouli, peppermint, rosemary, spearmint, spruce, tarragon

Fruit: avocado, banana, blackberry, cantaloupe, cherry, cranberry, gooseberry, grape / raisin, kiwi, lemon, papaya, passion fruit, pear, pineapple, plum / prune, raspberry, Saskatoon berry, tomato, watermelon

Grains: barley, buckwheat, cereal grain, corn, couscous, millet, oat, quinoa, rye, spelt, wheat, wheat bran, wheat germ

Herbs: alfalfa, aloe vera, angelica, anise seed, arnica, Ashwagandha, astragalus, balm of Gilead, bilberry, bistort, black cohosh, blue cohosh, borage, buchu, butcher's broom, Cannabis, caraway seed, chaparral, chickweed, cinnamon, comfrey, dandelion, eucalyptus, fennel, fenugreek, gentian, ginger, ginseng, goldenseal, gravel root, hawthorn, holy basil, Lady's slipper root, lavender, lemon balm, lemongrass, licorice root, lobelia, marshmallow, meadowsweet, melaleuca, milk thistle, mullein, nettle, oatstraw, olive leaf, oregano, plantain, pleurisy root, pokeweed, prickly ash, primrose, raspberry, red clover, rose hips, rosemary, sassafras, skullcap, slippery elm, spearmint, thyme, turkey rhubarb, turmeric, valerian, white oak bark, white pond lily, witch hazel, wormwood, yarrow, yellow dock

Legumes: bean (black), black-eyed pea, carob, garbanzo bean, kidney bean, lentil, navy bean.

Meat:

Beef: beef, beef kidney

Lake, ocean, river, sea: clams, fish: saltwater, halibut, herring, mackerel, salmon, sardines, tuna

Poultry: chicken, egg

Nuts, Oils, Seeds:

Nut: cashew, pecan, walnut

Oil: avocado oil, grapeseed oil, hemp seed oil, olive oil, sesame seed oil, walnut oil

Seed: cacao, flaxseed, hemp seed, mustard seed, sesame seed, sunflower seed

Vegetable: asparagus, beet, broccoli, Brussel sprouts, cabbage, cauliflower, celery, collards, cucumber, garlic, kale, kelp, lettuce (romaine), mushroom (white), onion (green and red), pea, pepper (bell), spinach, squash, sweet potato, Swiss chard, turnip

ANTI-MALARIAL

Herbs: Ashwagandha, olive leaf, oregano, Peruvian bark

ANTIMICROBIAL

Fruit: grape/raisin

Herbs: barberry, bayberry, blessed thistle, caraway seed, chamomile, chlorella, cilantro, echinacea, ginger, goldenseal, licorice root, melaleuca, olive leaf, oregano, peppermint, reishi mushroom, rose hips, rosemary, sage, turkey rhubarb, white oak bark

Nuts, Oils, Seeds:

Nut: coconut

Seed: pumpkin seed

ANTIOXIDANT

Amino Acids, Minerals, Omega Oils, Vitamins:

Amino Acid: l-glutamine, l-lysine, l-tyrosine

Mineral: germanium, molybdenum, selenium, silicon, sulfur, zinc

Vitamins: A, C, E, coenzyme Q10

Dairy: buttermilk, milk (cow), milk (goat)

Essential Oils: cinnamon, melaleuca/tea tree oil, oregano oil

Fruit: apple, apricot, avocado, blackberry, blueberry, cantaloupe, cherry, chokecherry, cranberry, currant (red), date, fig, goji berry, gooseberry, grape/raisin, grapefruit, guava, kiwi, lemon, lime, orange, papaya, passion fruit, peach, pear, pineapple, plum / prune, raspberry, rhubarb, Saskatoon berry, strawberry, tangerine, tomato, watermelon

Grains: barley, buckwheat, cereal grain, corn, couscous, millet, oat, quinoa, rice (brown), rye, spelt, wheat, wheat bran, wheat germ.

Herb: amaranth, Ashwagandha, balm of Gilead, basil, bilberry, burdock, cannabis, Chamomile, chlorella, cilantro, cloves, fennel, ginger, green tea, hawthorn, holy basil, Lemongrass, lobelia, marjoram, milk thistle, oregano, peppermint, reishi mushroom, rose hips, Spearmint, thyme, turmeric, white oak bark, yellow dock

Legume: bean (red), carob, garbanzo bean, kidney bean, lentil, lima bean, navy bean, peanut, pinto bean, soybean

Meat:

Cow: beef

Lake, ocean, river, sea: fish: fresh water, fish: oils, sardines, tuna

Lamb: lamb

Pork: pork

Poultry: chicken, egg

Nuts, Oils, Seeds:

Nut: almond, Brazil nut, cashew, coconut, hazelnut, macadamia nut, pecan, pine nut, pistachio, walnut

Oil: almond oil, avocado oil, coconut oil, grapeseed oil, hazelnut oil, hemp seed oil, olive oil, sesame seed oil, Siberian pine nut oil, walnut oil

Seed: chia seed, cacao, hemp seed, pumpkin seed, sesame seed, sunflower seed

Vegetable: artichoke, asparagus, beet, beet greens, broccoli, Brussel sprouts, cabbage, carrots, cauliflower, celery, collards, corn, cucumber, dulse, garlic, kale, kelp, kohlrabi, lettuce (iceberg and romaine), mushroom (white), mustard greens, onion (red), pea, pepper (bell), potato, radish, rutabaga, spinach, squash, sweet potato, Swiss chard, turnip

ANTI-PARASITIC

Essential Oils: bergamot, chamomile (roman), cinnamon, melaleuca/tea tree oil, myrtle, nutmeg, oregano oil, spruce

Herbs: agrimony, black walnut, blessed thistle, cascara sagrada, cilantro, cloves, gravel root, licorice root

Nuts, Oils, Seeds: Seed: pumpkin seed

ANTI-PERSPIRANT

Herbs: black walnut

ANTI-PYRETIC

Herbs: ginger

ANTISCORBUTIC

Fruit: lemon, lime.

Herbs: cleaver, yellow dock

ANTISEPTIC

Fruits: cranberry, tangerine

Essential Oils: bergamot, cedarwood, chamomile, cinnamon, clary sage, cypress, eucalyptus, fennel, fir, frankincense, geranium, ginger, grapefruit, juniper berry, lavender, lemon, lemongrass, marjoram, melaleuca/tea tree oil, myrrh, myrtle, nutmeg, orange, oregano oil, patchouli, peppermint, pina, sage, sandalwood, spruce, tangerine, tarragon, thyme, ylang ylang

Herbs: amaranth, balm of Gilead, barberry, birch, black walnut, borage, borage, buchu, burdock, butcher's broom, chaparral, chickweed, cilantro, cloves, echinacea, eucalyptus, garlic, gentian, hawthorn, horseradish, hyssop, Irish moss, juniper, kelp, lavender, lobelia, marshmallow, melaleuca, mullein, myrrh, oatstraw, oregano, plantain, pleurisy root, prickly ash, rose hips, rosemary, senna, slippery elm, spearmint, thyme, white oak bark, wild indigo

ANTISPASMODIC

Essential Oils: bergamot, chamomile (Blue), chamomile (Roman), clary sage, fennel, juniper berry, lavender, marjoram, myrtle, orange, peppermint, rosemary, sage, spearmint, spruce, tangerine, tarragon, thyme, ylang ylang

Fruit: tangerine

Herbs: barberry, basil, black cohosh, black walnut, blessed thistle, blue cohosh, burdock, calendula, cannabis, cayenne, chamomile, cilantro, cloves, cramp bark, fennel, fenugreek, garlic, ginger, hops, hyssop, Irish moss, Lady's slipper root, Lavender, lemongrass, licorice root, lobelia, marjoram, mullein, nettle, oregano, Peruvian bark, plantain, prickly ash, primrose, red clover, rosemary, skullcap, slippery elm, spearmint, valerian

ANTI-SUPPRESSANT

Essential Oils: chamomile

ANTITOXIN

Essential Oils: fennel, lavender

Herbs: lavender

ANTI-TUMOUR

Essential Oils: cloves, frankincense, reishi mushroom

Fruit: peach

Herbs: goldenseal, turkey rhubarb

ANTIVIRAL

Amino Acids, Minerals, Omega Oils, Vitamins:

Mineral: germanium

Essential Oils: cinnamon, clary sage, cloves, eucalyptus, lemon, melaleuca/tea tree oil, Myrrh, oregano oil, ravensara, rosewood, sage, tarragon, thyme

Fruit: lemon

Herbs: agrimony, aloe vera, astragalus, bearberry, bilberry, burdock, cloves, echinacea, eucalyptus, holy basil, hyssop, juniper, lemon balm, licorice root, melaleuca, mullein, myrrh, oregano, Pau d'arco, peppermint, pleurisy root, pokeweed, reishi mushroom, rose hips, white oak bark, yarrow, yellow dock

Nuts, Oils, Seeds:

Nut: coconut

Seed: pumpkin seed

Vegetables: kelp, onion (green)

ANXIETY

Herbs: cilantro, lavender

APERIENT

Herbs: cleaver

ASTRINGENT

Essential Oils: cedarwood, cinnamon, clary sage, cypress, frankincense, geranium, helichrysium/strawflower, juniper berry, lemon, myrrh, myrtle, patchouli, sandalwood

Fruit: blackberry, blueberry, lemon

Herbs: agrimony, aloe vera, amaranth, balm of Gilead, bayberry, bearberry, birch, bistort, borage, buchu, calendula, cayenne, comfrey, cramp bark, cranesbill, dandelion, gentian, goldenseal, gravel root, Irish moss, kelp, lemongrass, lobelia, marshmallow, meadowsweet, mullein, myrrh, nettle, prickly ash, primrose, raspberry, rose hips, rosemary, sage, senna, skullcap, turkey rhubarb, white oak bark, white pond lily, wild indigo, witch hazel, wormwood, yarrow, yellow dock

Nuts, Oils, Seeds:

Oil: Hazelnut Oil

CARMINATIVE

Herbs: angelica, anise seed, buchu, catnip, cayenne, chamomile, chaparral, cilantro, ginger, hyssop

CATHARTIC

Herbs: balm of Gilead, birch, blessed thistle, borage, butcher's broom, cilantro, dandelion, holy basil, juniper, licorice root, marjoram, marshmallow, mullein, myrrh, parsley, peppermint, plantain, pleurisy root, prickly ash, raspberry, senna, slippery elm, spearmint

CATHARTIC

Herbs: kelp, licorice root, mandrake, marshmallow, pleurisy root, sage, senna, turkey rhubarb, yellow dock

DECONGESTANT

Essential Oils: cypress, fennel, fir, frankincense, ginger, orange

Herbs: eucalyptus, rosemary

DEMULCENT

Herbs: aloe vera, amaranth, angelica, balm of Gilead, black walnut, calendula, chaparral, comfrey, eyebright, marshmallow, mullein, primrose, wild indigo, yarrow, yellow dock

DIAPHORETIC

Essential Oils: frankincense, marjoram, patchouli, spearmint

Herbs: arnica, astragalus, blessed thistle, buchu, catnip, cayenne, chamomile, dandelion, echinacea, garlic, ginger, horseradish, hyssop, Lady's slipper root, Mandrake, marshmallow, oatstraw, pleurisy root, prickly ash, sage, spearmint, yarrow

DIURETIC

Essential Oils: cedarwood, cypress, eucalyptus, fennel, geranium, grapefruit, juniper berry, patchouli, sage

Herbs: arnica, balm of Gilead, bayberry, bearberry, bilberry, birch, bistort, black cohosh, Burdock, butcher's broom, chamomile, chaparral, chickweed, cleaver, cramp bark, cranesbill, fennel, fenugreek, garlic, gravel root, green tea, hops, horseradish, juniper, Lady's slipper root, marjoram, meadowsweet, mullein, nettle, parsley, plantain, rose hips, spearmint, sage, sassafras, skullcap, spearmint, white poplar, yarrow

Essential Oils: frankincense, marjoram, patchouli, spearmint, radish

EMETIC

Herbs: angelica, mandrake, marshmallow, plantain

EMMENAGOGUE

Herbs: black cohosh, borage, catnip, chamomile, juniper, raspberry, sage, white poplar, wormwood

EMOLLIENT

Herbs: aloe vera, arnica, balm of Gilead, borage, calendula, chickweed, eyebright, hyssop, marshmallow, sage

EXPECTORANT

Essential Oils: marjoram, melaleuca/tea tree oil, myrtle, peppermint, ravensara, sage

Herbs: aloe vera, anise seed, arnica, Herbs: aloe vera, arnica, balm of Gilead, black cohosh, burdock, chaparral, comfrey, cramp bark, garlic, ginseng, hyssop, licorice root, marshmallow, melaleuca, myrrh, nettle, plantain, pleurisy root, rose hips

Vegetables: onion (green)

FUNGICIDE

Herbs: melaleuca, olive leaf, oregano

HEPATIC

Herbs: cascara sagrada, dandelion, ginseng, mandrake, thyme, turkey rhubarb, yellow dock

Vegetable: beet, beet greens, corn

LAXATIVE

Essential Oils: ginger, nutmeg, tarragon

NERVINE

Dairy: cheese: (goat), milk (Cow)

Essential Oils: cedarwood, chamomile (Roman), clary sage, thyme

Herbs: Angelica, black cohosh, cannabis, catnip, chamomile, chlorella, cilantro, cramp bark, ginseng, gravel root, holy basil, hops, Lady's slipper root, licorice root, mandrake, mullein, oatstraw, plantain, reishi mushroom, rosemary, skullcap, valerian

Vegetable: beet greens

PAIN RELIEVER: SEE ANODYNE

PARTURIENT

Herbs: raspberry

PECTORAL

Herbs: aloe vera, angelica, calendula, chaparral, chickweed, eyebright, garlic, hyssop, Lady's slipper root, mullein, sage

PESTICIDE

Herbs: holy basil, lemongrass

PULMONARY

Herbs: ginseng, marjoram

PURGATIVE

Herbs: turkey rhubarb, wormwood

RELAXANT

Amino Acids, Minerals, Omega Oils, Vitamins:

Vitamins: B5

Dairy: cheese (goat), milk (Cow), milk (goat)

Essential Oils: clary sage, fir, frankincense, geranium, lavender, lemongrass, marjoram, orange, patchouli, sage, sandalwood, spearmint, tangerine, ylang ylang

Herbs: agrimony, alfalfa, Ashwagandha, catnip, cinnamon, cleaver, gravel root, Lady's slipper root, lavender, lemongrass, lobelia, milk thistle, reishi mushroom

Meat:

Beef: beef liver

Poultry: turkey

RESTORATIVE

Essential Oils: cypress, fir, lemon, lemongrass, peppermint, spearmint

Herbs: lemongrass, peppermint, spearmint

RUBEFACIENT

Herbs: horseradish, prickly ash

SOOTHING

Herbs: cleaver

STIMULANT

Essential Oils: birch, eucalyptus, ginger, grapefruit, juniper berry, melaleuca/tea tree oil, oregano oil, peppermint, spearmint, tarragon, thyme

Herbs: Ashwagandha, aloe vera, arnica, balm of Gilead, barberry, bayberry, birch, borage, buchu, burdock, butcher's broom, cannabis, catnip, cayenne, chamomile, cilantro, dandelion, fenugreek, garlic, ginseng, gravel root, horseradish, hyssop, juniper, kelp, lemon balm, licorice root, marjoram, melaleuca, myrrh, oatstraw, peppermint, Peruvian bark, Plantain, prickly ash, raspberry, Red Clover, reishi mushroom, sage, lemongrass, peppermint, spearmint, white oak bark, white poplar, yarrow

STOMACHIC

Herbs: alfalfa, aloe vera, balm of Gilead, basil, cannabis, cascara sagrada, chamomile, cilantro, cloves, dandelion, fennel, fenugreek, gentian, ginseng, goldenseal, holy basil, hops, Irish moss, juniper, kelp, Lady's slipper root, lemon balm, lemongrass, Lobelia, marjoram, marshmallow, meadowsweet, mullein, peppermint, plantain, prickly ash, rose hips, rosemary, slippery elm, turkey rhubarb, valerian, white oak bark, white poplar, wormwood, yellow dock

TONIC

Herbs: angelica, balm of Gilead, basil, bayberry, bearberry, birch, black cohosh, borage, burdock, calendula, cascara sagrada, cannabis, cayenne, chamomile, chaparral, cilantro, cleaver, cloves, comfrey, cramp bark, cranesbill, dandelion, fennel, fenugreek, garlic, gentian, ginger, goldenseal, gravel root, hawthorn, hops,

Lady's slipper root, lemon balm, lemongrass, lobelia, mandrake, parsley, pleurisy root, Red Clover, rose hips, rosemary, sage, sassafras, Skullcap, Lemongrass, peppermint, spearmint, turkey rhubarb, valerian, white oak bark, white poplar, witch hazel, wormwood, yarrow, yellow dock

VERMICIDE

Herbs: lobelia, mandrake, olive leaf, Pau d'arco, senna, thyme, valerian, white oak bark, wormwood

Ailments and Alternative Options

Please keep in mind: This book is not to be used as a diagnosis or as a prescription of any kind. The information is for those who are curious as to how the earth medicines can work with our body for better health and well-being.

Caution: The information from each essential oil, fruit, grain, herb, nut/oil/seed and vegetable must also be taken into consideration, as some of them have cautionary notes and specific warnings for who can consume some of the earth medicines and foods.

ABDOMEN

Amino Acids, Minerals, Omega Oils, Vitamins: Vitamins: B1

ACID REFLUX

Herbs: fennel

Acne: See Skin: Acne

ADDICTIONS

Amino Acids, Minerals, Omega Oils, Vitamins: Amino Acid: l-glutamine

ADDISON'S DISEASE

Herb: licorice root

ADHD

Nuts, Oils, Seeds: Seed: hemp seed

ADRENAL FATIGUE

Essential Oils: sage, spruce

Herbs: licorice root

Meat: Lake, ocean, river, sea: fish oils

ADRENAL GLANDS

Amino Acids, Minerals, Omega Oils, Vitamins:

Amino Acid: l-tyrosine

Vitamins: A, B2, B5, B12

Dairy: butter, cheese: cow, cheese: goat, milk: cow, milk: goat

Grains: buckwheat, couscous, millet, oat, quinoa, rice (brown and white), rye, spelt, wheat, wheat bran, wheat germ

Herbs: astragalus, borage, ginseng, kelp, licorice root, milk thistle, slippery elm

Meat:

Beef: beef, calf liver, beef kidney, beef liver

Lake, ocean, river, sea: fish: fresh water, fish oils

Pork: pork

Poultry: chicken, egg

Nuts, Oils, Seeds:

Seed: chia seed

AGE SPOTS: SEE SKIN

AGING

Amino Acids, Minerals, Omega Oils, Vitamins:

Vitamin: coenzyme Q10

Fruit: blackberry, cranberry, plum/prune

Nuts, Oils, Seeds: Oil: hemp seed oil

Vegetable: rutabaga.

AIDS

Amino Acids, Minerals, Omega Oils, Vitamins:

Mineral: germanium, selenium

Dairy: whey

Herbs: astragalus, bearberry, cannabis, chaparral, echinacea, garlic, licorice root, olive leaf, Pau d'arco, red clover, reishi mushroom, turmeric

Nuts, Oils, Seeds: Nut: coconut

ALCOHOLISM

Amino Acids, Minerals, Omega Oils, Vitamins:

Amino Acid: l-glutamine, l-lysine

Essential Oils: ginger

Herbs: alfalfa, cayenne, ginger, primrose, valerian

ALLERGIES

Amino Acids, Minerals, Omega Oils, Vitamins:

Mineral: germanium

Vitamin: C, coenzyme Q10

Essential Oils: lavender, patchouli, pina

Fruit: grape / raisin

Herbs: alfalfa, aloe vera, eyebright, lavender, licorice root, mandrake, parsley, reishi mushroom

Vegetable: onion (green)

ALZHEIMER'S

Amino Acids, Minerals, Omega Oils, Vitamins:

Vitamins: choline

Fruit: grape / raisin, rhubarb, tomato

Herbs: cilantro, sage

Legume: peanut

Nuts, Oils, Seeds:

oil: coconut oil, sesame seed oil

Amino Acids, Minerals, Omega Oils, Vitamins:

Amino Acid: Better Absorption

Vitamins: B6

ANEMIA

Amino Acids, Minerals, Omega Oils, Vitamins:

Amino Acid: l-lysine

Mineral: copper, iron, manganese

Vitamins: A, B5, B12, C

Dairy: cheese (cow), cheese (goat), milk (cow), milk (goat)

Essential Oils: lemon

Fruit: date, plum /prune

Grains: barley.

Herbs: calendula, fennel, ginseng, hawthorn, horsetail, Pau d'arco, thyme, yellow dock

Legumes: black-eyed peas, garbanzo beans, kidney beans, lentil

Meat:

Beef: beef kidney, beef liver

Lake, ocean, river, sea: clams, fish: fresh water

Lamb: lamb

Pork: pork

Nuts, Oils, Seeds:

Nut: Brazil nut, hazelnut

Vegetable: beet, beet greens, dulse, kohlrabi, spinach, turnip

ANGER

Essential Oils: cedarwood, myrtle

ANGINA

Amino Acids, Minerals, Omega Oils, Vitamins:

Vitamin: E

Essential Oils: ginger, orange

Herbs: hawthorn.

ANOREXIA

Essential Oils: tarragon

Herbs: gentian

ANTIBODIES

Amino Acids, Minerals, Omega Oils, Vitamins:

Vitamins: B1, B5

ANXIETY

Amino Acids, Minerals, Omega Oils, Vitamins:

Amino Acid: l-taurine

Mineral: manganese, phosphorus

Vitamins: B3, B5, inositol

Essential Oils: bergamot, cedarwood, chamomile (roman), lavender, lemon, marjoram, patchouli, ylang ylang

Fruits: tangerine

Herbs: chamomile, cinnamon, skullcap

Meat:

Beef: beef, beef liver

Lake, ocean, river, sea: clams, fish: saltwater, halibut, herring, mackerel, salmon, sardines, tuna

Lamb

Pork

APHRODISIAC

Essential Oils: sandalwood, thyme

APPENDICITIS

Essential Oils: melaleuca/tea tree, patchouli

Herbs: alfalfa, melaleuca, slippery elm

Appetite: to reduce

Amino Acids, Minerals, Omega Oils, Vitamins:

Amino Acid: l-tyrosine

Vitamins: B1

Herbs: fennel, green tea, red clover

Legume: lentil

Nuts, Oils, Seeds:

Nut: pine nut

Oil: Siberian pine nut oil

Nuts, Oils, Seeds: Seed: chia seed

APPETITE: TO STIMULANT

Essential Oils: bergamot, ginger, grapefruit, myrrh, nutmeg, orange, spearmint, tarragon

Herbs: angelica, blessed thistle, cannabis, chamomile, ginseng, milk thistle, oregano, Parsley, wormwood, yarrow

Meat:

Beef: beef liver

Vegetable: onion (green), spinach

ARTERIES

Amino Acids, Minerals, Omega Oils, Vitamins:

Mineral: silicon

Vitamins: folate, inositol

Fruit: grape/raisin

Essential Oils: lemongrass, marjoram, ylang ylang

Grains: buckwheat, cereal grain, couscous, millet, oat, rice (white), rye, spelt, wheat, wheat bran, wheat germ

Herbs: butcher's broom, kelp, Pau d'arco, skullcap

Legumes: kidney bean, navy bean

Nuts, Oils, Seeds:

Nut: Brazil nut, hazelnut, pecan, pine nut

Oil: hemp seed oil, sesame seed oil, Siberian pine nut oil, sunflower seed

Vegetable: kale, lettuce (romaine)

ARTERIES: PLAQUE BUILD-UP

Fruit: grape / raisin

Grain: millet, quinoa

Herbs: milk thistle

Vegetables: kale

ARTERIOSCLEROSIS

Herbs: ginseng

ARTHRITIS

Amino Acids, Minerals, Omega Oils, Vitamins:

Amino Acid: l-glutamine

Mineral: germanium

Omega Oil: omega 3, omega 6

Vitamins: B3, B6, paba, C

Essential Oils: bay, birch oil, cloves, cypress, lavender, marjoram, peppermint, pina, rosemary, sage, spruce, tarragon

Fruit: cherry, kiwi, lemon, papaya, passion fruit, pineapple, raspberry, Saskatoon berry

Herbs: alfalfa, angelica, astragalus, barberry, burdock, cayenne, chamomile, chaparral, horsetail, lobelia, oatstraw, olive leaf, oregano, prickly ash, primrose, turmeric

Meat:

Beef: beef, beef kidney

Lake, ocean, river, sea: clams

Lamb

Poultry: chicken, egg

Nuts, Oils, Seeds:

Nut: pecan

Oil: avocado oil, grapeseed oil

Seed: hemp seed, mustard seed, sesame seed

Vegetables: mushroom (white), onion (green), pea, sweet potato, Swiss chard, turnip

ARTHRITIS: RHEUMATOID

Essential Oils: bay, birch

Herbs: alfalfa, aloe vera juice, cannabis, cayenne, chaparral, devil's claw, balm of Gilead, burdock, nettle, Pau d'arco, pleurisy root, pokeweed

ASIAN FLU

Herbs: peppermint

ASTHMA

Amino Acids, Minerals, Omega Oils, Vitamins:

Omega Oil: omega 3, omega 6

Vitamin: coenzyme Q10

Essential Oils: cedarwood, chamomile (Roman), cypress, eucalyptus, fir, frankincense, lavender, lemon, oregano oil, peppermint, pina, sage, thyme

Fruit: mango, passion fruit

Grain: rye

Herbs: alfalfa leaf, black cohosh root, bearberry, chickweed, comfrey, cramp bark, eucalyptus, garlic, green tea, hyssop, juniper, kelp, lavender, licorice root, lobelia, mandrake, marjoram, marshmallow, mullein, myrrh, nettle, oregano, parsley, Pau d'arco, pleurisy root, red clover, reishi mushroom, slippery elm, thyme, white pond lily

Meat: lamb

Nuts, Oils, Seeds:

Nut: cashew

Seed: hemp seed, mustard seed, sesame seed, sunflower seed

Vegetables: onion (green), radish, squash, sweet potato

ATHEROSCLEROSIS

Vegetable: mustard greens

ATHLETIC ENDURANCE

Vegetable: potato

ATHLETES FOOT

Essential Oils: melaleuca/tea tree

Herbs: Chickweed, melaleuca, oregano, thyme

Vegetables: onion (red)

ATTENTION DISORDER

Amino Acids, Minerals, Omega Oils, Vitamins:

Omega Oil: omega 3, omega 6

AUTOIMMUNE DISEASE

Amino Acids, Minerals, Omega Oils, Vitamins: l-glutamine

Fruit: blackberry

BAD BREATH

Essential Oils: cloves, frankincense, spearmint

Herbs: caraway seed, cloves, wormwood

BACK PAIN

Herbs: gravel root

BACTERIA: SEE INFECTIONS

BEE STINGS

Herbs: oregano, rose hips

Vegetable: onion (red)

BED SORES

Herbs: melaleuca, myrrh

BED-WETTING

Herbs: bearberry, marjoram, oatstraw, parsley, plantain, white poplar

BELCHING

Essential Oils: tarragon

BILE

Amino Acids, Minerals, Omega Oils, Vitamins:

Mineral: sulfur

Herb: dandelion root

BI-POLAR

Amino Acids, Minerals, Omega Oils, Vitamins:

Vitamins: choline

BITES: INSECT

Essential Oils: frankincense

Herbs: basil, calendula, holy basil, melaleuca, oregano, rose hips, white oak bark, witch hazel, wormwood

BITES: SNAKE
Essential Oils: frankincense

Herbs: basil, echinacea

BLADDER: CANCER
Vegetables: broccoli

BLADDER: CLEANSER
Fruit: cranberry

Herbs: yellow dock

BLADDER: GRAVEL
Herbs: valerian

BLADDER: INFECTION
Essential Oils: lemongrass

Herbs: blue cohosh, buchu, horsetail, Irish moss, juniper, marshmallow, oregano, plantain

BLADDER: INFLAMMATION
Herbs: bearberry, spearmint, white oak bark, yarrow

BLADDER: SUPPORT
Fruit: cherry, chokecherry, cranberry

Herbs: balm of Gilead, basil, bearberry, birch, butcher's broom, cleaver, dandelion, gravel root, green tea, Irish moss, juniper, lemongrass, marjoram, nettle, oatstraw, Peruvian bark, plantain, rose hips, sassafras, skullcap, slippery elm, white poplar, yarrow

BLADDER: TONE: AFTER GIVING BIRTH
Herbs: mullein

BLADDER: ULCERATED
Herbs: white oak bark

BLEEDING: TO STOP THE BLEEDING
Essential Oils: lemon

Herbs: bayberry, bistort, cayenne, cranesbill, ginseng, witch hazel, wormwood

BLEPHARITIS
Herbs: eyebright

BLOOD CELL FORMATION
Amino Acids, Minerals, Omega Oils, Vitamins:

Mineral: copper, potassium

Vitamin: biotin

BLOOD: CELL SUPPORT
Amino Acids, Minerals, Omega Oils, Vitamins:

Mineral: germanium, molybdenum

Vitamins: A

Fruit: blackberry

Vegetable: mustard greens

BLOOD: CIRCULATION
Amino Acids, Minerals, Omega Oils, Vitamins:

Vitamins: B1, B3, folate

Essential Oils: chamomile: roman, cinnamon, cypress, helichrysium/strawflower, lemon, marjoram, melaleuca/tea tree, nutmeg, orange, sage, thyme

Fruit: passion fruit, pineapple, rhubarb

Herbs: aloe vera, bayberry, bilberry, black cohosh, blessed thistle, butcher's broom, cayenne, chlorella, calendula, catnip, cayenne, chamomile, chickweed, cinnamon, cloves, garlic, ginger, ginseng, hyssop, lobelia, melaleuca, myrrh, nettle, prickly ash, reishi mushroom, rose hips, rosemary, turmeric, valerian, wild indigo, wormwood, yarrow

Legumes: navy bean, soybean

Meat:

Beef: beef kidney, beef liver

Lake, Ocean, River, Sea: clams, fish oils

Pork

Poultry: chicken, egg, egg yolk

Nuts, Oils, Seeds:

Nut: almond

Vegetable: dulse, kohlrabi, onion (Green), squash

BLOOD: CHOLESTEROL TO LOWER

Amino Acids, Minerals, Omega Oils, Vitamins:

Omega Oil: omega 3, omega 6

Fruit: papaya

Herbs: Ashwagandha, bilberry, black cohosh, black walnut, butcher's broom, dandelion, fenugreek, ginger, ginseng, green tea, hawthorn, holy basil, milk thistle, myrrh, reishi mushroom, thyme, turmeric

Legumes: bean (black), lima bean

Nuts, Oils, Seeds:

Nut: almond, Brazil nut, coconut

Oil: avocado oil, coconut oil, grapeseed oil, Siberian pine nut oil

Seed: sesame seed, sunflower seed

Vegetable: artichoke, cauliflower, collards, pepper (Bell), squash, squash

BLOOD: CLEANSER AND SUPPORT

Amino Acids, Minerals, Omega Oils, Vitamins:

Amino Acid: l-taurine

Mineral: molybdenum, sulfur

Vitamins: B2, B3

Dairy: cheese (cow), cheese (goat), milk (cow), milk (goat)

Fruit: apple, apricot, avocado, goji berry, gooseberry, grape/raisin, lemon, lime, orange, papaya, passion fruit, peach, pear, raspberry, strawberry, tomato, watermelon

Grains: barley, cereal grain, corn, couscous, millet, oat, quinoa, rice (brown and white), spelt, wheat, wheat bran, wheat germ

Herbs: alfalfa, agrimony, anise seed, balm of Gilead, barberry, birch, black cohosh, blessed thistle, burdock, butcher's broom, cannabis, calendula, cayenne, chlorella, dandelion root, helichrysium/strawflower, red clover, lemon, caraway seed, chaparral, chickweed, cilantro, comfrey, dandelion, echinacea, eyebright, fennel, gentian, ginger, green tea, hawthorn, holy basil, Irish moss, kelp, lemongrass, licorice root, lobelia, mandrake, marshmallow, mullein, nettle, oatstraw, olive leaf, oregano, parsley, Pau d'arco, Peruvian bark, plantain, pokeweed, prickly ash, raspberry, red clover, rose hips, rosemary, sage, sassafras, slippery elm, spearmint, turmeric, white oak bark, wild indigo, yarrow, yellow dock, yellow dock

Legumes: bean (red), carob, garbanzo bean, kidney bean, lima bean, navy bean

Meat:

Beef: beef, beef liver, calf liver

Lake, ocean, river, sea: fish: saltwater, halibut, herring, mackerel, salmon, sardines, tuna

Lamb

Pork

Poultry: egg, turkey

Nuts, Oils, Seeds:

Nut: almond, Brazil nut, hazelnut, macadamia nut, pecan, pine nut

Oil: almond oil

Seed: chia seed, cacao, pumpkin seed, sesame seed, sunflower seed

Vegetable: beet, beet greens, broccoli, Brussel sprout, celery, collards, corn, dulse, garlic, kale, kelp, lettuce (iceberg), mushroom (white), mustard greens, pepper (bell), radish, rutabaga, squash, Swiss chard, squash

BLOOD: CLOTTING TO PROMOTE

Amino Acids, Minerals, Omega Oils, Vitamins:

Mineral: calcium, phosphorus

Vitamin: E, K

Fruit: cranberry, currant (red)

Dairy: buckwheat, oat

Herbs: green tea, horsetail, juniper, reishi mushroom

Meat:

Beef: beef: calf liver

Lamb

Vegetable: sweet potato

BLOOD: CLOTTING TO REDUCE

Nuts, Oils, Seeds:

Oil: hemp seed oil (reduce), walnut oil

BLOOD: HEMORRHAGING

Herbs: mullein, nettle, Pau d'arco, plantain, white oak bark

BLOOD: HDL, LDL REGULATE

Fruit: cranberry

Nuts, Oils, Seeds:

Oil: cotton seed oil, olive oil, sesame seed oil

BLOOD POISONING

Herbs: marshmallow, plantain, pleurisy root

BLOOD PRESSURE: TOO LOW

Essential Oils: rosemary, sage

Herbs: cayenne, cloves, parsley, pleurisy root

BLOOD PRESSURE: TOO HIGH

Amino Acids, Minerals, Omega Oils, Vitamins:

Mineral: selenium

Omega Oil: omega 3, omega 6

Vitamin: coenzyme Q10

Dairy: whey

Essential Oils: frankincense, lavender, marjoram, ylang ylang

Fruit: banana, passion fruit

Grains: buckwheat

Herbs: alfalfa, aloe vera, astragalus, barberry, black cohosh root, blue cohosh, borage oil, cayenne, evening primrose, fennel, green tea, kelp, lavender, lemongrass, nettle, parsley, primrose, reishi mushroom, skullcap

Legumes: black-eyed peas, lentil

Nuts, Oils, Seeds:

Nut: pecan

Seed: cacao, hemp seed, mustard seed, sesame seed

Vegetable: bean (snap), dulse, lettuce (romaine), rutabaga, squash, Swiss chard

BLOOD PRESSURE: TO REGULATE

Amino Acids, Minerals, Omega Oils, Vitamins:

Mineral: potassium, selenium, sodium

Fruit: cherry, grapefruit, guava, raspberry

Herbs: astragalus, black walnut, cayenne, ginseng, hyssop, juniper, rosemary, yarrow

Legumes: kidney bean, navy bean, pinto bean

Nuts, Oils, Seeds:

Nut: walnut

Vegetable: asparagus, Brussel sprout, kohlrabi, onion (red), parsnip, potato, radish

Blood: Red Blood Cells

Amino Acids, Minerals, Omega Oils, Vitamins:

Mineral: iron

Vitamin: B12, folate, inositol, paba

Fruit: date

Meat: clams

Nuts, Oils, Seeds:

Nut: pecan

BLOOD SUGAR: REGULATE

Amino Acids, Minerals, Omega Oils, Vitamins:

Amino Acid: l-glutamine

Mineral: chromium, manganese, vanadium

Vitamin: biotin

Dairy: whey

Essential Oils: cinnamon

Fruit: blueberry, blueberry, cherry, currant (red), fig, kiwi, raspberry, Saskatoon berry, strawberry

Grains: buckwheat, rye

Herbs: alfalfa, Ashwagandha, cinnamon, bearberry, bilberry, black walnut, buchu, burdock, cilantro, cinnamon, fenugreek, garlic, goldenseal, kelp, marshmallow, Pau d'arco, reishi mushroom

Legumes: bean (Black and White), garbanzo bean, kidney bean, lima bean, navy bean, pinto bean

Nuts, Oils, Seeds:

Nut: walnut

Oil: hemp seed oil

Seed: chia seed, flaxseed

Vegetable: asparagus, bean (lima and snap), cabbage, corn, garlic, pea, Spinach, Sweet potato, Swiss chard

BLOOD SUGAR: TO HIGH

Herbs: holy basil, milk thistle

BLOOD SUGAR: TOO LOW

Herbs: goldenseal, green tea, licorice root, skullcap

BLOOD: THINNER

Herbs: bilberry

BLOOD: WHITE BLOOD CELLS – TO BUILD UP

Amino Acids, Minerals, Omega Oils, Vitamins:

Vitamins: folate

Herbs: echinacea

Blood: White Blood Cells – to slow down

Herbs: garlic

BOILS: SEE SKIN

BONE: BROKEN

Dairy: cheese (cow), milk (cow), milk (goat), whey, yogurt

Essential Oils: ginger or ginger root,

Herbs: arnica, horsetail, Irish moss

BONE: DEVELOPMENT / GROWTH

Amino Acids, Minerals, Omega Oils, Vitamins:

Amino Acid: l-lysine

Mineral: manganese, phosphorus, silicon, vanadium, zinc

Vitamins: A

Dairy: butter, cheese (cow), cheese (goat), milk (cow), milk (goat), yogurt

Legumes: garbanzo beans

Meat:

Beef: beef, beef Liver

Pork: pork

BONE: HEALTH

Amino Acids, Minerals, Omega Oils, Vitamins:

Mineral: molybdenum

Vitamin: C, E

Dairy: butter

Fruit: peach, pineapple, rhubarb, tangerine

Vegetables: artichoke, squash

BONES, JOINTS, CARTILAGE, TENDONS: SUPPORT

Amino Acids, Minerals, Omega Oils, Vitamins:

Amino Acid: l-glutamine

Mineral: boron, calcium

Vitamins: B6, C, D

Dairy: butter, cheese (cow), milk (cow), milk (goat), whey, yogurt

Essential Oils: spruce

Fruit: avocado, blackberry, cantaloupe, mango, passion fruit, tomato

Grains: buckwheat, millet, oat, quinoa, wheat, wheat bran, wheat Germ

Herbs: arnica, bilberry, blue cohosh, horsetail, Irish moss, marshmallow, mullein, nettle, oatstraw, Pau d'arco, raspberry, skullcap

Legumes: bean (red), navy bean, soybean

Meat:

Beef: beef: calf liver, beef liver

Lake, ocean, river, sea: fish: oils, herring

Poultry: turkey

Nuts, Oils, Seeds:

Nut: cashew, coconut, hazelnut, walnut

Oil: avocado oil

Seed: sesame seed

Vegetable: bean (snap), dulse, kohlrabi, lettuce (romaine), mushroom (white), radish, squash, Swiss chard, squash

BONE MARROW

Amino Acids, Minerals, Omega Oils, Vitamins:

Vitamins: folate

BONE: RHEUMATIC PAIN

Herbs: black cohosh, burdock, cannabis, gravel root, cannabis, hawthorn, hops, horseradish, Irish moss, lavender, lobelia, mandrake, mullein, nettle, oatstraw, pleurisy root, pokeweed, prickly ash, sassafras, skullcap, slippery elm, wild indigo, wormwood, yarrow, yellow dock

BONE SPURS

Essential Oils: birch

Herbs: turmeric,

Minerals: calcium and magnesium

Vitamins: vitamin B Complex with extra vitamin B6.

BOWEL: BLEEDING

Herbs: chickweed, mullein, yarrow, yellow dock

Minerals: magnesium

BOWEL: INFLAMMATION

Herbs: milk thistle, Pau d'arco, red clover

BOWEL: SUPPORT

Amino Acids, Minerals, Omega Oils, Vitamins:

Mineral: magnesium

Minerals, Omega Oils, Vitamins:

Vitamins: inositol

Fruit: banana, cherry, date, fig, guava, kiwi, passion fruit, pear, plum/prune, rhubarb, watermelon

Grains: buckwheat, cereal grain, corn, couscous, millet, oat, rice (brown and white), rye, spelt, wheat, wheat bran, wheat germ

Herbs: amaranth, balm of Gilead, barberry, bearberry, bilberry, bistort, cascara sagrada, chaparral, chlorella, fennel, fenugreek, gentian, ginger, Irish moss, kelp, mandrake, meadowsweet, melaleuca, oatstraw, Pau d'arco, peppermint, Peruvian bark, red clover, rose hips, slippery elm, valerian, yarrow, yellow dock, rutabaga

Legumes: beans (white), black-eyed pea, garbanzo bean, kidney bean, navy bean, pinto bean

Nuts, Oils, Seeds:

Nut: hazelnut

Oil: sesame seed oil

Seed: chia seed, cacao, flaxseed

Vegetable: radish, rutabaga, sweet potato

BRAIN CELLS

Fruit: rhubarb

Vegetable: potato

BRAIN DEVELOPMENT AND FUNCTION

Amino Acids, Minerals, Omega Oils, Vitamins:

Amino Acid: l-taurine

Mineral: boron

Vitamins: B6, folate

BRAIN: MEMORY

Fruit: cherry

Herb: sage

Nuts, Oils, Seeds: oil: walnut oil

BRAIN: SUPPORT

Amino Acids, Minerals, Omega Oils, Vitamins:

Amino Acid: l-glutamine

Mineral: boron, iodine

Vitamins: B1, folate, inositol

Fruit: goji berry

Herbs: Ashwagandha, fennel, ginger, rosemary

Legumes: kidney beans, lentil

Meat:

Beef: beef, beef kidney, beef liver,

Lake, ocean, river, sea: fish: fresh water, fish: oils, fish: saltwater, halibut, herring, mackerel, salmon, sardines, tuna

Poultry: egg, egg yolk, pork, turkey

Nuts, Oils, Seeds:

Nut: pecan

Oil: grapeseed oil, sesame seed oil, walnut oil

Seed: sunflower seed

Vegetables: artichoke, bean (lima), Brussel sprout, dulse, pumpkin

BREAST CANCER / PREVENTION

Fruit: blackberry, mango, peach, tomato

Herb: milk thistle

Legume: lima bean

Vegetables: broccoli, mushroom (white)

BREASTFEEDING: LACTATION INFLAMMATION

Herb: chickweed

BREASTFEEDING: STOP LACTATION

Herb: sage

BREAST: INFLAMED

Herbs: white pond lily, wild indigo

BREAST: SORE NIPPLES

Herbs: cranesbill, yarrow

BREAST: TUMOURS

Herbs: cleaver, dandelion, milk thistle

BREAST: SUPPORT

Fruit: cherry

Grain: rye

Nuts, Oils, Seeds:

Nut: walnut

Oil: olive oil

Seed: hemp seed

BREATH FRESHENER

Herbs: myrrh, parsley

BRIGHT'S DISEASE

Herbs: cranesbill

BRONCHIAL CONGESTION

Essential Oils: eucalyptus, melaleuca/tea tree

Herbs: aloe vera, balm of Gilead, bayberry, garlic, horsetail, licorice root, mullein, sage, sassafras, yarrow

BRONCHITIS

Essential Oils: basil, bergamot, cedarwood, clary sage, cloves, cypress, eucalyptus, fir, frankincense, lavender, marjoram, melaleuca/tea tree, myrrh, myrtle, orange, Oregano Oil, peppermint, pina, ravensara, rosemary, sage, sandalwood, spruce, thyme

Herbs: angelica, balm of Gilead, bearberry, borage, caraway seed, catnip, chickweed, echinacea, eucalyptus, fennel, ginseng, horsetail, hyssop, Irish moss, lavender, lobelia, melaleuca, myrrh, oregano, Pau d'arco, plantain. pleurisy root, red clover, sage, sassafras, slippery elm, spearmint, thyme, valerian, yarrow, yellow dock

BRUISES: SEE SKIN

BURNING SENSATION

Amino Acids, Minerals, Omega Oils, Vitamins:

Vitamins: B6

BURNS: SEE SKIN

BURSITIS

Essential Oils: cypress, marjoram

Herbs: alfalfa, oatstraw

CALCIUM ABSORPTION

Amino Acids, Minerals, Omega Oils, Vitamins:

Amino Acid: l-lysine

CANCER PREVENTION

Amino Acids, Minerals, Omega Oils, Vitamins:

Mineral: calcium, germanium, molybdenum, selenium

Vitamins: A, C

Dairy: whey

Essential Oils: frankincense

Fruit: blackberry, blueberry, cantaloupe, cranberry, currant (red), ate, fig, goji berry, gooseberry, guava, lemon, passion fruit, peach, plum / prune, raspberry, strawberry, tomato, watermelon

Grain: rye

Herbs: alfalfa, astragalus, bilberry, black walnut, cannabis, chaparral, eucalyptus, fennel, garlic, Irish moss, mandrake, milk thistle, parsley, Pau d'arco, reishi mushroom, rose hips, rosemary, sassafras, turmeric, white oak bark, yarrow, yellow dock

Legumes: carob, garbanzo beans, lentil, pinto bean, soybean

Nuts, Oils, Seeds:

Nut: almond, Brazil nut, hazelnut, pistachio, walnut

oil: almond oil, grapeseed oil, hazelnut oil, sesame seed oil, walnut oil

Seed: cacao, flaxseed, hemp seed, pumpkin seed

Vegetable: cabbage, collards, collards, garlic, kale, lettuce (romaine), mustard greens, onion (red), potato, pumpkin, radish, turnip

CANDIDA

Amino Acids, Minerals, Omega Oils, Vitamins:

Mineral: germanium

Dairy: yogurt

Essential Oils: bergamot, eucalyptus, frankincense, melaleuca/tea tree, myrtle, rosewood, sandalwood, spearmint, spruce, thyme

Grains: barley

Herbs: chickweed, garlic, melaleuca, oregano, Pau d'arco

Nuts, Oils, Seeds:

Nut: coconut

Oil: coconut oil

Seed: flaxseed

Vegetable: garlic

CARBUNCLES

Essential Oils: frankincense, lavender

Herbs: chickweed, marshmallow

CARDIAC SPASM: SEE HEART

CARDIOVASCULAR: SEE HEART SUPPORT

CARDIOVASCULAR DISEASE

Amino Acids, Minerals, Omega Oils, Vitamins:

Mineral: calcium, silicon

Vitamin: E

Nuts, Oils, Seeds:

Oil: almond oil, coconut oil

Seed: sunflower seed

CARPAL TUNNEL SYNDROME

Herbs: butcher's broom

CARTILAGE
Amino Acids, Minerals, Omega Oils, Vitamins:

Mineral: manganese

CATARACTS
Herbs: bilberry, eyebright

Nuts, Oils, Seeds:

Nut: pistachio

Oil: avocado oil

Vegetable: carrots, kale. pepper (bell), spinach

CATARRH
Essential Oils: myrrh, sage, sandalwood

Herbs: lobelia, pokeweed

CELIAC DISEASE
Nuts, Oils, Seeds: Nut: almond, Brazil nut, pine nut

CELLULITE
Essential Oils: cedarwood, fennel, grapefruit, lemongrass, patchouli, rosemary, sage, Tangerine

Herbs: cedarwood, fennel

Nuts, Seeds, Oil: Oil: coconut oil

CEREBRAL SYSTEM STIMULANT
Amino Acids, Minerals, Omega Oils, Vitamins:

Amino Acid: l-glutamine

Essential Oils: nutmeg,

CERVICITIS
Herbs: meadowsweet

CERVICAL CANCER: PREVENTION
Fruit: blackberry

CIRRHOSIS
Herbs: milk thistle

CHEMICAL POISONING
Herbs: ginseng, white oak bark

CHEMOTHERAPY: TO REDUCE EFFECTS
Amino Acids, Minerals, Omega Oils, Vitamins:

Vitamin: coenzyme Q10

Herbs: white oak bark

CHEST INFECTIONS
Herbs: hyssop

CHEST: CONGESTION
Essential Oils: fir

Herbs: hyssop, marjoram, yarrow

CHEST: PAIN
Amino Acids, Minerals, Omega Oils, Vitamins:

Vitamins: B1

CHICKEN POX
Essential Oils: blue chamomile, calamine, lavender

Herbs: yarrow

CHILBLAINS: ULCERS ON THE FEET
Herbs: horseradish

CHILDBIRTH
Herbs: blue cohosh, raspberry, white poplar, yarrow

Childbirth: Stop Cramping and Pain Afterwards

Herbs: sassafras

Childbirth: Vaginal Inflammation after giving birth

Herbs: witch hazel

CHILLS
Herbs: spearmint

Vegetable: onion (green)

CHOLERA
Essential Oils: rosemary

Herbs: bistort, cranesbill, olive leaf

CHOLESTEROL: TO LOWER
Amino Acids, Minerals, Omega Oils, Vitamins:

Mineral: calcium

Omega Oil: omega 9

Vitamins: B3, C

Essential Oils: clary sage, helichrysium/strawflower, orange

Fruit: currant (red), date, orange, Saskatoon berry, tomato

Grains: buckwheat, cereal grain

Herbs: alfalfa, aloe vera, butcher's broom, kale, kelp, lettuce (romaine)

Legumes: bean (white), garbanzo bean, kidney bean, navy bean, pinto bean

Meat:

Lamb

Nuts, Oils, Seeds:

Nut: pecan, pine nut, pistachio

Oil: avocado oil, hemp seed oil

Seed: chia seed, flaxseed, sesame seed, sunflower seed

Vegetable: onion (green and red), parsnip, rutabaga, spinach

CHLAMYDIA
Herbs: olive leaf

CHRONIC FATIGUE
Herbs: bilberry, echinacea, olive leaf, reishi mushroom, skullcap

CHRONIC PAIN

Fruit: cherry

Vegetable: turnip

CIRCULATION: SEE BLOOD CIRCULATION

COLDS

Fruit: lemon, oranges, pineapple

Essential Oils: basil, cinnamon, eucalyptus, fir, ginger, lemon, marjoram, melaleuca/tea Tree, orange, rosemary

Herbs: angelica, astragalus, chickweed, echinacea, oregano oil, peppermint, basil, eyebright, juniper, lemon balm, meadowsweet (adults only, and not pregnant women), melaleuca, olive leaf, oregano, rose hips, slippery elm, spearmint, wild indigo, wormwood, yarrow

Vegetables: onion (green)

COLD SORES

Amino Acids, Minerals, Omega Oils, Vitamins:

Amino Acid: l-lysine

Essential Oils: melaleuca/tea tree

Herbs: melaleuca, oregano, peppermint

COLLAGEN FORMATION

Amino Acids, Minerals, Omega Oils, Vitamins:

Mineral: zinc

COLIC

Essential Oils: bergamot, chamomile: blue, fennel, marjoram

Herbs: angelica, anise seed, blue cohosh, caraway seed, chamomile, cinnamon, fennel, Lady's slipper root, lemongrass, lobelia, marjoram, peppermint, prickly ash, raspberry, senna, spearmint

COLITIS: PREVENTION (INFLAMMATION OF THE COLON LINING)

Essential Oils: helichrysium/strawflower, peppermint, tarragon, thyme

Herbs: cloves, kelp, Pau d'arco, reishi mushroom, slippery elm, collards

Legumes: beans (black)

COLON CANCER: PREVENTATIVE
Dairy: buttermilk
Fruit: apple, blackberry, date, grape/raisin, kiwi, mango, orange, papaya
Legume: peanut
Vegetables: broccoli, corn, kelp, onion (green)

COLON: CLEANSER
Herbs: licorice root, myrrh, Pau d'arco, yellow dock
Nuts, Oils, Seeds: flaxseed

COLON: SUPPORT
Amino Acids, Minerals, Omega Oils, Vitamins:
Vitamin: C
Fruit: date, Saskatoon berry
Legumes: bean (black), garbanzo bean, lima bean, peanut
Nuts, Oils, Seeds:
Nut: almond
Oil: almond Oil
Seed: flaxseed, pumpkin feed, fesame feed, funflower feed
Vegetables: broccoli, carrots, lettuce (romaine)

COLON: SWELLING
Herbs: buchu, catnip, cloves, ginger

CONCENTRATION
Amino Acids, Minerals, Omega Oils, Vitamins:
Amino Acid: l-lysine
Essential Oils: basil

CONCUSSIONS
Amino Acids, Minerals, Omega Oils, Vitamins:
Omega Oil: omega 3, omega 6, omega 9

Herbs: arnica

CONSTIPATION

Amino Acids, Minerals, Omega Oils, Vitamins:

Mineral: magnesium, potassium

Essential Oils: cedarwood, ginger, marjoram, orange, spearmint, tangerine

Fruit: cherry, guava, plum/prune, rhubarb

Herbs: aloe vera juice, barberry, bayberry bark, cannabis, cascara sagrada, balm of Gilead, cascara sagrada, chlorella, cleaver, dandelion, fenugreek, gentian, kelp, lobelia, mandrake, marshmallow, oatstraw, senna, slippery elm, wormwood

Legumes: black-eyed pea, lentil, navy bean

Nuts, Oils, Seeds:

Nut: hazelnut

Seed: flaxseed

Vegetable: onion (red), parsnip, rutabaga, squash

CONSTIPATION DURING PREGNANCY:

Essential Oils: cedarwood, fennel, ginger, ginger root, juniper.

CONSUMPTION

Herbs: mullein

CONTAGIOUS DISEASES

Essential Oils: ginger, ginger root,

Herbs: aloe vera, licorice root, slippery elm,

CONVULSIONS

Amino Acids, Minerals, Omega Oils, Vitamins:

Mineral: manganese

Vitamins: B6, D

Essential Oils: chamomile: blue, lavender

Herbs: anise seed, catnip, cramp bark, lavender, lobelia, marjoram, skullcap, valerian

CORONARY DISEASE

Nuts, Oils, Seeds:

Oil: almond oil, sesame seed oil

CORONARY SUPPORT

Nuts, Oils, Seeds:

Nut: macadamia nut

Oil: sesame seed oil

COUGHS

Essential Oils: cinnamon, cypress, eucalyptus, frankincense, oregano, melaleuca/tea tree

Fruit: pineapple

Herbs: angelica, balm of Gilead, chickweed, oregano, cinnamon, comfrey, echinacea, eyebright, fennel, horseradish, lemongrass, lobelia, marjoram, melaleuca, mullein, oregano, plantain, pleurisy root, red clover, slippery elm, spearmint, thyme, valerian

CRABS

Herbs: thyme

CRAMPS

Essential Oils: birch, cypress, lavender

Herbs: butcher's broom, chamomile flowers, marjoram

Vegetable: squash

CRAMPS: ALSO SEE MUSCLE CRAMPS

CRAMPS: LEG

Essential Oils: birch, cypress

Herbs: butcher's broom, chamomile

CROHN'S' DISEASE

Herbs: cannabis, slippery elm

Nuts, Oils, Seeds: Seed: flaxseed

Vegetable: Brussel sprout, collards

CROUP
Herbs: eucalyptus, lobelia, pleurisy root, slippery elm, thyme

CUSHING DISEASE
Herb: licorice root

CYST & CYSTITIS
Essential Oils: cedarwood, chamomile: blue, eucalyptus, fennel, myrtle, oregano oil, peppermint, spearmint, thyme

CYSTIC FIBROSIS
Herbs: Lady's slipper root

DIAPER RASH: SEE SKIN

DANDRUFF
Essential Oils: cedarwood, lavender, patchouli, rosemary

Herbs: chaparral, oregano

Nuts, Oils, Seeds:

Oil: Siberian pine nut oil

DECONGESTANT
Essential Oils: chamomile: blue, cinnamon, cypress, melaleuca/tea tree, myrtle, patchouli, peppermint, pina, sandalwood

Herbs: bayberry, juniper

DEHYDRATION
Amino Acids, Minerals, Omega Oils, Vitamins:

Amino Acid: l-taurine

DELIRIUM
Herb: skullcap

DEMENTIA
Amino Acids, Minerals, Omega Oils, Vitamins:

Vitamins: choline

Herbs: wild indigo

DEPRESSION

Amino Acids, Minerals, Omega Oils, Vitamins:

Amino Acid: l-glutamine, l-tyrosine

Omega Oil: omega 3, omega 6

Vitamins: B1, B3, B5, B12, biotin, inositol, paba, C

Dairy: cheese, goats milk, milk, whey, yogurt

Essential Oils: basil, bergamot, chamomile, clary sage, grapefruit, juniper berry, lavender, melaleuca/tea tree, patchouli, rosewood, sandalwood, spearmint, spruce, tangerine, thyme, ylang ylang

Fruit: tangerine

Herbs: Ashwagandha, hawthorn, kelp, lavender, milk thistle, rosemary, wild indigo

Legumes: beans (red), carob, garbanzo beans

Meat:

Beef: beef: liver, chicken

Lake, ocean, river, sea: fish: fresh water, fish: saltwater, halibut, herring, mackerel, salmon,

Lamb

Pork

Poultry: egg, egg yolk, lamb, pork, turkey

Nuts, Oils, Seeds:

Oil: olive oil

Seed: cacao, sunflower seed

Vegetable: parsnip

DERMATITIS: SEE SKIN: DERMATITIS

DESPONDENCY

Herbs: valerian

DETOX

Essential Oils: helichrysium/strawflower, juniper berry

DIABETES: BLOOD SUGAR REGULATORS / PREVENTION

Amino Acids, Minerals, Omega Oils, Vitamins:

Mineral: chromium

Omega Oil: omega 3, omega 6

Vitamin: C

Fruit: blueberry, cranberry, gooseberry, mango, raspberry, tangerine

Essential Oils: cinnamon, eucalyptus, geranium, pina, rosemary, ylang ylang

Herbs: bilberry, bistort, blue cohosh, buchu, burdock, kelp, marshmallow

Legume: kidney bean, lentil, lima bean, navy bean, pinto bean, soybean

Nuts, Oils, Seeds:

Nut: cashew, pecan, pistachio

Oil: sesame seed oil

Seed: hemp seed, pumpkin seed, sesame seed, sunflower seed

Vegetable: bean (snap), mushroom (white), parsnip, pepper (bell), spinach, squash

DIABETES: TYPE 2

Essential Oil: milk thistle

Fruit: pear

Grain: rye

Nuts, Oils, Seeds:

Nut: walnut

Oil: almond oil, avocado oil

Vegetable: collards, pea, sweet potato, Swiss chard

DIAPER RASH

Amino Acids, Minerals, Omega Oils, Vitamins:

Mineral: zinc

Essential Oils: lavender

Herbs: calendula, lavender

DIARRHEA

Amino Acids, Minerals, Omega Oils, Vitamins:

Mineral: iodine

Vitamins: B3

Essential Oils: cloves, eucalyptus, frankincense, geranium, ginger, melaleuca/tea tree, myrrh, myrtle, nutmeg, orange, patchouli, peppermint, sandalwood, spearmint, tangerine

Herbs: agrimony, amaranth, barberry, bearberry, bilberry, bistort, catnip, chaparral, Cloves, comfrey, cranesbill, gentian, goldenseal, Irish moss, mandrake, marjoram, Marshmallow, meadowsweet, myrrh, nettle, peppermint, plantain, prickly ash, raspberry, rose hips, sassafras, thyme, turkey rhubarb, white oak bark, white poplar, wild indigo, witch hazel, yarrow

Vegetable: onion (green), vegetable (squash)

DIGESTION / DIGESTIVE TRACT

Amino Acids, Minerals, Omega Oils, Vitamins:

Amino Acid: l-taurine

Omega Oil: omega 3, omega 6

Vitamin: paba

Fruit: blackberry, blueberry, kiwi, lemon, mango, papaya, passion fruit, pear, pineapple, raspberry, rhubarb, tangerine

Herbs: cayenne, cilantro, cinnamon, cloves, comfrey, gentian, ginseng, holy basil, kelp, lemon balm, lemongrass, marjoram, marshmallow, melaleuca, prickly ash, spearmint, turkey rhubarb

Legumes: beans (black and red), black-eyed peas, kidney beans, lentil, soybean

Nuts, Oils, Seeds:

Nut: coconut, hazelnut oil

Seed: flaxseed, hemp seed

Vegetable: artichoke, heart (cardiovascular), collards, cucumber, dulse, garlic, kale, mustard greens, onion (red), parsnip, pea, rutabaga, spinach, sweet potato, squash

DIPHTHERIA

Essential Oils: frankincense

Herbs: eucalyptus

DISINFECTANT

Essential Oils: melaleuca/tea tree, sage, myrrh

DIURETIC

Essential Oils: cedarwood, cypress, eucalyptus, fennel, frankincense, geranium, tarragon

DIZZINESS

Herbs: rose hips, spearmint

DNA PROTECTION

Amino Acids, Minerals, Omega Oils, Vitamins:

Mineral: calcium, folate

Dairy: cheese: goat, milk: goat

Fruit: kiwi, lemon

Grains: cereal grain

Legume: navy bean

Nuts, Oils, Seeds:

Oil: olive oil

Vegetable: mushroom (white), onion (green)

DROPSY

The swelling of soft tissues due to the accumulation of excess water (sore feet at night).

Herb: bayberry, marjoram, birch, blessed thistle, blue cohosh, borage, butcher's broom, dandelion, gravel root, hawthorn, horseradish, horsetail, marjoram, plantain, sassafras, spearmint, wormwood

DRUG ADDICTIONS/WITHDRAWAL

Herbs: ginseng, licorice root, valerian

DRAVET'S SYNDROME: A DEBILITATING FORM OF EPILEPSY THAT AFFECTS CHILDREN.

Herbs: cannabis

DYSENTERY

Essential Oils: myrrh, myrtle, oregano oil

Herbs: bistort, cranesbill, marshmallow, plantain, pleurisy root, raspberry, sassafras, skullcap, witch hazel

DYSPEPSIA

Essential Oils: grapefruit, orange

Herbs: barberry, fennel, gentian, yellow dock

EARS: TO INCREASE HEARING

Herbs: angelica, ginseng

EARACHES

Essential Oils: basil

Herbs: cloves, eyebright, goldenseal, lobelia, melaleuca, mullein, rose hips, wormwood

Nuts, Oils, Seeds:

Oil: hazelnut oil

EAR INFECTIONS

Herbs: black cohosh, butcher's broom, calendula, cloves, garlic, lobelia, melaleuca, oregano, rose hip

Nuts, Oils, Seeds: Oil: almond oil

EATING DISORDERS

Essential Oils: grapefruit

Herbs: butcher's broom

EBOLA VIRUS

Herb: olive leaf

E. COLI

Herb: olive leaf

Eczema: see Skin: Eczema

EDEMA

Amino Acids, Minerals, Omega Oils, Vitamins:

Amino Acid: l-taurine

Mineral: potassium

Essential Oils: lemongrass

Herbs: astragalus, butcher's broom, dandelion root

EMPHYSEMA

Herbs: astragalus, licorice root, marshmallow, pleurisy root

EMOTIONAL DISTRESS

Essential Oils: chamomile (blue)

Herbs: agrimony, reishi mushroom

ENDOCRINE: GLANDS, SYSTEM

Amino Acids, Minerals, Omega Oils, Vitamins:

Vitamin: E

Meat:

beef: calf liver

Vegetables: garlic, onion (red)

ENEMA

Herbs: hops

ENERGY PRODUCTION

Amino Acids, Minerals, Omega Oils, Vitamins:

Mineral: boron, calcium, copper, iron, magnesium, phosphorus

Vitamins: B2, B5, folate

Diary: whey

Fruit: banana, raspberry

Essential Oils: basil, fir

Legumes: kidney bean, lentil, navy bean

Meat:

beef: calf liver

Nuts, Oils, Seeds:

Nut: cashew, pistachio

Seed: chia seed

Vegetables: bean (lima), squash

ENZYME: ACTIVATOR

Amino Acids, Minerals, Omega Oils, Vitamins:

Mineral: molybdenum

Vitamin: C

ENZYME: DIGESTIVE

Fruit: pineapple

EPILEPSY

Amino Acids, Minerals, Omega Oils, Vitamins:

Amino Acid: l-taurine

Essential Oils: basil

Herbs: anise seed, black cohosh, blue cohosh, cloves, hyssop, lady's slipper root, lobelia, plantain, skullcap, valerian

ESTROGEN BALANCING

Fruit: blackberry

Nuts, Oils, Seeds: Seed: flaxseed

Vegetable: cucumber

EXHAUSTION: FATIGUE

Amino Acids, Minerals, Omega Oils, Vitamins:

Mineral: iodine, iron, selenium, zinc

Vitamins: B1, B3, C

Essential Oils: cinnamon, clary sage, peppermint, thyme

Herbs: agrimony, angelica, astragalus, lemon balm, oregano, skullcap

Legume: lentil

Meat: beef, beef kidney

EXPECTORANT

Essential Oils: fennel, frankincense, ginger

EYES

Amino Acids, Minerals, Omega Oils, Vitamins:

Amino Acid: l-lysine

Mineral: manganese

Vitamins: B1, B2, C

Essential Oils: lemongrass, peppermint

Fruit: apricot, blackberry, cantaloupe, chokecherry, date, lemon, mango, papaya, passion fruit, pineapple, raspberry, tangerine, tomato

Herbs: angelica, arnica, bilberry, balm of Gilead, bayberry, bilberry, black walnut, blessed thistle, borage, caraway seed, chaparral, eyebright, evening primrose (helps all eye disorders), fennel, garlic, ginseng, horsetail, marshmallow

Legumes: beans (red), black-eyed peas, carob

Meat:

Beef: beef kidney, beef liver

Lake, ocean, river, sea: fish oils

Pork

Poultry: chicken, egg, egg yolk

Nuts, Oils, Seeds:

Nut: pistachio

Oil: avocado oil

Vegetable: beet greens, broccoli, carrots, dulse, lettuce (romaine), onion (green), Pepper (bell), pumpkin, rutabaga, squash, Swiss chard

EYES: INFECTIONS

Herbs: calendula, caraway seed, eyebright, peppermint

EYES: LIDS ULCERATED

Herb: yellow dock

EYES: MACULAR DISEASE

Fruit: chokecherry

EYES: NIGHT VISION/VISION

Amino Acids, Minerals, Omega Oils, Vitamins:

Mineral: zinc

Vitamins: A

Dairy: cheese: cow, milk (cow), milk (goat)

Fruit: cantalope

Meat:

Beef: calf liver

Vegetable: squash

EYES: SORE / INFLAMMATION

Amino Acids, Minerals, Omega Oils, Vitamins:

Amino Acids: l-lysine

Herbs: plantain, raspberry, red clover, white oak bark, white poplar, witch hazel, wormwood

EYES: NIGHT VISION

Diary: cheese (goat)

Meat:

Beef: calf liver

Vegetable: squash

EYE: WASH

Herbs: raspberry

FAINTING

Essential Oils: basil, lavender, nutmeg

Herbs: cramp bark

Fatigue: see exhaustion

FETUS DEVELOPMENT / GROWTH

Amino Acids, Minerals, Omega Oils, Vitamins:

Mineral: chromium, magnesium, selenium

Vitamins: B2, biotin

Legume: soybean

Meat:

Beef: liver

Lamb: lamb

Pork: pork

Nuts, Oils, Seeds:

Nut: hazelnut

Vegetable: artichoke, beet

FEVERS: TO REDUCE

Essential Oils: basil, eucalyptus, lemon, lemongrass, peppermint, spearmint

Herbs: agrimony, barberry, basil, birch, blessed thistle, borage, calendula, chamomile, ginger, ginseng, hyssop, lemongrass, mandrake, olive leaf, Peruvian bark, plantain, prickly ash, raspberry, rose hips, skullcap, spearmint, white oak bark, white poplar, wild indigo, wormwood, yarrow

FIBROMYALGIA

Fruit: cherry

Herbs: astragalus, olive leaf, oregano

FIBROSIS

Amino Acids, Minerals, Omega Oils, Vitamins:

Amino Acid: l-glutamine

Essential Oils: sage

FINGER NAILS

Amino Acids, Minerals, Omega Oils, Vitamins:

Vitamins: folate

FISTULAS

This is an abnormal passage that leads from an abscess or hollow organ or part to the body surface or from one hollow organ or part to another. This can be caused by tissue damage during surgery.

Herb: Pau d'arco

FITS

Herbs: blue cohosh, cramp bark

FLATULENCE

Essential Oils: fennel, ginger, lavender, orange, spearmint, tarragon

Herb: fennel

FLATWORM

Herb: olive leaf

FLU

Essential Oils: clove, peppermint, thyme

Herbs: cinnamon, echinacea, juniper, lemon balm, lemongrass, meadowsweet (adults only, and not pregnant women), myrrh, olive leaf, oregano, pleurisy root, rose hips, slippery elm, spearmint, yarrow

FLUID RETENTION

Essential Oils: cypress, grapefruit, lavender, lemongrass, rosemary, tangerine

FOOD POISONING:

Herbs: goldenseal, lobelia

Other: Activated Charcoal and drink with a lot of water

FRIEDREICH'S ATAXIA

Amino Acids, Minerals, Omega Oils, Vitamins:

Vitamins: choline

FRIGIDITY

Essential Oils: clary sage

FROST BITE

Herbs: cayenne

FROZEN SHOULDER

Fruit: cherry

FRUSTRATION

Essential Oils: ylang ylang

Fungicide: see Infections: Fungus

GALL BLADDER

Essential Oils: chamomile: blue, geranium, helichrysum/strawflower, lavender, tangerine

Grains: buckwheat

Herbs: agrimony, barberry, blessed thistle, borage, burdock, calendula, cascara sagrada, ginger, kelp, milk thistle, parsley, pokeweed, red clover, sage, senna, wormwood

GALL STONE PREVENTION
Essential Oils: eucalyptus, grapefruit, lemon, nutmeg

Grains: buckwheat, rye

Herbs: buchu, hops, lavender, mandrake, senna

Legume: peanut

Nuts, Oils, Seeds:

Nut: Cashew, Hazelnut Oil

GANGRENE
Amino Acids, Minerals, Omega Oils, Vitamins:

Vitamin: E

Herbs: marshmallow, white oak bark, wild indigo

GANGRENE: DIABETIC
Herbs: melaleuca

GIARDIA
Herbs: olive leaf, oregano

Nuts, Oils, Seeds:

Nut: coconut

GAS
Herbs: fennel, marjoram, slippery elm, spearmint

GASTRITIS CHRONIC
Essential Oils: chamomile (blue)

Nuts, Oils, Seeds:

Oil: Siberian pine nut oil

GASTROENTERITIS
Herbs: chaparral, goldenseal, marshmallow

GASTROINTESTINAL TRACT
Amino Acids, Minerals, Omega Oils, Vitamins:

Vitamins: B3

Nuts, Oils, Seeds:

Seed: mustard seed

GENITALS: INFECTION

Herbs: white poplar

GENITALS: RASHES

Essential Oils: clary sage

Herbs: chickweed

GILLES DE LA TOURETTE'S DISEASE

Amino Acids, Minerals, Omega Oils, Vitamins:

Vitamins: choline

GINGIVITIS

Essential Oils: chamomile, melaleuca/tea tree

GLANDS: INFLAMED / SWOLLEN

Herbs: goldenseal, mullein, pokeweed, white oak bark

GLANDULAR SUPPORT

Essential Oils: sage

Herbs: alfalfa, caraway seed, Irish moss, licorice root, mandrake, marshmallow, mullein, yarrow

Nuts, Oils, Seeds:

Seed: chia seed

GOITRE

Amino Acids, Minerals, Omega Oils, Vitamins:

Mineral: iodine

Herbs: pokeweed

GONORRHEA

Essential Oils: bergamot, eucalyptus, frankincense

Herbs: bearberry, Pau d'arco, white poplar

GOUT

Essential Oil: basil, birch, fennel, lemon

Fruit: cherry

Herbs: alfalfa, bilberry, birch, burdock root, burdock, gravel root, horsetail, Irish moss, Juniper berry, nettle, oatstraw, senna, wormwood

Vegetable: sweet potato, squash

GRAVES' DISEASE

Herbs: lemon balm

GRIPE

Essential Oil: sage

Herbs: fennel, hyssop

GUM DISEASE

Amino Acids, Minerals, Omega Oils, Vitamins:

Mineral: calcium, molybdenum

Essential Oils: melaleuca/tea tree

Nuts, Oils, Seeds:

Oil: avocado oil

HAIR: DAMAGE / LOSS / SUPPORT

Amino Acids, Minerals, Omega Oils, Vitamins:

Amino Acid: l-lysine

Mineral: copper, iron, silicon, zinc

Vitamin: biotin, folate, inositol

Dairy: cheese (goat), milk (cow), milk (goat)

Essential Oils: cedarwood, lavender, nutmeg, rosemary, ylang ylang

Fruit: gooseberry

Grains: buckwheat, couscous, millet, oat, quinoa, rice: (brown and white), rye, spelt, Wheat, wheat bran, wheat germ

Herbs: agrimony, chaparral, horsetail, oatstraw, fennel, lavender, nettle, rosemary, sage, wormwood, yarrow

Meat:

Beef: beef kidney

Nuts, Oils, Seeds:

Nut: coconut

Oil: avocado oil, coconut oil, grapeseed oil, hazelnut oil, hemp seed oil

Seed: flaxseed

HAIR: GREY (TO RESTORE COLOUR)

Amino Acids, Minerals, Omega Oils, Vitamins:

Vitamin: paba

Fruit: tangerine

HAIR: MOISTURIZE

Herb: Irish moss

HAY FEVER

Herbs: goldenseal, mandrake, marjoram, mullein, nettle

Vegetable: onion (green)

HEADACHES

Amino Acids, Minerals, Omega Oils, Vitamins:

Vitamins: B3

Essential Oils: basil, coves. frankincense, grapefruit, lavender, lemongrass, marjoram, peppermint (digestive headaches), rosemary, spearmint, thyme

Fruit: banana, cherry

Herbs: angelica, arnica, balm of Gilead, basil, black cohosh, blessed thistle, borage, butcher's broom, cannabis, catnip, chamomile, Ginger, holy basil, kelp, Lady's slipper root, lavender, lemon balm, lemongrass, lobelia, mandrake, marjoram, marshmallow, oregano, peppermint, rosemary, skullcap, slippery elm, spearmint, thyme, white poplar, witch hazel, wormwood, yarrow

Vegetable: onion (green)

HEAD: COLDS

Herbs: echinacea

HEAD: CONGESTION

Herb: valerian

HEARTBURN

Herb: white poplar

HEART: CARDIAC SPASM

Essential Oil: orange

Herb: hawthorn

HEART: CARDIOVASCULAR SYSTEM

Amino Acids, Minerals, Omega Oils, Vitamins:

Mineral: silicon, vanadium

Omega Oil: omega 3, omega 6

Vitamin: E

Essential Oils: grapefruit, lemongrass, orange

Fruit: currant (red), papaya, raspberry, rhubarb, Saskatoon berry, strawberry, tomato

Grains: buckwheat, oat, quinoa, rye, spelt, wheat, wheat bran, wheat germ

Herbs: black cohosh, gentian, ginger, hawthorn, hops, Pau d'arco, pleurisy Root, Primrose, Reiki mushroom, skullcap, slippery elm, wormwood

Legumes: beans (black), garbanzo beans, kidney beans, peanut, pinto bean

Meat:

Beef: beef: calf liver, beef liver

Lake, ocean, river, sea: clams, fish: fresh water, fish oils, herring, mackerel, salmon, sardines, tuna

Nuts, Oils, Seeds:

Nut: cashew, pecan, walnut

Oil: grapeseed oil, hemp seed oil, olive oil, sesame seed oil, walnut oil

Seed: cacao, sunflower seed

Vegetables: beet, Brussel sprout, cabbage, carrots, cauliflower, celery, collards, garlic, kale, kelp, mushroom (white), mustard greens, pea

HEART: DISEASE PREVENTION

Amino Acids, Minerals, Omega Oils, Vitamins:

Vitamins: B3

Fruit: blackberry, goji berry, grape/raisin

Legumes: bean (black and white), pinto bean

Nuts, Oils, Seeds:

Seed: hemp seed, mustard seed

Vegetable: Brussel sprout, pea

HEART: PALPITATION

Essential Oils: orange, ylang ylang

HEART: REDUCE FAST HEART RATE

Fruit: guava

Herbs: barberry, valerian

HEART: SUPPORT

Amino Acids, Minerals, Omega Oils, Vitamins:

Amino Acid: l-taurine

Mineral: calcium, magnesium, manganese, phosphorus, potassium, selenium

Vitamins: B1, C, E, coenzyme Q10

Dairy: buttermilk

Fruit: apple, apricot, avocado, banana, blueberry, cranberry, date, fig, grapefruit, lemon, mango, orange, peach, pear, pineapple, raspberry, rhubarb, strawberry, tangerine, watermelon

Grains: cereal grain, corn, couscous, rice (brown and white)

Herbs: anise seed, bearberry, bilberry, black cohosh, blessed thistle, borage, butcher's broom, calendula, chickweed, cilantro, dandelion, fenugreek, garlic, gentian, ginger, ginseng, hawthorn, kelp, Lady's slipper root, Lemongrass, licorice root, lobelia, oatstraw, parsley, Pau d'arco, peppermint, Peruvian bark, reishi mushroom, skullcap, turmeric

Legumes: bean (red), black-eyed pea, carob, garbanzo bean, kidney bean, lentil, lima bean, navy bean, peanut, pinto bean, soybean

Meat:

Lake, ocean, river, sea: clam

Lamb

Poultry: egg

Nuts, Oils, Seeds:

Nut: almond, cashew, coconut, macadamia nut, pecan, pistachio

Oil: almond oil, avocado oil, grapeseed oil, hemp oil, olive oil, olive oil, sesame seed oil, alnut oil

Seed: chia seed, cacao, hemp seed

Vegetable: bean (lima and snap), broccoli, Brussel sprout, corn, dulse, garlic, lettuce (romaine), mushroom (white), onion (green and red), parsnip, pepper (bell), potato, radish, rutabaga, squash, squash

HEARTBURN

Essential Oils: ginger, lemon, peppermint

Herbs: aloe vera, angelica, chamomile, gentian, milk thistle

HEART MUSCLES

Amino Acids, Minerals, Omega Oils, Vitamins:

Vitamins: inositol

HEAVY METAL POISONING

Herb: chlorella, cilantro, cranesbill

Vegetable: sweet potato

HEMATOMA

Essential Oils: helichrysium/strawflower

HEMORRHOIDS: TO REDUCE INFLAMMATION

Essential Oils: clary sage, cypress, frankincense, melaleuca/tea tree, myrtle, patchouli, peppermint, sandalwood

Herbs: agrimony, alfalfa, bistort, butcher's broom, calendula, catnip, chamomile, cranesbill, goldenseal, melaleuca, mullein, myrrh, plantain, slippery elm, white oak bark, white pond lily, witch hazel

Nuts, Oils, Seeds:

Oil: Siberian pine nut oil

HEPATITIS

Essential Oils: myrrh, peppermint, rosemary

Herbs: burdock, Siberian ginseng, calendula, dandelion, gentian, lobelia, milk thistle, olive leaf, oregano, red clover

HERNIAS

Herb: Pau d'arco

HERPES

Amino Acids, Minerals, Omega Oils, Vitamins:

Amino Acid: l-lysine

Essential Oils: eucalyptus, frankincense, lavender, melaleuca/tea tree, ravensara

Grains: barley

Herbs: bearberry, gravel root, hyssop, lavender, lemon balm, licorice root, peppermint, raspberry, slippery elm

Nuts, Oils, Seeds:

Nut: coconut

Vegetable: kelp

HEAVY METALS

Herbs: chlorella, cilantro

HICCUPS

Essential Oils: basil, spearmint, tarragon

Herbs: black cohosh, blue cohosh

HIGH BLOOD PRESSURE: SEE BLOOD

HIRSUTISM (EXCESSIVE HAIR GROWTH)

Herbs: spearmint

HIV: SEE AIDS

HIVES

Vegetable: onion (green)

HODGKIN'S DISEASE

Herb: Pau d'arco

HOOKWORMS

Herbs: caraway seed, olive leaf

Hormone stabilizer: see Menstrual: hormone stabilizer

HOT FLASHES

Fruit: blackberry

Essential Oils: peppermint, sage

Herbs: black cohosh, borage, ginger, primrose, raspberry, red clover, sage

Nuts, Oils, Seeds: Seed: sunflower seed

HUNTINGTON'S DISEASE

Amino Acids, Minerals, Omega Oils, Vitamins:

Vitamins: choline

HYDROPHOBIA

This is fear of water. This fear can be extreme, rational and irrational. Hydrophobia can be one of the effects of rabies in a human.

Herbs: skullcap

HYPERACTIVITY

Amino Acids, Minerals, Omega Oils, Vitamins:

Amino Acid: l-taurine

Vitamins: B6

Herbs: skullcap

HYPERSENSITIVITY

Essential Oils: chamomile: blue

HYPERTENSION

Amino Acids, Minerals, Omega Oils, Vitamins:

Amino Acid: l-taurine

Mineral: manganese

Essential Oils: birch, cloves, peppermint, pina, sandalwood, ylang ylang

Herbs: skullcap

Meat: pork

Nuts, Oils, Seeds: Oil: olive oil

HYPOCHONDRIA

Amino Acids, Minerals, Omega Oils, Vitamins:

Vitamin: C

Herb: valerian

HYPOGLYCEMIA:
THIS IS CAUSED BY A LOW BLOOD SUGAR LEVEL AND IS SOMETIMES RELATED TO DIABETES.

Amino Acids, Minerals, Omega Oils, Vitamins:

Amino Acid: l-taurine

Mineral: chromium

Herb: skullcap

Legume: navy bean, pinto bean

Meat: pork

HYPOKALEMIA

Fruit: peach

HYPOTENSION

Essential Oils: oregano oil

Herb: peppermint

HYSTERIA

Amino Acids, Minerals, Omega Oils, Vitamins:

Vitamin: C

Essential Oils: lavender, melaleuca/tea tree

Herbs: catnip, cramp bark, Lady's slipper root, lavender, melaleuca, rosemary, skullcap, spearmint, valerian, yarrow

IBS (IRRITABLE BOWEL SYNDROME): PREVENTION
Legume: kidney beans

IMMUNE SYSTEM: SUPPORT
Amino Acids, Minerals, Omega Oils, Vitamins:

Mineral: copper, iron, manganese, selenium, silicon, zinc

Omega Oil: omega 9

Vitamins: B5, B6, folate, C, E, coenzyme Q10

Dairy: buttermilk

Essential Oils: cinnamon, frankincense, lemon, oregano oil, thyme

Fruit: apple, blackberry, blueberry, currant (red), goji berry, grapefruit, kiwi, lemon, lime, orange, passion fruit, pineapple, plum / prune, raspberry, Saskatoon berry, strawberry, tangerine, watermelon

Grains: buckwheat

Herbs: alfalfa, aloe vera, astragalus, anise seed, Ashwagandha, astragalus, bilberry, burdock, chlorella, cilantro, cinnamon, echinacea, ginseng, green tea, hawthorn, melaleuca, myrrh, oatstraw, oregano, Pau d'arco, red clover, wild indigo

Legumes: garbanzo beans, lentil

Meat:

Beef: beef: calf liver, beef

Lake, ocean, river, sea: fish: fresh water, fish: saltwater, halibut, herring, mackerel, salmon, sardines, tuna

Nuts, Oils, Seeds:

Nut: coconut, pine nut

Oil: coconut oil, hemp seed oil, Siberian pine nut oil

Seed: cacao, sunflower seed

Vegetables: cauliflower, corn, dulse, garlic, lettuce (romaine), mushroom (white), onion (green and red), parsnip, pepper (bell), pumpkin, rutabaga

IMPOTENCY
Amino Acids, Minerals, Omega Oils, Vitamins:

Mineral: zinc

Essential Oils: clary sage, clove, ginger, sandalwood, ylang ylang

Herbs: ginger, ginseng

INDIGESTION

Essential Oils: ginger, lavender, peppermint,

Herbs: basil, lavender, lemon balm, peppermint

Vegetable: onion (green and red)

INFECTIONS: BACTERIAL

Amino Acids, Minerals, Omega Oils, Vitamins:

Mineral: sulfur

Vitamins: A, C

Dairy: cheese: cow, cheese: goat, milk (cow), milk (goat)

Fruit: cranberry

Essential Oils: oregano, peppermint, pina, rosewood, sage

Herbs: black walnut, cinnamon, cloves, Pau d'arco, red clover, reishi mushroom, rose hips

Meat:

Beef: beef: calf liver

Poultry: egg

Nuts, Oils, Seeds:

Nut: pecan

Vegetables: onion (red)

INFECTIONS: FUNGAL

Essential Oils: melaleuca/tea tree, myrrh, oregano, patchouli, peppermint, rosewood, sage

Fruit: grape / raisin

Herbs: black walnut, garlic, melaleuca, olive leaf, oregano, Pau d'arco, pokeweed, raspberry, reishi mushroom

INFECTIONS: VIRAL

Amino Acids, Minerals, Omega Oils, Vitamins:

Mineral: germanium

Essential Oils: bergamot, cinnamon, clary sage, cloves, eucalyptus, lemon, lemongrass, melaleuca/tea tree, myrtle, nutmeg, ravensara, rosemary, rosewood, sage, thyme, melaleuca, Pau d'arco, reishi mushroom, rose hips

Nuts, Oils, Seeds:

Seed: pumpkin seed

INFECTIONS: YEAST

Herbs: melaleuca, Pau d'arco

INFECTIOUS DISEASES

Essential Oils: lemon

INFLAMMATION: SWELLING OF THE JOINTS OR ORGANS.

Essential Oils: frankincense, melaleuca/tea tree, myrtle, patchouli, peppermint

Fruit: pineapple (bromelain), cranberry

Herbs: barley grass, cats claw, devil's claw, echinacea, holy basil, turmeric, melaleuca

Legumes: black-eyed peas

Nuts, Oils, Seeds:

Oil: grapeseed oil, olive oil, sesame seed oil, walnut oil

INFLUENZA

Essential Oils: cypress, eucalyptus, fir, lavender, melaleuca/tea tree

Herbs: astragalus, chaparral, horseradish, lavender, lemon balm, melaleuca, olive leaf, peppermint, pleurisy root, raspberry

Nuts, Oils, Seeds:

Nut: coconut

Oil: Siberian pine nut oil

INFERTILITY

Amino Acids, Minerals, Omega Oils, Vitamins:

Vitamin: C

Herb: skullcap

IRRITABLE BOWL SYNDROME

Herb: peppermint

INSECT: BITES

Essential Oils: clary sage, frankincense, patchouli

Herbs: aloe vera, holy basil, plantain, rosemary, skullcap

INSECT: REPELLANT

Essential Oils: cedarwood, citronella, cloves, eucalyptus, geranium, patchouli

Herbs: melaleuca, wormwood

INSOMNIA

Amino Acids, Minerals, Omega Oils, Vitamins:

Mineral: magnesium

Vitamins: B3

Essential Oils: basil, chamomile, clary sage, cypress, geranium, lavender, lemon, marjoram, myrtle, orange, tangerine

Herbs: chamomile, garlic, hawthorn, Lady's slipper root, lavender, lemon balm, oatstraw, reishi mushroom, skullcap, valerian

Meat: Pork

Nuts, Oils, Seeds:

Nut: cashew, walnut

Vegetable: onion (green)

INTESTINE: CLEANSER

Essential Oils: basil, cypress, fennel, nutmeg

Herbs: anise seed, ginger, holy basil, Irish moss, lobelia, senna, white oak bark

Nuts, Oils, Seeds:

Seed: pumpkin seed

INTESTINE: CRAMPS & SPASMS

Essential Oils: clary sage, cloves, fennel, marjoram, tangerine, tarragon, lemongrass

INTESTINE: INFLAMMATION

Herbs: marshmallow

INTESTINE: INFECTIONS

Essential Oils: ylang ylang

Herbs: marshmallow

INTESTINE: PARASITES

Essential Oils: basil, bergamot, cloves, cypress, lemon, nutmeg

Herbs: amaranth, black walnut, melaleuca, wormwood

INTESTINES: WORMS

Herbs: black walnut, catnip, mandrake, valerian, white oak bark

INTESTINE: SUPPORT

Amino Acids, Minerals, Omega Oils, Vitamins:

Amino Acid: l-glutamine

Vitamins: B5, B12

Herbs: barberry, cascara sagrada, goldenseal, Irish moss, marjoram, sassafras, turkey rhubarb, valerian

Legumes: bean (black)

Nuts, Oils, Seeds:

Oil: hemp seed oil

Seed: chia seed

Vegetable: mustard greens

INTESTINAL FLORA

Amino Acids, Minerals, Omega Oils, Vitamins:

Vitamin: paba

INTESTINAL TRACT: GAS

Essential Oils: peppermint, thyme

Herb: goldenseal

Vegetable: cucumber

INTERNAL BLEEDING

Herbs: agrimony

INSOMNIA

Herbs: borage

IRON ABSORBTION

Amino Acids, Minerals, Omega Oils, Vitamins:

Vitamin: C

IRRITABILITY

Essential Oils: tangerine

IRRITABLE BOWEL

Amino Acids, Minerals, Omega Oils, Vitamins:

Mineral: magnesium

Herbs: caraway seed, valerian

Vegetable: Brussel sprout

JAUNDICE

Essential Oils: frankincense, geranium,

Herbs: barberry, bayberry, blessed thistle, borage, butcher's broom, dandelion, gentian, hops, mandrake, Parsley, Plantain, sage, senna, wormwood, yarrow, yellow dock

JET LAG:

Essential Oils: grapefruit

JOINTS: SORE

Amino Acids, Minerals, Omega Oils, Vitamins:

Mineral: manganese

Essential Oils: spruce

KIDNEY: INFECTION

Fruit: cherry, chokecherry, cranberry

Herbs: burdock, gentian, horsetail, juniper, marshmallow

KIDNEY INFLAMMATION

Herbs: mullein, nettle, parsley, spearmint

KIDNEY: STONE

Amino Acids, Minerals, Omega Oils, Vitamins:

Mineral: magnesium

Fruit: cranberry, lemon, orange

Essential Oils: fennel, juniper berry, cleaver

Herbs: comfrey, holy basil, Hops, juniper, oatstraw, rose hips, spearmint

Vegetable: radish

KIDNEY: SUPPORT

Amino Acids, Minerals, Omega Oils, Vitamins:

Mineral: chromium, magnesium, molybdenum, phosphorus, sodium, vanadium

Vitamin: D

Essential Oils: clary sage, cloves, geranium, grapefruit, lemongrass, spearmint, tarragon

Fruit: cherry, chokecherry, tomato, watermelon

Herbs: agrimony, alfalfa, balm of Gilead, basil, bearberry, bilberry, birch, bistort, black cohosh, borage, buchu, burdock, butcher's broom, caraway seed, cayenne, chaparral, cleaver, cranesbill, dandelion, fenugreek, gravel root, hawthorn, horseradish, horsetail, hyssop, Irish moss, juniper, k lemongrass, milk thistle, nettle, plantain, pleurisy root, red clover, slippery elm, white oak bark, wormwood, yarrow

Meat:

Beef: beef: calf liver

Lamb: lamb

Pork: pork

Poultry: egg

Nuts, Oils, Seeds:

Nut: coconut

KIDNEY: WATER RETENTION

Herbs: marjoram, plantain, rose hips, spearmint, wormwood

LABOUR: TO INDUCE LABOUR

Herbs: raspberry leaves

LACTATION: TO INCREASE

Essential Oils: fennel,

Herbs: blessed thistle, borage

Nuts, Oils, Seeds:

Oil: Siberian pine nut oil

LARYNGITIS

Essential Oils: cypress, frankincense, lavender, peppermint

Herbs: goldenseal, lavender, pokeweed

LAXATIVES

Essential Oils: ginger

Herbs: aloe vera, black walnut, blue cohosh, ginger, hops, licorice root, mullein, parsley, pokeweed tarragon, fennel, rose hips, turkey rhubarb

Nuts, Oils, Seeds:

Oil: almond oil

LEAD POISONING

Herb: mandrake

LEARNING DISABILITIES

Amino Acids, Minerals, Omega Oils, Vitamins:

Vitamins: B1, B2

LEG: CRAMPS

Amino Acids, Minerals, Omega Oils, Vitamins:

Mineral: magnesium

Vitamins: B6

LEG: RESTLESSNESS

Amino Acids, Minerals, Omega Oils, Vitamins: Amino Acid: l-tyrosine

LEG: ULCER

Amino Acids, Minerals, Omega Oils, Vitamins: Vitamin: E

Essential Oils: chamomile: blue, cloves

LEPROSY
Grains: barley

Herb: yellow dock

LEUCORRHEA
Herbs: bistort, blue cohosh, white oak bark, white pond lily, yarrow

LEUKEMIA
Herbs: chaparral, Pau d'arco, yellow dock

LICE
Essential Oils: melaleuca

Herbs: melaleuca, oregano, thyme

LIMB: ACKY AND TIRED
Essential Oils: tangerine

LIVER: CLEANSE / SUPPORT
Amino Acids, Minerals, Omega Oils, Vitamins:

Amino Acid: l-glutamine

Mineral: chromium, germanium, molybdenum, selenium, sodium, sulfur, zinc

Vitamins: B3, B6, inositol, C

Essential Oils: chamomile: blue, cypress, geranium, grapefruit, helichrysium/strawflower, peppermint, sage, tangerine

Fruit: apricot, cranberry, date, fig, goji berry, lemon, lime, orange, pear, raspberry, tomato, watermelon

Grains: buckwheat, corn, couscous, millet, oat, quinoa, rice: brown, rye, spelt, wheat, wheat bran, wheat germ

Herbs: agrimony, aloe vera, astragalus, barberry, bayberry, bearberry, bilberry, birch, bistort, black cohosh, black walnut, blessed thistle, borage, burdock, butcher's broom, calendula, cannabis, caraway seed, cascara sagrada, chaparral, chlorella, cilantro, cinnamon, comfrey, dandelion, echinacea, eyebright, garlic, gentian, ginger, ginseng, green tea, holy basil, hops, horseradish, horsetail, hyssop, Irish moss, kelp, lemongrass, licorice root, lobelia, mandrake, marjoram, marshmallow, Milk thistle, nettle, oatstraw, olive leaf, parsley, Pau d'arco, plantain, pokeweed, prickly ash, red clover, reishi mushroom, rose hips, rosemary, sage, sassafras, Slippery elm, thyme, turkey rhubarb, turmeric, white oak bark, wild indigo, wormwood, yarrow, yellow dock

Legumes: bean (black and red), carob, garbanzo beans, peanut

Meat:

Beef: beef: calf liver, beef

Lake, ocean, river, sea: salmon, tuna

Pork: pork

Nuts, Oils, Seeds:

Nut: almond, Brazil nut, coconut, hazelnut, macadamia nut, pine nut, walnut

Oil: Siberian pine nut oil

Seed: cacao, pumpkin seed, sesame seed

Vegetables: artichoke, beet, beet greens, broccoli, Brussel sprout, cauliflower, collards, corn, garlic, kale, kelp, lettuce (Iceberg), mustard greens, onion (red), pepper (bell), radish, squash

LOCKJAW

Herbs: cramp bark, lobelia

LUPUS

Herbs: Pau d'arco

LUNG

Amino Acids, Minerals, Omega Oils, Vitamins:

Mineral: phosphorus

Vitamins: inositol, coenzyme Q10

Essential Oils: basil, bergamot, cedarwood, fir

Fruit: cherry, tomato

Herbs: agrimony, aloe vera, angelica, anise seed, astragalus, barberry, basil, bayberry, blessed thistle, Borage, Calendula, caraway seed, catnip, cayenne, chaparral, cinnamon, comfrey, cramp bark, eucalyptus, eyebright, fennel, garlic, ginseng, green tea, hawthorn, holy basil, horseradish, Irish moss, juniper, kelp, Lady's slipper root, lemon balm, licorice root, mandrake, marjoram, marshmallow, myrrh, oatstraw, Pau d'arco, plantain, pokeweed, reishi mushroom, wild indigo (must be careful not to use large amounts), yarrow, yellow dock

Meat: lamb

Nuts, Oils, Seeds: Seed: sesame seed

Vegetable: pumpkin

LUNGS: BLEEDING

Herbs: chickweed, yellow dock

LUNG: CANCER

Fruit: tomato

LUNGS: DECONGESTION

Herbs: melaleuca, mullein, sage

LUNGS: HEMORRHAGING

Herbs: yarrow

LUNGS: INFECTION/INFLAMMATION

Herbs: marshmallow, myrrh, olive leaf, Pau d'arco, peppermint, pleurisy root, reishi mushroom

LUNGS: MUCOUS

Essential Oils: fir

Herbs: anise seed, balm of Gilead, bayberry, bearberry, burdock, chamomile, chaparral, cinnamon, fenugreek, garlic, ginger, goldenseal, holy basil, horseradish, hyssop, juniper, mullein, myrrh, nettle, plantain, pleurisy root, valerian, wild indigo

LUPUS

Fruit: cherry

Essential Oils: cloves

LYME DISEASE

Herbs: olive leaf, oregano

LYMPHATIC GLANDS

Herbs: pokeweed, yellow dock

LYMPHATIC SYSTEM

Essential Oils: cypress, grapefruit, helichrysium/strawflower, lavender, lemongrass, sage, tangerine

Herbs: black cohosh, burdock, chaparral, echinacea, lavender, mullein, pleurisy root

MACULAR DEGENERATION & SUPPORT

Fruit: mango

Nuts, Oils, Seeds: Oil: avocado oil

MALARIA

Essential Oils: ashwagandha, eucalyptus,

Herbs: eucalyptus, gentian, gravel root, holy basil, olive leaf, Peruvian bark

MEASLES

Essential Oils: eucalyptus, hyssop

Herbs: marjoram, pleurisy root, valerian, yarrow

MELANCHOLIA (DEPRESSION)

Herbs: wild indigo

MEMORY

Amino Acids, Minerals, Omega Oils, Vitamins:

Mineral: manganese

Vitamins: B1, choline

Essential Oils: cloves

Herbs: blessed thistle, blue cohosh, fennel, holy basil, rosemary

Legume: navy bean

Meat:

Beef: beef kidney, beef liver,

Lake, ocean, river, sea: fish: fresh water, fish: saltwater, halibut, herring, mackerel, salmon, sardines, sardines, tuna

Pork: pork

Poultry: egg, turkey

Nuts, Oils, Seeds:

Nut: walnut

Vegetable: spinach

MENIERE'S DISEASE

Herbs: butcher's broom

MENINGITIS

Essential Oils: frankincense, sage

Herbs: olive leaf, skullcap, wild indigo

MENOPAUSE

Essential Oils: clary sage, cloves, fennel, orange, sage

Herbs: black cohosh, ginseng, red clover

Legume: soybean

Nuts, Oils, Seeds:

Seed: mustard seed, sesame seed, sunflower seed

MENSTRUAL: BLOATING

Herbs: thyme

MENSTRUAL: CRAMPING:

Essential Oils: clary sage, cypress, lavender, marjoram, nutmeg

Fruit: raspberry

Herbs: black cohosh, angelica, basil, bistort, black cohosh, blue cohosh, butcher's broom, cannabis, calendula, catnip, chamomile, chaparral, cinnamon, cramp bark, Dandelion, fenugreek, ginger, ginseng, lavender, lobelia, primrose, raspberry, rosemary, sage, sassafras, senna, skullcap, slippery elm, spearmint, thyme, white oak bark, wormwood

Nuts, Oils, Seeds:

Seed: sesame seed

MENSTRUATION: DEPRESSION AND HORMONE REGULATOR

Amino Acids, Minerals, Omega Oils, Vitamins:

Vitamin: E

Fruit: blackberry

Essential Oils: chamomile, chamomile: blue, clary sage, lavender, myrtle, pina, sage, sandalwood, spruce

Herbs: black cohosh root, cannabis, fenugreek seed, tarragon, borage, dandelion, fenugreek, ginseng, licorice root, lobelia, skullcap

Meat: beef: beef: calf liver, beef kidney

Nuts, Oils, Seeds:

Oil: grapeseed oil, hemp seed oil

Seed: flaxseed, hemp seed

MENSTRUATION: HEAVY BLEEDING

Essential Oils: spearmint

Herbs: amaranth, bayberry, bearberry, chamomile, cinnamon, ginger, goldenseal, nettle, peppermint, plantain, primrose, raspberry, rosemary, witch hazel

MENSTRUATION: IRREGULAR PERIODS

Fruit: cantaloupe

Essential Oils: chamomile: blue, peppermint, rosemary, sage, spearmint

Herbs: black cohosh, calendula, catnip, horsetail, wormwood, yarrow

MENSTRUATION: PAIN

Essential Oils: cypress, grapefruit, lavender, ginseng

Herbs: cannabis, sassafras, slippery elm, spearmint, thyme, white oak bark

MENSTRUATION: SCANTY PERIODS AND STIMULATE MENSTRUATION

Essential Oils: basil, nutmeg

Herbs: myrrh, wormwood

MENTAL ALERTNESS / DEVELOPEMENT

Amino Acids, Minerals, Omega Oils, Vitamins:

Amino Acid: l-glutamine

Mineral: boron

Vitamins: B1

MENTAL DISABILITIES

Amino Acids, Minerals, Omega Oils, Vitamins: l-glutamine

MENTAL FATIGUE

Essential Oils: rosemary, ylang ylang

Herb: ginseng

MENTAL HEALTH / WELL-BEING

Amino Acids, Minerals, Omega Oils, Vitamins:

Amino Acid: l-lysine

Mineral: iodine, manganese

Vitamins: B3, B12, C, E

Dairy: cheese: cow, cheese: goat, milk: cow, milk: goat

Fruit: plum / prune

Meat:

Beef: beef kidney

Lake, ocean, river, sea: fish: saltwater, halibut, herring, mackerel, salmon, sardines, tuna

Lamb: lamb

MERCURY POISONING

Herb: cranesbill

METABOLISM: STIMULATE

Amino Acids, Minerals, Omega Oils, Vitamins:

Amino Acid: l-tyrosine

Mineral: boron, iodine, manganese, vanadium

Vitamins: B2, B5 (carbs, fats & proteins), biotin, folate, C

Dairy: cheese: cow, cheese: goat, milk: cow, milk: goat

Fruit: blueberry, cantaloupe, mango, rhubarb

Herbs: gentian, kelp, pokeweed, primrose, white oak bark

Legumes: soybean

Meat:

Beef: beef, beef: kidney

Lake, ocean, river, sea: fish oils

Pork

Poultry: chicken, egg, egg yolk, pork, fish oils

Nuts, Oils, Seeds:

Nut: pecan, pistachio

Oil: hemp seed oil, olive oil

Seed: chia seed

Vegetable: parsnip, rutabaga, squash

MIGRAINES:

Essential Oils: asil, eucalyptus, lavender, marjoram, peppermint,

Herb: ginger

Nuts, Oils, Seeds: Nut: cashew, mustard seed, sesame seed

MORNING SICKNESS

Herbs: ginger, kelp, raspberry, wormwood

MOTION SICKNESS

Herb: marjoram

MOUTH: CANKER SORES

Herbs: bayberry, bearberry, birch, bistort, cinnamon, cranesbill, myrrh, nettle, raspberry, white pond lily

MOUTH: GUMS – BLEEDING

Herbs: amaranth, birch, sage, witch hazel

Mouth: Gums- Disease

Herbs: barberry, bayberry, chamomile, cinnamon, goldenseal, melaleuca, myrrh, Peruvian bark, wild indigo

MOUTH: GUMS - SORE

Essential Oils: spearmint

Herbs: arnica, bayberry, bearberry, bistort, black walnut, buchu, calendula, chamomile, Chlorella, cinnamon, dandelion, goldenseal, melaleuca, oregano

MOUTH: INFECTIONS/BACTERIA

Herbs: barberry, chamomile, chlorella, cinnamon, fennel, goldenseal, lavender, licorice Root, oregano, prickly ash, rose hips, sage, thyme, wild indigo, yarrow

MOUTH: SORES

Amino Acids, Minerals, Omega Oils, Vitamins:

Mineral: iodine

Essential Oils: cinnamon, cinnamon bark, cloves, ginger, lavender, myrrh, nettle

Herbs: calendula, cinnamon, goldenseal, lavender, meadowsweet, prickly ash, rose hips, senna, wild indigo

MOUTH: SUPPORT

Vegetable: pumpkin (cancer prevention)

MUCUS BUILD-UP

Herb: chickweed, rose hips, white oak bark

MUCOUS MEMBRANES

Fruit: lemon

MULTIPLE SCLEROSIS (MS): AN AUTOIMMUNE DISEASE OF THE CENTRAL NERVOUS SYSTEM (BRAIN, SPINAL CORD).

Essential Oils: juniper berry

Herbs: cannabis, echinacea, primrose

Nuts, Oils, Seeds: Seed: hemp seed

MUMPS

Herbs: mullein, peppermint, pokeweed

MUSCLE: BUILDING

Amino Acids, Minerals, Omega Oils, Vitamins:

Mineral: calcium

Dairy: whey

Vegetable: potato

MUSCLE: BRUISES

Herbs: arnica, spearmint

MUSCLE: CRAMPS

Amino Acids, Minerals, Omega Oils, Vitamins:

Amino Acid: l-glutamine

Vitamin: D

Essential Oils: birch, cypress, marjoram, myrtle

Fruit: banana

Herbs: blue cohosh, catnip, chickweed, horsetail, Lady's slipper root, meadowsweet, prickly ash, skullcap, yarrow

Meat: poultry (turkey)

Nuts, Oils, Seeds:

Nut: cashew

Vegetable: pepper (bell)

MUSCLE: INFLAMMATION/ SWELLING (REDUCE)

Amino Acids, Minerals, Omega Oils, Vitamins:

Amino Acid: l-glutamine

MINERAL: MAGNESIUM

Dairy: whey

Essential Oils: chamomile (roman), lavender, lemongrass, ravensara, rosemary

Fruit: pear, pineapple, plum / prune, Saskatoon berry

Grains: buckwheat, corn, millet, oat, quinoa, rye, spelt

Herbs: arnica, Ashwagandha, basil, black cohosh, catnip, chaparral, chickweed, eucalyptus, gentian, ginseng, horsetail, hyssop, Lady's slipper root, licorice root, mullein, nettle, oregano, rosemary, spearmint, turkey rhubarb, turmeric, collards

Legumes: carob, navy bean

Meat:

Lake, ocean, river, sea: fish oils, halibut, herring

Poultry: chicken, egg

Vegetable: cucumber, Swiss chard

MUSCLE: LIGAMENTS

Herbs: arnica

MUSCLE: PAIN

Amino Acids, Minerals, Omega Oils, Vitamins:

Amino Acid: l-glutamine

Vitamin: biotin

Essential Oils: birch, cypress, eucalyptus, ginger, juniper berry, marjoram, orange

Fruit: cherry, Saskatoon berry

Herbs: angelica, balm of Gilead, black cohosh, cannabis, oregano, valerian, witch hazel, yarrow

MUSCLE: SPASM

Amino Acids, Minerals, Omega Oils, Vitamins:

Amino Acid: l-glutamine

Vitamins: choline

Essential Oils: chamomile: blue, myrtle, peppermint, ravensara, spruce, tarragon

Fruit: cherry

Herbs: black cohosh, blue cohosh, calendula, cloves, ginger, lobelia, skullcap, valerian

Nuts, Oils, Seeds:

Nut: cashew

Vegetables: celery, pepper (bell), sweet potato

MUSCLE: SPRAINS

Herb: arnica

MUSCLE: SUPPORT

Amino Acids, Minerals, Omega Oils, Vitamins:

Mineral: boron, magnesium, potassium, sodium

Vitamins: B1

Diary: whey

Fruit: peach

Grain: couscous, millet, oat, rice (brown)

Legumes: Bean (Black and Red), carob, garbanzo bean, kidney bean, lima bean, navy bean, pinto bean

Meat:

Lake, ocean, river, sea: herring, mackerel, salmon, sardines, tuna

Poultry: egg

Nuts, Oils, Seeds:

Seed: chia seed, hemp seed, sunflower seed

Vegetable: potato, rutabaga, squash

NAILS

Amino Acids, Minerals, Omega Oils, Vitamins:

Mineral: silicon

Herb: horse tail

NASAL CONGESTION

Herb: lemongrass

NARCOTIC POISONING

Herb: marjoram

NAUSEA

Essential Oils: cloves, fennel, ginger, lavender, nutmeg, peppermint, spearmint

Herbs: alfalfa, basil, cayenne, cinnamon, caraway seed, ginger, eucalyptus, gentian, ginger, ginseng, lavender, marjoram, peppermint, raspberry, sage, spearmint, white oak bark, wild indigo, wormwood

NERVE DISEASE

Fruit: grape/raisin

Nerves: Calming

Amino Acids, Minerals, Omega Oils, Vitamins:

Mineral: magnesium, manganese

Vitamins: B6, inositol

Essential Oils: basil, cedarwood, chamomile (roman), clary sage, cypress, geranium, juniper berry, lavender, oregano oil, sage, spearmint, tarragon

Grains: buckwheat, oat, quinoa, rye, spelt, wheat

Herbs: Ashwagandha, basil, black cohosh, blue cohosh, borage, cannabis, catnip, cayenne, chamomile, chlorella, cilantro, cinnamon, cramp bark, ginseng, gravel root, hawthorn, holy basil, hops, horsetail, hyssop, kelp, Lady's slipper root, lobelia, mandrake, milk thistle, mullein, oatstraw, red clover, reishi mushroom, rosemary, sage, skullcap, spearmint, valerian, wormwood, yarrow

Legumes: carob

Meat:

Lake, ocean, river, sea: herring, mackerel

Pork

Nuts, Oils, Seeds:

Seed: sunflower seed

Vegetables: beet greens, dulse, pumpkin, Swiss chard

NERVES: NERVE ENDINGS AND TRANSMISSION

Amino Acids, Minerals, Omega Oils, Vitamins:

Mineral: sodium

Vitamins: B1, B5

Essential Oil: thyme

NERVOUS SYSTEM: SUPPORT

Amino Acids, Minerals, Omega Oils, Vitamins:

Amino Acid: l-taurine, l-tyrosine

Mineral: calcium, copper, potassium

Vitamins: B2, B3, B6, B12, biotin, E

Fruit: peach

Grains: corn, couscous, millet, rice (Brown), wheat bran, wheat germ

Meat:

Beef: beef, beef liver,

Lake, ocean, river, sea: clams, fish: fresh water, fish oils, fish: saltwater, halibut, salmon, sardines, tuna

Poultry: chicken, egg, turkey

Nuts, Oils, Seeds:

Nut: cashew, walnut

Oil: hemp seed oil, sesame seed oil, Siberian pine nut oil, walnut oil

Vegetable: kohlrabi, potato, pumpkin, squash

NERVE TISSUE

Vegetable: sweet potato

NEURASTHENIA
Herb: skullcap

NEURALGIA
Herbs: blue cohosh, cramp bark

NEURALGIC PAIN (ACHES)
Essential Oils: chamomile (blue), valerian

NEURODEGENERATIVE DISEASES
Fruit: peach

NEUROLOGICAL DISEASES
Fruit: cranberry

NEUROLOGICAL SYSTEM
Fruit: cherry

NEW CASTLE DISEASE
Herbs: peppermint

NIGHTMARES
Herbs: marjoram

NIGHT SWEATS
Essential Oils: sage

Herbs: sage

NIPPLES: SORE
Herbs: myrrh

NURSING: PROMOTE LACTATION
Herbs: fennel

NURSING: STOP LACTATION
Herbs: black walnut

Nose: Stop Nose Bleeds

Herbs: alfalfa, amaranth, horsetail, nettle, witch hazel

ORGAN SUPPORT

Legumes: carob

Vegetables: cauliflower, onion (red)

Nuts, Oils, Seeds: Seed: cacao

OSTEOARTHRITIS

Herbs: bilberry

Vegetables: kelp

OSTEOPOROSIS

Amino Acids, Minerals, Omega Oils, Vitamins:

Mineral: boron, copper

Omega Oil: omega 3, omega 6

Vitamin: D

Essential Oils: birch

Fruit: kiwi

Herbs: cilantro, horsetail

Nuts, Oils, Seeds:

Nut: Brazil nut, pecan

Oil: avocado oil

Seed: flaxseed, sesame seed, sunflower seed

Vegetable: squash

OSTEOMYELITIS

Herbs: Pau d'arco

OVARIAN CANCER: PREVENTION

Vegetables: broccoli

PAIN RELIEVER

Amino Acids, Minerals, Omega Oils, Vitamins:

Vitamin: P

Essential Oils: chamomile (blue), cloves

Herbs: chamomile, Pau d'arco

PALSY:
PALSY IS A FORM OF PARALYSIS THAT IS FOLLOWED BY INVOLUNTARY TREMORS.

Herbs: lobelia, cloves

PANCREAS: PROMOTE INSULIN PRODUCTION

Herbs: raspberry

PANCREAS: SUPPORT

Essential Oils: cypress, helichrysium/strawflower

Herbs: bearberry, cascara sagrada, cayenne, dandelion, holy basil, juniper, oatstraw, reishi mushroom

Legumes: bean (black)

Nuts, Oils, Seeds:

Nut: coconut

Oil: almond oil, Siberian pine nut oil

Vegetable: asparagus, bean (lima)

PARALYSIS

Herbs: eucalyptus, oatstraw, prickly ash

PARANOIA

Herbs: reishi mushroom

PARASITES

Essential Oils: chamomile (Roman), fennel, melaleuca/tea tree, oregano, patchouli, tangerine, tarragon, thyme

Fruit: pineapple

Herb: agrimony, black walnut, blessed thistle, cascara sagrada, catnip, garlic, lobelia, oregano, Pau d'arco, wormwood

Nuts, Oils, Seeds: Seed: pumpkin seed

PARASYMPATHETIC SYSTEM

Essential Oil: lemongrass, marjoram

PARKINSON'S DISEASE

Herbs: skullcap

PEPTIC ULCERS

Herbs: Irish moss, marshmallow

PESTICIDE

Fruit: banana (mosquitoes)

Herbs: lemongrass

PHLEBITIS

Essential Oils: lavender

PH LEVELS

Amino Acids, Minerals, Omega Oils, Vitamins:

Mineral: sodium

PINWORM

Essential Oils: oregano

Herb: garlic, wormwood, blessed thistle, garlic, white oak bark

PITUITARY GLAND

Amino Acids, Minerals, Omega Oils, Vitamins:

Vitamin: E

Herb: aloe vera, buchu, comfrey, kelp

Meat:

Lake, ocean, river, sea: halibut, herring, mackerel, salmon, sardines, tuna

PLAQUE
Essential Oils: cloves, sage

Herbs: sage

PLEURISY
Essential Oils: cypress, lobelia

PMS: SEE MENSTURATION

PNEUMONIA
Essential Oils: frankincense, oregano oil

Herbs: astragalus, lobelia, mullein, olive leaf, pleurisy root

POISON IVY
Herbs: lobelia, sassafras, slippery elm

POISON OAK
Herbs: bearberry, lobelia, sassafras

POISONOUS MUSHROOMS
Herbs: wormwood

POLIO VIRUS 1
Herbs: raspberry

POST MENOPAUSE
Grain: rye

PREGNANCY: FOLATE
Legume: garbanzo beans

Vegetable: lettuce (romaine)

PREGNANCY: SUPPORTIVE
Herbs: catnip, nettle, raspberry

PERSPIRATION
Herbs: oatstraw, pleurisy root, prickly ash, sage, yarrow

PLEURISY
Herbs: pleurisy root

PROBIOTIC
Dairy: yogurt

PROSTATE CANCER
Fruit: tomato

Meat: lamb

PROSTATE INFLAMMATION
Herbs: licorice root, nettle

PROSTATE SUPPORT
Amino Acids, Minerals, Omega Oils, Vitamins:

Mineral: selenium, zinc

Essential Oils: peppermint, spruce, thyme

Fruit: currant (red), grape / raisin, guava, tomato

Grains: barley, buckwheat, oat, rye, wheat

Herb: angelica, black cohosh, buchu, chaparral, gravel root, horsetail, juniper, kelp, milk thistle, nettle, parsley, Pau d'arco

Nuts, Oils, Seeds:

Nut: walnut

Seed: pumpkin seed

Vegetable: broccoli, Brussel sprouts, mushroom (white), pumpkin, squash

PSORIASIS: SEE SKIN

PTSD
Herbs: cannabis

PULMONARY SUPPORT

Essential Oils: myrtle, sage, sandalwood

Herbs: chickweed, kale

RABIES

Herbs: lobelia

RADIATION POISONING

Amino Acids, Minerals, Omega Oils, Vitamins:

Amino Acid: l-glutamine

Vitamin: coenzyme Q10

Herbs: ginseng

RAYNAUD'S DISEASE

Herbs: butcher's broom

RASHES

Herbs: olive leaf

RECTAL

Nuts, Oils, Seeds: Oil: almond oil

RECTAL PROLAPSE: CHILDREN

Nuts, Oils, Seeds:

Oil: almond oil

RELAXANT: SEDATIVE

Fruit: cherry, passion fruit

Essential Oils: basil, bergamot, cedarwood, clary sage, fir, frankincense, geranium, lavender, lemongrass, marjoram, orange, spruce

Herbs: borage, lavender, oatstraw, red clover, rosemary

REPRODUCTIVE GLANDS

Herbs: ginseng, white poplar

REPRODUCTIVE ORGANS

Amino Acids, Minerals, Omega Oils, Vitamins:

Amino Acid: l-lysine

Mineral: zinc

Essential Oils: rosemary

Herbs: rosemary

RESPIRATORY DISCOMFORT

Amino Acids, Minerals, Omega Oils, Vitamins:

Vitamin: coenzyme Q10

Fruit: kiwi

Essential Oils: cedarwood, eucalyptus, lemon, lemongrass, sage, sandalwood

Herbs: basil, licorice root, plantain, pleurisy root, pokeweed, red clover, reishi mushroom, slippery elm

RESPIRATORY: INFECTION

Essential Oils: basil, bergamot, eucalyptus, melaleuca/tea tree, oregano

Herbs: burdock, melaleuca/tea tree, reishi mushroom, slippery elm, onion (green)

RESPIRATORY: MUCUS

Essential Oils: fir

Herbs: burdock, pleurisy root

RESPIRATORY: SUPPORT

Amino Acids, Minerals, Omega Oils, Vitamins:

Vitamins: B2, B3

Fruit: kiwi, pineapple

Nuts, Oils, Seeds: Oil: Siberian pine nut oil

RESPIRATORY TRACT

Vegetable: onion (green)

RESTLESSNESS

Herbs: skullcap, valerian

REYNAUD'S DISEASE

Herbs: bilberry

RHEUMATOID ARTHRITIS

Essential Oils: birch, cinnamon, cloves, cypress, ginger, juniper berry, lavender, lemon, marjoram, nutmeg, oregano, pina, sage, spruce, tarragon, thyme

Fruit: kiwi

Herbs: agrimony, cayenne, chickweed, basil, black cohosh, buchu, cayenne, chaparral, Gravel root, hawthorn, hops, horseradish, Irish moss, lavender, lobelia, mandrake, nettle, oatstraw, Pau d'arco, pleurisy root, pokeweed, prickly ash, sassafras, senna, skullcap, slippery elm, wild indigo, yarrow, yellow dock

Nuts, Oils, Seeds:

Seed: hemp seed, mustard seed, sesame seed, sunflower seed

Vegetable: Brussel sprout, collards, squash

RICKETS:
THIS HAPPENS WHEN A PERSON DOES NOT GET ENOUGH VITAMIN D, CALCIUM AND PHOSPHOROUS.

Mineral: calcium, phosphorous

Vitamin: D

Herbs: red clover, skullcap

RINGWORM:

Essential Oils: geranium, melaleuca/tea tree, oregano oil

Herbs: aloe vera, borage, goldenseal, holy basil, lobelia, melaleuca, oregano

RHEUMATIC FEVER

Amino Acids, Minerals, Omega Oils, Vitamins: Vitamin: E

RNA SUPPORT

Amino Acids, Minerals, Omega Oils, Vitamins:

Mineral: calcium

ROCKY MOUNTAIN SPOTTED FEVER

Herbs: olive leaf

ROOT CANAL
Herbs: sassafras

ROSACEA
Nuts, Oils, Seeds: Seed: flaxseed

ROUNDWORM
Herbs: olive leaf

SCABIES
Herbs: caraway seed, oregano, pokeweed

SCARLET FEVER
Herbs: bayberry, hyssop, lobelia, pleurisy root, valerian

SKELETAL MUSCLES
Amino Acids, Minerals, Omega Oils, Vitamins:

Vitamins: inositol

SCIATICA
Essential Oil: tarragon

Herbs: burdock

SCURVY
Amino Acids, Minerals, Omega Oils, Vitamins:

Vitamin: C

Essential Oil: ginger

Fruit: gooseberry, lemon, lime

Herbs: balm of Gilead, bayberry, bilberry, burdock, horseradish, yellow dock

SEDATIVE: SEE RELAXANT

SEIZER
Amino Acids, Minerals, Omega Oils, Vitamins:

Amino Acid: l-taurine

Mineral: magnesium

Vitamin: D

SEXUAL: HORMONES, STIMULANT

Amino Acids, Minerals, Omega Oils, Vitamins:

Vitamin: E

Herbs: ginseng

Nuts, Oils, Seeds:

Nut: pistachio

SEXUALLY TRANSMITTED DISEASES

Herbs: Pau d'arco

SHINGLES

Essential Oils: geranium

Herbs: olive leaf

SHOCK:

Essential Oils: melaleuca/tea tree, peppermint, ylang ylang

Herbs: lobelia

SINUS: INFECTIONS/SINUSITIS

Essential Oils: eucalyptus, helichrysium/strawflower, melaleuca/tea tree, myrtle, peppermint, ravensara, rosemary, sage

Herb: anise seed, black cohosh root, buchu, cayenne, pina, eucalyptus, horseradish, marjoram, marshmallow, meadowsweet, mullein, oregano, peppermint

SINUS: SUPPORT

Herbs: myrrh, witch hazel

Skin: Abscesses

Herbs: myrrh, pokeweed

SKIN: ACNE

Amino Acids, Minerals, Omega Oils, Vitamins:

Mineral: zinc

Essential Oils: cedarwood, chamomile (blue), helichrysium/strawflower, juniper berry, melaleuca/tea tree, myrtle, sandalwood

Herb: agrimony, aloe vera, black walnut, burdock root, chaparral, horse tail, melaleuca, oregano, rosewood

Nuts, Oils, Seeds:

Oil: hazelnut oil

Seed: flaxseed

Vegetable: lettuce (romaine)

SKIN: AGE SPOTS

Herbs: dandelion root, ginseng, licorice root

Skin: Bacteria

Herbs: barberry, burdock, gentian, yarrow

SKIN: BOILS

Herbs: black walnut, burdock, dandelion, garlic, lemongrass, marshmallow, melaleuca, milk thistle, myrrh, oatstraw, olive leaf, sassafras, slippery elm

SKIN: BRUISES

Amino Acids, Minerals, Omega Oils, Vitamins:

Vitamin: P

Essential Oils: marjoram, myrtle

Herbs: arnica, hyssop, mullein, rose hips, witch hazel, yarrow

SKIN: BURNS

Amino Acids, Minerals, Omega Oils, Vitamins:

Amino Acid: l-glutamine

Vitamin: E

Essential Oils: eucalyptus, lavender, melaleuca/tea tree

Fruit: papaya

Herbs: aloe vera, balm of Gilead, calendula, horsetail, lavender, marshmallow, melaleuca, plantain, red clover, slippery elm, thyme, witch hazel, yarrow

Vegetable: onion (red)

SKIN: CANCER

Fruit: tangerine

Grain: millet

Herbs: cleaver, Pau d'arco, pokeweed

SKIN: CANKER SORES

Herbs: amaranth

SKIN: CARE

Amino Acids, Minerals, Omega Oils, Vitamins:

Mineral: copper, silicon

Omega Oil: omega 3, omega 6

Vitamins: A, B2, B3, inositol

Essential Oils: peppermint, ylang ylang

Fruit: apricot, avocado, cantaloupe, chokecherry, gooseberry, guava, lemon, mango, passion fruit, peach, raspberry, tangerine

Grain: couscous, oat, quinoa, rice (brown and white), rye, spelt, wheat, wheat bran, wheat germ

Herbs: chamomile, hyssop, kelp, pleurisy root

Legumes: bean (red), black-eyed peas, carob

Meat:

Beef: beef: calf liver, beef liver

Lake, ocean, river, sea: clams, dish: fresh water, halibut, herring, mackerel, salmon, sardines, tuna

Lamb: lamb

Poultry: egg, egg yolk, turkey

Nuts, Oils, Seeds:

Nut: cashew, coconut, hazelnut, pecan, pine nut

Oil: almond oil, avocado oil, coconut oil, grapeseed oil, hazelnut oil, hemp seed oil, sesame seed oil

Seed: chia seed, flaxseed, hemp seed, pumpkin seed

Vegetable: cucumber, radish, rutabaga

SKIN: CIRRHOSIS

Herbs: milk thistle, olive leaf

SKIN: CUTS

Herbs: bayberry, cayenne, cleaver, comfrey, cranesbill, fennel, hyssop, meadowsweet, melaleuca, myrrh, plantain, white oak bark, wild indigo, witch hazel

SKIN: CORNS

Herbs: sassafras

SKIN: DERMATITIS

Essential Oils: helichrysium/strawflower, juniper berry, patchouli

Herbs: Pau d'arco

Nuts, Oils, Seeds: Nut: coconut

SKIN: DIAPER RASH

Herbs: mullein, slippery elm

SKIN: DISORDERS

Herb: cedarwood, chaparral, cranesbill, plantain, primrose, white oak bark

SKIN: DISEASES

Amino Acids, Minerals, Omega Oils, Vitamins:

Vitamin: paba

Essential Oils: cedarwood, cloves, geranium, orange

Herbs: balm of Gilead, black walnut, dandelion, gentian, oatstraw, sassafras, senna

SKIN: DRY/ITCHY

Essential Oils: clary sage, cypress, geranium, orange, peppermint, rosewood, spearmint

Grain: oat

Herbs: balm of Gilead, chaparral, hyssop, marshmallow, pleurisy root, primrose

Nuts, Oils, Seeds:

Nut: Brazil nut

Oil: almond oil, coconut oil, hemp seed oil

Seed: flaxseed, hemp seed

SKIN: ECZEMA

Essential Oils: cedarwood, chamomile, chamomile (Blue), helichrysium/strawflower, juniper berry, lavender, melaleuca/tea tree, patchouli, peppermint, rosewood, spearmint

Grains: oat

Herbs: aloe vera, birch, burdock, calendula, chamomile, chaparral, goldenseal, kelp, lavender, lobelia, melaleuca, myrrh, nettle, Pau d'arco, red clover, rosemary, thyme, white oak bark, white poplar, yellow dock

Nuts, Oils, Seeds:

Nut: coconut

Oil: almond oil

SKIN: HERPES

Herbs: black walnut, myrrh, slippery elm

SKIN: HIVES

Herbs: ginger, nettle, yellow dock

SKIN: INFECTIONS / INFLAMMATION /RASHES

Amino Acids, Minerals, Omega Oils, Vitamins:

Amino Acid: l-glutamine

Mineral: zinc

Vitamin: biotin

Essential Oils: cloves, eucalyptus, myrrh, patchouli, sage, sandalwood, thyme

Fruit: lemon

Grain: oat

Herbs: angelica, balm of Gilead, bearberry, black walnut, borage, burdock, calendula, chamomile, chaparral, chickweed, comfrey, eucalyptus, garlic, goldenseal, horsetail, melaleuca, nettle, olive leaf, plantain, rose hips, rosemary, sassafras, slippery elm, thyme, white oak bark, white poplar, wild indigo, yellow dock

Nuts, Oils, Seeds:

Nut: coconut

Seed: hemp seed

Vegetable: radish

SKIN: OILY

Essential Oils: fennel, geranium

SKIN: PARASITES

Herb: melaleuca

SKIN: PIMPLES

Herbs: myrrh

SKIN: PSORIASIS

Essential Oils: bergamot, geranium, helichrysium/strawflower, lavender, melaleuca/tea tree, thyme

Herbs: burdock, cleaver, comfrey, dandelion, melaleuca, oregano, Pau d'arco, pokeweed, red clover, rose hips, sassafras, thyme

Nuts, Oils, Seeds:

Nut: coconut

Oil: avocado oil, hemp seed oil

SKIN: REGENERATIVE

Fruit: tangerine

Essential Oils: orange, patchouli

Herbs: comfrey, fennel, Irish moss, marshmallow, primrose, rose hips, rosemary, white pond lily

Vegetables: cucumber, lettuce (romaine)

SKIN: SCARS

Essential Oils: lavender

Herbs: lavender

Nuts, Oils, Seeds: Oil: Siberian pine nut oil

SKIN: SLIVERS

Herbs: garlic, hawthorn

Skin: Stretchmark/Tightening

Essential Oils: grapefruit, lavender, myrrh, patchouli, sage

Herbs: lavender, lemongrass

SKIN: SUNBURN

Herbs: balm of Gilead, calendula, chaparral, cleaver, comfrey, melaleuca

SKIN: ULCERS

Amino Acids, Minerals, Omega Oils, Vitamins:

Amino Acid: l-glutamine

Herbs: amaranth, chickweed, goldenseal, myrrh, Pau d'arco, prickly ash

Skin: Wounds (regeneration)

Amino Acids, Minerals, Omega Oils, Vitamins:

Vitamin: C, E

Essential Oils: geranium, juniper berry, lavender, lemongrass

Fruit: tangerine

Herbs: amaranth, angelica, balm of Gilead, black walnut, catnip, cayenne, comfrey, cranesbill, eucalyptus, ginger, horsetail, lemongrass, lobelia, marshmallow, mullein, oatstraw, prickly ash, rosemary, slippery elm, wild indigo, witch hazel, wormwood

Nuts, Oils, Seeds:

Oil: avocado oil, hazelnut oil, Siberian pine nut oil

Vegetable: squash

SKIN: WOUNDS INFECTED

Amino Acids, Minerals, Omega Oils, Vitamins:

Vitamin: C

Essential Oils: chamomile (blue), cloves, eucalyptus, frankincense, juniper berry, tarragon

Herbs: agrimony, angelica, arnica, black walnut, catnip, echinacea, ginger, goldenseal, mullein, myrrh, oatstraw, oregano, plantain, prickly ash, slippery elm, thyme, white oak bark, white poplar, wild indigo

Nuts, Oils, Seeds:

Oil: hazelnut oil

SKIN: WRINKLES

Essential Oils: grapefruit

Herbs: aloe vera, cranesbill, kelp

SLEEP

Fruit: passion fruit

Herb: catnip, chamomile, lavender, mullein, skullcap

Nuts, Oils, Seeds:

Nut: walnut

Seed: mustard seed, sesame seed

SMOKERS COUGH

Herbs: Pau d'arco

SNAKE BITES

Essential Oils: patchouli

Herbs: sage, skullcap

SNORING

Nuts, Oils, Seeds: Oil: hazelnut oil

SPASMS

Essential Oils: cypress

SPINAL MENINGITIS

Herbs: skullcap

SPLEEN

Essential Oils: cloves

Herbs: agrimony, astragalus, bearberry, black cohosh, cayenne, horseradish, milk thistle, Pau d'arco, pokeweed, white oak bark, yellow dock

SPLINTERS

Herbs: agrimony

SPORT INJURIES
Amino Acids, Minerals, Omega Oils, Vitamins:
Amino Acid: l-glutamine

SPORT TRAINING
Amino Acids, Minerals, Omega Oils, Vitamins:
Amino Acid: l-glutamine

SPRAINS
Amino Acids, Minerals, Omega Oils, Vitamins:
Amino Acid: l-glutamine
Essential Oils: ginger, marjoram, sage
Herbs: agrimony, witch hazel, wormwood

STAPH INFECTION
Essential Oils: frankincense, thyme

STERILITY
Essential Oils: geranium

STIMULANT
Essential Oils: birch, eucalyptus, ginger, oregano oil, ravensara, sage
Herbs: agrimony, alfalfa

STOMACH: CANCER
Vegetable: pea

STOMACH: CLEANSER
Essential Oils: basil, cloves
Herbs: agrimony, blessed thistle, goldenseal, licorice root
Vegetable: cabbage

STOMACH: CRAMPS
Essential Oils: helichrysium/strawflower

Herbs: alfalfa, aloe vera, basil, blessed thistle, cramp bark, fennel, hops, hyssop, Lady's slipper root, pleurisy root, reishi mushroom, rose hips, thyme

Vegetable: kohlrabi

STOMACH: CYSTS

Herbs: astragalus

STOMACH: DIGESTION

Essential Oils: basil, bergamot, cannabis, chamomile (Blue), cinnamon, clary sage, cloves, fennel, frankincense, geranium, ginger, grapefruit, helichrysium/strawflower, juniper berry, lemon, lemongrass, peppermint, melaleuca/tea tree, myrrh, nutmeg, orange, oregano oil, patchouli, peppermint, pina, sage, spearmint, tangerine, tarragon, thyme

Herbs: alfalfa, aloe vera, angelica, anise seed, astragalus, black walnut, borage, buchu, burdock, catnip, cayenne, chamomile flowers, cayenne, chamomile, cilantro, dandelion, eucalyptus, garlic, ginger, holy basil, horseradish, juniper, lavender, mandrake, milk thistle, oatstraw, oregano, parsley, peppermint, Peruvian bark, pleurisy root, prickly ash, reishi mushroom, rosemary, sage, slippery elm, spearmint, turkey rhubarb, white oak bark, white pond lily, wormwood, yellow dock

Vegetable: broccoli, Brussel sprout, cabbage, carrots, cauliflower

STOMACH: GAS & GASTRITIS

Fruit: blackberry, rhubarb

Herbs: ginger, hyssop, Irish moss, kelp, marjoram, mullein, myrrh, Pau d'arco, peppermint, plantain, pleurisy root, prickly ash, rose hips, spearmint, thyme, white poplar

Nuts, Oils, Seeds:

Oil: Siberian pine nut oil

Vegetable: kohlrabi

STOMACH: INFECTIONS

Essential Oils: melaleuca/tea tree, oregano

Herbs: goldenseal, melaleuca, prickly ash

STOMACH: SPASMS

Essential Oils: orange

Herbs: anise seed, blessed thistle, lobelia, pleurisy root, turkey rhubarb, white poplar

STOMACH SUPPORT

Dairy: yogurt

Fruit: cherry

Herbs: chickweed, cilantro, ginseng, holy basil, Irish moss, licorice root, marjoram, myrrh, parsley, pokeweed, valerian, white oak bark, yarrow

Vegetable: cabbage, celery, mustard greens, pea, squash

STOMACH: ULCERS

Herbs: eyebright, plantain, reishi mushroom, sage

Vegetable: celery

STREP THROAT

Herbs: white oak bark

STRESS

Amino Acids, Minerals, Omega Oils, Vitamins:

Vitamin: C

Essential Oils: chamomile, geranium, grapefruit, lavender, marjoram, rosewood, spruce, ylang ylang, tangerine

Herb: Ashwagandha, catnip, ginseng

Nuts, Oils, Seeds:

Nut: coconut, pecan

Vegetable: Swiss chard

STROKE PREVENTION

Amino Acids, Minerals, Omega Oils, Vitamins:

Vitamin: coenzyme Q10

Dairy: buttermilk

Fruit: apple, grape / raisin

Legume: peanut, pinto bean

Nuts, Oils, Seeds:

Nut: macadamia nut, pine nut

Oil: olive oil

Seed: sesame seed

SUBSTANCE ABUSE

Amino Acids, Minerals, Omega Oils, Vitamins:

Amino Acid: l-glutamine

ST. VITUS'S DANCE: JERKING MOTIONS

Herbs: skullcap, valerian

SWEAT GLANDS

Vegetable: onion (green)

SUNSTROKE

Essential Oils: lavender

Fruit: coconut milk

SYMPATHETIC NERVOUS SYSTEM

Herbs: gravel root

SYPHILIS

Essential Oils: frankincense

Grains: barley

Herbs: burdock, lobelia, Pau d'arco, prickly ash, sassafras, slippery elm, white poplar

TAPE WORMS

Herbs: aloe vera, black walnut, gravel root, olive leaf

TARDIVE DYSKINESIA

Amino Acids, Minerals, Omega Oils, Vitamins:

Vitamins: choline

TEETH: CAVITY PROTECTION

Fruit: cranberry

TEETH: GROWTH AND SUPPORT

Amino Acids, Minerals, Omega Oils, Vitamins:

Mineral: calcium, phosphorus, vanadium

Vitamins: A, B6, D

Dairy: butter, cheese (cow), cheese (goat), milk (cow), milk (goat)

Fruit: cantaloupe, cranberry, peach

Herbs: black walnut, green tea, holy basil, horsetail, lobelia, raspberry, sage

Meat:

Beef: beef: calf liver, beef liver

Lake, ocean, river, sea: fish oils

Lamb: lamb

Pork: pork

Poultry: egg

Vegetable: squash

TEETH: INFECTIONS

Fruit: cranberry

Herbs: cinnamon, cloves, melaleuca, thyme

Nuts, Oils, Seeds: Nut: coconut

TENDINITIS

Essential Oils: basil, birch

TESTICLES: SWELLING

Herbs: chickweed, mullein

TETANUS

Herbs: lobelia

THROAT: INFECTION

Essential Oils: cinnamon, clary sage, cypress, lavender, melaleuca/tea tree, oregano, peppermint, spearmint

Herbs: lavender, melaleuca, rosemary, white oak bark

THROAT: INFLAMMATION

Herbs: arnica, melaleuca, pokeweed, witch hazel

THROAT: MUCOUS

Herbs: wild indigo

THROAT: SORE

Essential Oils: chamomile, cinnamon, clary sage, cypress, fir, geranium, ginger, lemon, lemongrass

Herbs: anise seed, balm of Gilead, barberry, bayberry, black walnut, blue cohosh, cayenne, eucalyptus, eyebright, fenugreek, goldenseal, holy basil, hops, hyssop, lavender, licorice root, marshmallow, melaleuca, mullein, myrrh, oregano, peppermint, pokeweed, rose hips, slippery elm, white oak bark

Vegetable: onion (green)

THROMBOPHLEBITIS

Herbs: butcher's broom

THRUSH

Essential Oils: lavender

Herbs: Goldenseal, lavender, melaleuca

THYMUS GLAND

Essential Oils: spruce

Herbs: Irish moss

TYPHUS

Herbs: pleurisy root

THYROID: HYPER

Essential Oils: lavender, myrrh, myrtle, spruce

Herb: kelp

Amino Acids, Minerals, Omega Oils, Vitamins:

Mineral: selenium

THYROID: SUPPORT

Amino Acids, Minerals, Omega Oils, Vitamins:

Amino Acid: l-tyrosine

Mineral: iodine, selenium

Vitamins: B2

Dairy: butter, cheese (cow), cheese (goat), milk (goat)

Herbs: kelp, pokeweed, skullcap, yellow dock, dulse, kelp

Meat:

Beef: liver

Lake, ocean, river, sea: herring

Pork: pork

Poultry: chicken, egg, egg yolk

Nuts, Oils, Seeds:

Nut: coconut

Seed: chia seed

TOBACCO POISONING

Herbs: sassafras

TONSILLITIS

Essential Oils: bergamot, frankincense, ginger, melaleuca/tea tree

Herbs: black walnut, calendula, lobelia, melaleuca, mullein, pokeweed

Nuts, Oils, Seeds:

Oil: Siberian pine nut oil

TOOTHACHE / TOOTH INFECTION

Essential Oils: chamomile, cinnamon, cloves, melaleuca/tea tree, peppermint

Herbs: angelica, calendula, cinnamon, marjoram, oregano, prickly ash, sage, wild indigo

TRAVEL SICKNESS

Essential Oils: peppermint

TREMORS

Amino Acids, Minerals, Omega Oils, Vitamins:

Mineral: phosphorus

Herbs: Lady's slipper root, skullcap

TUBERCULOSIS

Essential Oils: cloves, cypress, eucalyptus, frankincense, lavender, oregano, peppermint, thyme

Grains: barley

Herbs: black walnut, chaparral, cloves, Irish moss, lavender, mullein, myrrh, oregano, plantain, pleurisy root, slippery elm, white pond lily, witch hazel

TUMOURS: PREVENTION AND REDUCE

Fruit: peach

Herbs: chaparral, chickweed, fennel, Pau d'arco, reishi mushroom, rosemary, slippery elm, witch hazel, yellow dock

Legumes: bean (black), lentil

Nuts, Oils, Seeds:

Nut: walnut

Oil: olive oil

Vegetable: asparagus

TYPHOID FEVER

Essential Oils: cinnamon, frankincense, lavender

Herbs: bilberry, echinacea, eucalyptus, Lady's slipper root, mandrake, wild indigo

ULCERS

Essential Oils: birch, chamomile (Blue), clary sage, frankincense, geranium, myrrh, peppermint,

Herbs: amaranth, astragalus, bayberry, ginseng, sassafras, slippery elm, wild indigo, yarrow, yellow dock

Nuts, Oils, Seeds: Oil: Siberian pine nut oil

ULCERS: EXTERNAL

Herbs: eucalyptus, ginseng, white oak bark

ULCERS: INFLAMED

Herbs: valerian, white oak bark

UTERUS:

Herbs: astragalus, bayberry, black cohosh, cramp bark, goldenseal, gravel root, kelp, mandrake, white oak bark

UTERUS: AFTER BIRTHING CRAMPS

Herbs: blue cohosh

UTERUS: HEMORRHAGING

Herbs: goldenseal

UTERUS: INFECTIONS

Herbs: cinnamon

URETHRITIS

Essential Oils: myrtle

Herbs: buchu

URIC ACID

Essential Oil: basil, birch, fennel, lemon

Herbs: alfalfa, bilberry, birch, burdock root, burdock, gravel root, horsetail, Irish moss, juniper berry, nettle, oatstraw, senna, wormwood

URINARY: BLEEDING

Herbs: marshmallow, white oak bark

URINARY: INFECTIONS

Fruit: cranberry

Essential Oils: cedarwood, juniper berry, thyme

Herbs: bearberry, bilberry, gentian

URINARY: STONES

Essential Oils: fennel, geranium

Herbs: gravel root

URINARY: SUPPORT

Essential Oils: sage

Fruit: cranberry

Herbs: bearberry, black walnut, gravel root (urogenital irritation), slippery elm

Vegetable: radish

URINARY TRACT
Fruit: cranberry

URETER INFECTIONS:
Essential Oils: lemon

UTERINE CANCER
Herbs: white pond lily

UTERUS: INFLAMMATION
Herbs: white pond lily

UTERUS: PROLAPSED / TIPPED
Herbs: black walnut

UTERUS: SUPPORT
Herbs: white pond lily

UV PROTECTION
Amino Acids, Minerals, Omega Oils, Vitamins:

Vitamin: paba

Fruit: guava

Grain: couscous, millet, rye

Nuts, Oils, Seeds:

Oil: hazelnut oil

VAGINITIS
Essential Oils: cinnamon, melaleuca/tea tree, rosemary, rosewood, spearmint, thyme

Herbs: meadowsweet, melaleuca, olive leaf, slippery elm

VAGY NERVE
Herbs: peppermint

VARICOSE ULCERS
Herbs: Pau d'arco

VARICOSE VEINS

Essential Oils: cypress, lemon, lemongrass, peppermint

Herbs: Bilberry, butcher's broom, calendula, Irish moss, marshmallow, Pau d'arco, sassafras, white oak bark

Nuts, Oils, Seeds:

Oil: hemp seed oil

VASCULAR SYSTEM: SEE HEART

VEINS

Herbs: prickly ash

Legumes: kidney beans, navy bean

VENEREAL DISEASE

Herbs: chaparral, mullein, parsley, white oak bark, witch hazel

VENEREAL WARTS

Herbs: mandrake

VERTIGO

Herbs: butcher's broom, eyebright

VIRUS: SEE INFECTIONS

VISION: SEE EYES

VOMITING

Essential Oils: basil, cloves, nutmeg, peppermint, spearmint

Herbs: basil, cinnamon, ginseng, lobelia, mandrake, raspberry, spearmint, white oak bark

WARTS

Amino Acids, Minerals, Omega Oils, Vitamins:

Mineral: selenium

Essential Oils: cypress, frankincense, melaleuca/tea tree

Herbs: black walnut, cloves, mandrake, melaleuca, mullein, olive leaf, oregano, Pau d'arco, thyme

WATER RETENTION

Essential Oils: patchouli

Herbs: kelp

WEIGHT GAIN

Amino Acids, Minerals, Omega Oils, Vitamins:

Mineral: iodine

WEIGHT REDUCTION

Amino Acids, Minerals, Omega Oils, Vitamins:

Amino Acid: l-tyrosine

Mineral: chromium

Vitamins: B2

Essential Oils: grapefruit, patchouli

Fruit: lemon, pineapple, raspberry, tangerine

Herbs: evening primrose, chaparral, primrose, sassafras, wormwood

Legume: peanut

Nuts, Oils, Seeds:

Nut: coconut, pecan, pine nut, pistachio

Oil: almond oil, coconut oil, Siberian pine nut oil

Seed: chia seed, flaxseed, hemp seed

Vegetable: Brussel sprout, cauliflower, kohlrabi, lettuce (romaine), parsnip, rutabaga, Swiss chard

WHEEZING

Herbs: red clover

WHOPPING COUGH

Essential Oils: basil, clary sage, cypress, lavender, melaleuca/tea tree

Herbs: basil, horseradish, lavender, lobelia, melaleuca, oregano

WORMS

Essential Oils: oregano

Herbs: amaranth, basil, black walnut, borage, eucalyptus, horseradish, oregano, mandrake, olive leaf, parsley, senna, thyme, wormwood

Nuts, Oils, Seeds:

Seed: pumpkin seed

Vegetable: radish

WOUNDS: SEE SKIN

YEAST INFECTION

Amino Acids, Minerals, Omega Oils, Vitamins:

Vitamin: paba

Dairy: yogurt

Essential Oils: melaleuca/tea tree

Herbs: olive leaf, oregano, sage, witch hazel

Nuts, Oils, Seeds:

Nut: coconut

VAGINAL SWELLING: AFTER GIVING BIRTH

Herbs: witch hazel

CHAPTER 16

Safe and Natural Ways to Keep a Healthy Home

THROUGHOUT THIS BOOK, THERE ARE SEVERAL WAYS THAT WE CAN HEAL OUR BODIES naturally. With our food, using different ways of holistic treatments, and the use of energy work. Even though many ways have been mentioned, we also need to think of the other things we do in our homes and how we treat our bodies and the air around us. Several times the mention of unhealthy chemicals has come up in the chapters. When we take a good look at what we are using, it is surprising what we are using in our homes and businesses each day.

There are so many chemicals in the personal care products that we use today. Toxins that can cause allergy reactions such as blistering of skin, eczema, lung distress, migraines and so much more. These chemicals get absorbed into our skin pores and contaminate the organs in our body. They put a lot of stress on the liver, kidneys, lungs, bowels and skin. These are all the organs that help to detox our bodies. Before we get into some wonderful ideas of things to use in our homes, we need to really look at the list of the top twelve toxins that are found in the products from the stores.

12 TOP TOXIN LIST

Aging is not just the way we look, but, more importantly, it the degenerative diseases that are caused by chemicals that prematurely change our life.

The following diseases can be caused by the chemicals that are in the products that we use each day.

| Breast Cancer | Heart Disease | Depression |
| Hormone Disruption | Obesity | Memory Loss |

Birth Defects   ADD

The following are the worst of the worst, toxic, carcinogenic list commonly found in most skin and personal care products. Each is directly linked to one or more of the above conditions.

1. Benzoyl Peroxide: Frequently used in acne products, the MSDS states, "Facilitates action of known carcinogens. Possible tumour promoter. May act as mutagen: produces DNA damage in human and other mammalian cells in some concentrations. This is also toxic by inhalation. May be harmful if swallowed and in contact with skin. Eye, skin and respiratory irritant."

2. DEA (Diethanolamine), MEA (Monoethanolamine) & TEA (Triethanolamine): This foam booster is a skin/eye irritant and causes contact dermatitis. It is easily absorbed through skin to accumulate in body organs, even the brain. Repeated use results in major increase of liver and kidney cancer. Found in shea butter.

3. Dioxin: Won't appear on an ingredient list. Often contained in antibacterial ingredients like triciosan, emulsifiers, PEG's, and ethoxylated cleansers like sodium laureth sulfate. Dioxin causes cancer, reduced immunity, nervous system disorders, miscarriages and birth deformity. It's a hormone disrupting chemical with toxic effects measured in the parts per trillion – one drop in 300 Olympic sized swimming pools. Our bodies have no defense against its damage. The most visible example was Yushchenko, the Ukrainian president, who suffered from dioxin poisoning and looked old overnight.

4. DMDM Hydantoin & Urea (Imidazolidinyl): Just two of many preservatives that often release formaldehyde, which may cause joint pain, cancer, skin reactions, allergies, depression, headaches, chest pains, ear infections, chronic fatigue, dizziness, and loss of sleep. Exposure may irritate the respiratory system, trigger heart palpitations or asthma and aggravate coughs and colds.

5. FD&C Colour & Pigments: Synthetic colours from coal tar contain heavy metal salts that deposit toxins in the skin, causing skin sensitivity and irritation. Absorption can cause depletion of oxygen and death. Animal studies show almost all are carcinogenic.

6. Parabens: (Methyl, Butyl, Ethyl, Propyl): Used as preservatives and aren't always labelled "parabens." They're used in deodorant and antiperspirants and have been found is breast cancer tumours. Parabens, as xenoestrogens (hormone disruptors), may contribute to sterility in male mice and humans. Estrogen-like activity causes hormone imbalance in females and early puberty. It is found in: body lotioins, liquid hand soap, overnight tanning lotions, shea butters and shower gels.

7. PEG (Polyethylene Glycol): Made by ethoxylating Propylene Glycol. Dangerous levels of dioxin have been found as a by-product of the ethoxylation process. PEGs are in everything, including personal care products, baby care products and sunscreens. Found in body butter.

8. Phthalates: Xenoestrogens are commonly found in many products, usually not listed on labels. Health effects include damage to liver/kidneys, birth defects, decreased sperm counts and early breast development in girls and boys.

9. Propylene Glycol (PG) & Butylene Glycol: Petroleum plastics act as surfactants (wetting agents, solvents). EPA considers PG so toxic it requires protective gloves, clothing, goggles and disposal by burying. Because PG penetrates skin so quickly, EPA warns against skin contact to prevent brain, liver and kidney abnormalities. There is no warning label on products where concentration is greater than in most industrial applications. Found in baby lotions, body butters, body lotions, body moisturizers and some anti-frizz hair products.

10. Sodium Lauryl Sulfate (SLS) and Sodium Laureth Sulfate (SLES): Detergents and surfactants that pose serious health threats. Used in car washes, as garage floor cleaners, engine degreasers and 90% of personal care products that foam. Animals exposed to SLS experienced eye damage, depression, laboured breathing, diarrhea, severe skin irritation and even death. SLS may also damage the skin's immune system by causing layers to separate, inflame and age. Found in liquid hand soap, shower gel, 2 in 1 shampoos, and baby body wash.

11. Sunscreen Chemicals: avobenzone, benzphenone, ethoxycinnamate, PABA are commonly used ingredients that are known free radical generators and are believed to damage DNA or lead to cancers. Found in shower gels.

12. Triclosan: Synthetic "antibacterial" ingredient with chemical structure similar to Agent Orange. EPA registers it as a pesticide, posing risks to human health and environment. Classified as a chlorophenol, chemicals suspected of causing cancer in humans. Tufts University School of Medicine says Triclosan is capable of forcing emergence of super bugs it cannot kill.

All information taken from The Toxin Alarm TM Guide – courtesy of The ToxicFree R Foundation

NATURAL AND ORGANIC PRODUCTS

Naturally grown and organic self-care products provide our bodies with the energy, nutrients and protection that we need to maintain our health. With the use of social media, books and research we can find many ways to create our own products that don't damage our bodies.

What we are going to do in this chapter is share some ideas that you can use in your own home. We will explore both products and ideas for our bodies and our homes to provide a healthier environment. When my children were little, I had to find ways of cleaning the house in a safe manner as both my oldest child and I were chemically sensitive. If you can use the ingredients that are organic, you will have an extra advantage. If not, just getting started is a huge benefit for your whole family. You will notice a difference and can have fun creating and/or using natural health products.

Air

Air fresheners, colognes and perfumes are one of the strongest triggers for headaches and allergies. Many of these products can have an effect on our neurological system and cause extensive damage to the lungs. These products were created to cover the smell from body odour, smoke and other odours that occur in our home and offices. They do not clean the air. These chemicals coat our sense of smell in our noses and then get absorbed into our skin and lungs. They are a cover up like a lot of drugs on the market, and again, don't clean the air or get rid of the bacteria.

Cleaning the air: We can start with using natural products like essential oils to clean the air or as a personal scent for our body. In Chapter 14 we cover the essential oils and the abilities that they have to clean bacteria from the air and the therapeutic effect they can have on our health. An example is if the air in the house is stinky from cooking. We can use a diffuser for the essential oils to be distributed in the room. The essential oil will add a natural aromatic scent, diffuse the bacteria, relax our body and provide other healing benefits.

Colds, flus and other contagious diseases:

-The use of oils like oregano oil, tea tree oil and clove oils will help to clean the bacteria in the air. These oils would be excellent to use in the whole house and especially in the room that the sick person is residing in.

- Cutting an onion in half and placing it in the sleeping area of the person that is not feeling well will bring about a speedy recovery as the onion will absorb the bacteria from the person. This is more powerful than using Lysol.

- I have personally placed into a pot of water cinnamon, cloves, nutmeg and ginger oils and dried herbs when holding workshops so that if someone shows up who is not feeling a hundred percent, the air is much cleaner for all of us.

Lungs:

-When our lungs are in distress from bronchial discomforts and coughs, it is better to diffuse eucalyptus oil, tea tree oil, cinnamon oil, clove oil or oregano oil into the air. These all will keep the air clean for everyone in the room and provide the healing properties needed.

Paint Fumes:

- Freshly painted rooms can be minimized by clove oil in a diffuser or even have it sitting in a bowl with or without water.

Please try to remember to use a latex friendly based paint.

These are some ideas that you can use for the air and provide a healthier environment and assist others in it so that they will not get sick.

Furnace Filters: In Canada and in other parts of the world we have furnaces to keep us warm in the colder months. We need to change the filters during the year, and every so often we need to have the air ducts cleaned.

When we had the furnace and ducts done a couple of years ago, the company doing the job would not let clients see what came out of the ducts. The reason was that sometimes there are bugs and smaller dead animals in the ducts along with remains of other things that get sucked into the ducts and furnace. These all are unhealthy to be breathing in. Imagine what would be circulating in the home if the filter was not there, or the filter was clogged and the air was not circulating properly. Or what gets stuck in the ducts through holes or other improperly sealed connections.

We can experience headaches, nausea, lousy sleeping patterns, sore throats and more when the air is not clean in the home. If there are smokers or pets in the house, you may want to change that filter more often. When it is just me, the filter will get changed about every two months in the winter.

Mold in the Air: Mold can cause havoc to a person's health. Symptoms can be headaches, skin irritations, bronchial congestion, asthma, liver, bowels, runny nose, itchy eyes and can also affect the nervous system. Mold is a fungus that is found where there is a lot of moisture: leaky basements, improperly sealed and insulated walls and windows.

Mold continues to grow in the damp atmosphere on anything: books, food, carpet, clothing and wood. The pores of the mold then spread when the objects are moved and not thoroughly dried out. Example: If a basement has had a serious water damage done to it, anything that is in the area needs to be thoroughly cleaned and dried out. There should also be the monitoring of other areas in the basement to see if there are any signs that the mold may have started and spread. You can see dark areas in drywall, mold on paper and books or on window sills. The mold can grow on ceiling panels and even in the air ducts. It would be safer to keep the area with the water damage clear of any objects for a while till you are certain that the humidity has gone right down.

Cleaning of Mold: A detergent with tea tree oil or other strong and natural disinfectant. If you are uncertain of natural solutions and want something stronger bleach with water is a very strong solution, but **please** use rubber gloves and a mask (N-95 respirator) to do the task (you don't want to burn your lungs and get sick from the bleach). For expensive furniture, you may want to consult an expert on the proper cleaning methods for the wood and materials.

Use a circulating fan to help dry up the area immediately after the water damage has occurred, and equipment can be purchased to absorb any additional water. If uncertain, contact your nearest restoration company. Mold is dangerous and can cause serious damage to our bodies and organs.

Flowers are a wonderful way to brighten a home, especially during the summer. My granddaughter would get up in the morning with a bit of a cough and sounded congested. By lunch time she was just fine. When my grandson was born, around that same time some wonderful people sent in some flowers to the hospital for my daughter. Unknowingly, the new grandson was sensitive to the flowers and sneezed quite a bit at the hospital along with getting a mucous discharge in his eyes. The allergy was pointed out by the baby's doctor a week later, and it all fell into place. I had also realized that my granddaughter was bringing fresh flowers into the house from the gardens, and this was causing her congestion at night.

PLEASE DO KEEP THIS IN MIND:

On September 22**nd**, 2008, it was mentioned on the news, (Calgary, Alberta) how perfumes worn by pregnant mothers and colognes and aftershave lotions can affect unborn children, especially boys. Studies are showing that baby boys are not developing properly, and the genital area is being affected. I truly believe that the perfumes and colognes worn by males and females can affect both sexes of unborn children and could lead to other sensitivities in both the child and mother.

Whenever someone goes into a room with a perfume, hair spray or cologne on, other people can get headaches and even have problems with their breathing as the airways tighten. Many clinics, courtrooms and other public areas are banning the use and wearing of perfumes and colognes.

Please, even if you have the most wonderful scented perfume or cologne, think of the others who are in your area. We do not need to change our scent to be womanly or manly.

We can safely clean our air with the essential oils that are mentioned in Chapter 14.

Allergies

Our bodies react to foods and environmental substances. We get headaches, migraines, rashes and runny nose. Several years ago, it was said that a child who was always frail would stay that way, and they were always sick. I wonder now how many of these frail children and adults were suffering from allergies that were in their homes or in the food they ate. After a conversation with one of my children about an instance that happened many years ago when they were little, I realized what had started the allergy she had.

I believed that the house they stayed in (dusty and cat hair everywhere) was what caused an asthma attack for my daughter, that had never happened prior in her life. When I returned from my weekend trip away, I was shocked to walk in the relative's door and see an inhaler stuffed in my daughter's face. This asthma attack was from both the cat dandruff and stress. Another friend became sensitive to several food products when he became stressed over a mortgage that he really did not want to take on.

Allergies can fade away when we start to look after our well-being. When we eliminate the toxins in our area, we can heal those allergies quite significantly. My friend, after a year or so, could eat eggs and the other products again, but did learn to work on the stress and not let it control his life.

Allergies can also be released with energy work, including the process of acupressure or acupuncture. I believe we can release the energy blocks that our bodies are holding onto. I do believe that many allergies can be dealt with, without going through allergy shots (shots do work well, but other unknown stuff is injected into us) and we can live a lot more comfortable in our surroundings. Each of the following sections in this chapter will provide healthier options to keeping a healthy home and body.

Body & Organ Detoxing

We can naturally detox our bodies each day, no matter what environment we work in or live in. There is always something in our space that has been manufactured with chemicals. Even living in a tent, you will get the outgassing of the material and camping supplies, gas fumes from vehicles and sometimes toxins from the wood we are burning or the propane or gas from cooking stoves.

In 2010, the town I was living in was outgassing huge piles of boulders from a site that used a chemical for treating railway ties and other wood. This chemical also was proven to cause cancer in the people who worked for the company. When the land remediation was done, they did not say how the chemical was being extracted, but I could smell it in the air. When I realized what was going on, I got the dandelion tea out and started to drink a cup of it each day along with taking milk thistle capsules. Over the years I found many ways that I can help to detox my body, and it all starts with our liver.

There are times when I do get the urge to do a detox that is more than what I am normally doing daily with the food I eat and aromatherapy. I will not wait to start the procedure for the recommended times. My body speaks loudly when it needs to get my attention.

Some of the reasons that we are drawn to do a detox are candida, constipation, diarrhea, environmental sensitivities and difficulties with our other organs such as our skin, kidneys and lungs. It is better and safer to do a detox for our body before our organs start to shut down or are stricken by diseases like cancer. When we look after our body naturally, we can avoid the harsher ways that are being used such and chemotherapy.

Detoxing our bodies and changing our food diet at the same time can be beneficial in two ways:

1. When we choose to do a full body detox, we can clean our liver and our colon, which in turn has a good effect on the other organs in our body and helps to increase our energy.

2. Changing our diets to eliminate wheat, dairy, alcohol, vinegars and sugars during the detox not only aids in the cleansing but can make us aware of what could be causing health problems.

DETOXING PROGRAMS:

Homeopathic: The homeopathic system is the use of the essence of herbs that are placed into little tablets. These tablets have little or no taste to them.

Herbs: The herbs can be used in tablet form, liquid form (elixirs) or in their natural state.

Fruits, herbs and vegetables: These foods when consumed properly can provide ongoing support for all our organs.

There are many detox programs on the market, and you need to find the one that is suitable for your needs at the time. What we need to do is talk to either a naturopath, herbalist or a person working in a health store. There are different detox packages put together for different goals. Following are some of the programs available in the health stores.

a. Candida requires a strict diet of no wheat, dairy, alcohol, vinegars or sugars. The person would consider to also take a probiotic during the cleanse. Candida in many cases in caused by the overuse of antibiotics during the person's life and causes the body to get yeast infections that creates other discomforts in the body. Consult your health store for candida cleansing and some may have a list that you can go through to see if you have the various symptoms.

b. Environmental sensitivities can cause a lot of damage to the liver and other organs in the body. One must be careful when doing a detox, some of the herbs many be too strong for the system at the time. Consider doing a homeopathic detox and start very slowly. The homeopathic detoxes are gentle yet very effective.

c. Bowels: whether constipated or experiencing constant diarrhea, you want the right cleansing program to address the right issue. There are programs for each that provide the right minerals and herbs to help heal the organ and provide the strength for the colon to function better.

d. General Cleansing Program: There are some detox programs, for example, Wild Rose Detox (which I really like and have used) that requires that you eliminate wheat, dairy, alcohol, vinegars and sugars during the detox. This and others with the same requirement are working with your colon and liver.

When you are finished with the program that you are using, it is better to slowly introduce the wheat, and dairy back into your diet. You may find that your body will react to these foods, and is letting you know that the foods are not healthy for you to consume. There are other cleansing programs that do not have the diet recommendations and can be a lot easier to do when leading a busy life, and these too will work with cleansing the body. Look for the one that you feel comfortable with.

I personally believe that no matter what program you decide to go with, start off slowly with the detox. For me, my system is sensitive and no matter what I take in herbs, vitamins or minerals, I always take half of what is required for the first day or two and let my system adjust before proceeding. This way, if you have a bad reaction to a herb or homeopathic, you can stop before going further. Do keep in mind that as we do a detox the action of the natural ways can create a headache or affect our bowels as the toxins are being eliminated, but if you find the effects are extreme, you may want to adjust or change the product that you are using.

Again, sometimes we don't need the full amount that is recommended on labels. The label requirements are a guideline. We all have different systems, we all have been exposed to different things and many of us react to things stronger than others. Keep in mind that if your homeopathic practitioner, doctor or naturopath has recommended something, there is a reason behind it.

Caution: Always mention if you are taking medications prescribed by a doctor. Some medications do not work with herbs.

Bug Spray Alternatives

There are two major mosquito spray products for the human body to use, yet studies have shown that the ingredients in these sprays can be linked to allergies, immune toxicity, cancer, developmental and reproductive problems, problems for the organs, irritation for the skin, eyes, lungs and bad for skin absorption.

The products contain: N,n-Diethyl-Meta-Toluamide, Related Isomers, Inert Ingredients (95%), ethyl alcohol and fragrance. We all know that even the fragrances placed into products are bad for our neurological development. Then there is a warning not to use the bug sprays near acetate, rayon or varnished surfaces like cars. Now, if this will eat through manufactured products, what happens when our body absorbs the product? On a scale of 1 – 10 (highest) on the hazard list on the Skin Deep site, it rates at a 7.

How about using an essential oil? I did a search on lavender (as I was told it is a good bug spray for the body). Lavender came in low (1 – 2) for toxicity and is very beneficial as it has many healing properties. The only way that I could see an oil being toxic is if it was grown with herbicides and pesticides. How about eucalyptus or lemongrass? These oils are natural bug repellants and would have more benefits internally (though used externally) than other options. If you are going into an area where one is exposed to lots of mosquitoes, you can eat bananas before going on the journey to keep mosquitoes away. Another benefit is that those around you won't be subjected to chemicals in their air space.

Following are some natural bug spray ideas. Have fun creating the combination you want to use.

FOR EACH GALLON OF WATER ADD 4 – 8 DROPS OF EACH OIL:

Fleas	citronella, lavender, lemongrass, tansy
Flies	citronella, lavender, peppermint, tansy
Lice	cedarwood, peppermint, spearmint, tea tree oil

Mosquitoes	lavender, lemongrass, tansy citronella
Ticks	lemongrass, sage, thyme

Building Materials

For over seven years I worked for a family business doing hardwood flooring. During this time, I did a lot of research on building products and safer options. I believe that California was the first state to stop the use of paints that had a high toxin level because of the paint and urethanes that would outgas during the curing stage. This was a good start to informing the public on the toxicity of what we are placing in our homes.

Even if you don't mind the smell of the fumes from building products, they can still affect you. This also includes any lacquers, varnishes or stains for woodwork. The oil based products can take several months to cure, and during this time cause headaches, affects the liver, skin and bladder. While having to work in an office that was freshly painted by the landlords I got lethargic, queasy, and headachy. Try to look for the products that are more environmentally safe. Our business promoted the water based hardwood urethane, and we made sure the workers still wore masks during the application of the product.

Options for cleaning the air after using paints in a room:

- Place some vanilla extract in a bowl in the middle of the room that was just painted and keep a window open for the air flow.

- Essential oil diffuser in the room: cinnamon oil, clove oil, or any of the oils that will clean up the bacterial in the air.

When you place new carpets, linoleum, particle board and pine wood into a house, make sure to keep a window open as these products contain glues, petroleum products and resins that can make the occupants sick. Each time I walk into a show home, my muscles get tense, and I get nauseous and have a headache. The fumes are from all the new products in the house. This can take months to outgas if there is no fresh air flow.

All this stuff has chemicals and don't really start to outgas until they are unpacked and placed into your home. Many of these chemicals will have an effect on your nervous system, your digestion, your skin and your lungs and muscles. If we are running a business, we need to remember that those working for us also deserve the consideration of clean air.

Colds and Flus

When the fall time and winter is upon us, we again hear encouragement on radio and TV to get the flu shot. But is this the right decision for you? Before you make your decision be sure you are informed about the pros and cons of the flu shot.

Research has shown the flu shot can reduce the risk of upper respiratory illness by 25%. It helps reduce serious illness in the elderly and in individuals who are immune compromised. For those who care for others in this high risk group, the flu shot can help reduce the risk of spreading the flu.

However, the flu shot is not for everybody as the flu is not typically a serious infection in the general population. The flu shot protects against two to three strains of the flu. These strains are predicted up to six months in advance. Therefore the flu shot will not protect you against all strains of the flu. The flu vaccination contains mercury as a preservative. Mercury is toxic to the brain, nerve cells and arterial linings and has been linked to an increase in the risk of Alzheimer's disease, dementia, memory loss, depression, anxiety, ADD, heart disease, hypertension and birth defects.

Flu shots can be essential for some of the population, but my personal thinking is that they are not necessary for everyone. When colds, flus, tonsillitis, bronchitis, and all the fall and winter time ailments are upon us, it is time to rethink what we are eating for the season. The first thing we must remember is to get the proper sleep and rest when we start to feel a bit sluggish or even that wee tickle in the throat. Eat properly: fresh foods with the vitamins and minerals that the human body needs to function properly.

Some of the natural remedies in our cupboards are cinnamon, green tea, echinacea, garlic, honey, citrus fruits, oregano oil, oregano tea, cranberries and cranberry juice. Following are just a few ideas of how you can maintain a healthy body with what you use in your home and the foods that you are eating.

ESSENTIAL OILS:

Essential oils like tea tree oil, clove oil and eucalyptus oil are excellent to have around for aromatherapy to clean the bacteria from the air. The oils can be sprayed into the air or used in a cold air diffuser. The oils have antibacterial, antiseptic and antiviral properties that will provide a clean environment where the bugs have a hard time to survive in. We can use the oils at home, in our car and at work in our work space to keep the area clean and safely sanitized.

Tea tree oil is excellent to add to clean water or right on the cloth to wipe down door handles, sinks and toilets. This is safer than the hand sanitizers that have other chemicals in them. Eucalyptus oil and oregano oil can be used for cleaning too.

Oregano oil taken internally can help bring a virus to an end quick or help to build up the immune system so that a person does not catch the virus that is going around. I personally take a few drops of the oil in water and drink it down really fast.

Here are some examples from the book and what the oils can do for us during the cold and flu season.

Cloves (Eugenia caryophyllata)

Known best for its antibiotic and antiviral properties.

Therapeutic Action: antibacterial, anti-cancerous, antifungal, anti-tumour, antiviral, insect repellant, pain reliever

Eucalyptus (Eucalyptus globulus)

Eucalyptus oil and leaves have been used in saunas and hot tubs for years. The oil from the leaves and young twigs helps to clear out the sinuses and ward off virus and infections in the lungs.

Therapeutic Action: analgesic, antiseptic, anti-viral, diuretic, insect repellant, stimulant

FOODS:

Herbs, fruits, legumes, vegetables and even dark chocolate are some of the foods that help to build up our immune system. When we eat for our health, we have less chance of getting sick. We are looking for foods that are high in antioxidants and have antiviral and antibacterial properties. We can use more of these foods during this period and increase the amount of the herbs we use too. The foods mentioned are lumped into one section as we can cook and prepare our meals with all the ingredients and have fun doing it too.

Examples for herbs, fruits, legumes and vegetables:

Herb: Garlic (Allium sativa)

Known as poor man's treacle

Garlic is high in antioxidants.

Fruit: Lemons

- Lemons have more healing properties than the other citrus fruits.

- Grapefruit, lemons, limes and oranges have a high level of bioflavonoids that is found in the white membrane between the fruit and skin. This is a source has a very high amount of vitamin C.

- The absorbic acid (vitamin C) in the lemon makes it a powerful antioxidant that helps the body build up an immunity to o prevent viruses and diseases such as scurvy.

Legume: Pinto Beans

Pinto beans are high antioxidant properties. Pinto beans are low in fat and contain no saturated fat, trans fats or cholesterol. They are high in protein, fibre, iron, folic acid and potassium. Pinto beans also assist in lowering heart disease and cut the risk of high blood pressure and stroke. Pinto beans help with diabetes and cancer.

Vegetable: Kale

Kale is high in antioxidant properties

A serving of 2/3 cup of cooked kale meets your daily intake for vitamin K, and has a good source of lutein, vitamin A, C, fibre, folate, calcium and manganese. Kale contains anti-cancer compounds.

This is just a sample: See Chapter 15 for more options for antioxidants.

PROBIOTICS:

Probiotics are excellent to keep in the fridge, and there are some that are shelf stable.

Probiotics bring the good bacteria back into our system and make it harder for the bad bacteria from viruses to make us sick. This is also recommended to use after using antibiotics prescribed by doctors. The prescribed antibiotics kill off both the good and bad bacteria. People wonder why they are constantly on antibiotics during the winter from viral infections in the lungs and chest. When all the good bacteria had been destroyed by the prescribed antibiotic and then the person goes back into the same environment with a weak immune system, they get sick again.

Natural antibiotics like cinnamon do not kill off the good bacteria and will help to protect our body safely. If we are in a situation where the prescribed antibiotics are necessary, we need to take the probiotics during or after taking the prescription. The probiotics have strands of good bacteria that we need to get back into our body right away. Then we can also eat a healthy diet with some of the above foods that are mentioned.

Symptoms and how I approach them: (Please remember that everyone is different and that I am using this as an example.)

Nausea:
Ginger grated in tea.

Probiotics will help to bring up the good bacteria.

Clove ground up and added to water.

Sinuses:
Tea tree oil in a diffuser.

Eucalyptus oil in a pot of hot water to breathe in. I also pour a bit of the oil on a piece of cloth so that I can breathe in the fumes from the oil.

Peppermint oil on the bottom of my feet.

Sore throat:
Oregano oil in water two to three times a day. Seems to coat the throat and lessen coughing. Tastes awful but works.

Cinnamon mixed with some honey is another way to soothe the throat and heal at the same time.

Adding cinnamon to my drinks will help with all the above and be a good preventative and safe medicine.

What I have noticed over the years is that when a person tries to just fight off a flu virus without eating properly and not use something that will help deter the virus, it gets worse and many times the person will get hospitalized. The virus festers and gets stronger and is harder to ward off. If the natural products do not work within a day or two, and I have caught a contagious flu, I will resort to using a store bought anti-diarrhea and anti-nausea product for a day or two to stop the virus from festering then I will go back to the natural forms. This is a lot better than going onto the prescribed antibiotics and having to rebuild the whole immune system again.

OTHER IDEAS:

Cod Liver Oil:
Not so shocking that our grandparents were right. A tablespoon of cod liver oil every day in the winter months is a good idea. Cod liver oil is high in vitamins A and D. This is extremely good for our immune system in the months where we lack the sunshine vitamin: vitamin D.

Vitamins and Minerals:
Even if you take a good quality multivitamin, increasing your antioxidant intake (vitamin A, C, E and selenium) will help to strengthen the immune system.

HOMEOPATHIC:

Engystol will help to strengthen the immune system. There are other flu and virus remedies available in your health store. These are very safe. One practitioner I know has used these products for several years for both herself and her children, and they have not once gotten a virus.

Colloidal Silver

Colloidal silver did not seem to fit in the other chapters yet it is a powerful natural healer. This product can be found in a liquid or a gel form. People have taken colloidal silver for years as an antibiotic. As with any herb or essential oil, too much can have a reverse effect.

A few years ago, I used the colloidal silver for our family dog (as he would not take anything else and had a lump along his neck and was really sick) and with the fish in our fish tank. It has cleared up infections for mother pets that are trying to nurse the new litter of kittens or puppies.

During testing, colloidal silver destroyed on contact: MRSA, staph, E-coli, enterococcus, candida, pseudomonas and aspergillus.

Colloidal silver has been used for acne, allergies, athletes foot, boils, candida, canker sores, chronic cough, colds, diabetes, ear infections, eye infections, fatigue, flu, food poisoning, hepatitis, lesions, lupus, malaria, ringworm, shingles, warts, yeast infections and more.

The liquid can be applied directly to sores and taken internally. Use the colloidal silver to wash the wound, and you can soak the gauze in it to apply to a wound. The ointment is great for applying to external wounds on both humans and animals. Colloidal silver can be added to water to use as a household disinfectant.

Note: When Colloidal silver is made, it should be made with de-mineralized water so that it will not form silver compounds to cause argyria (greying of skin and nails).

There are a few websites on the internet that will share the dosages and provide many ways of using this amazing product for both your home and personal well-being.

Depression and Stress

Depression and stress: These two seem to go hand in hand. Experience showed that my high stress level led me to a mild depression a few years ago. This depression caused nausea, I was unable to eat properly, had anxiety and my bowels were not working right. I was scared to be away from a washroom. This was my real first awakening to the idea that we needed to replace in our body what had been used up. When a person is going through a depression or high levels of stress, the vitamin B levels become depleted.

After being prescribed antidepressants by the doctor, I looked at the bottle and did not open it. It was placed on a shelf. I did not want to take the prescription and had memories of conversations with other people and what they went through when taking antidepressants. I went back to the drug store the next day and talked to one of the assistants there. She led me to the vitamin Bs. The vitamin B50 complex ended up being a saving grace for my health and well-being. The depression greatly lessened and my outlook was a lot stronger. With this I started doing a lot more research into the herbs and vitamins and minerals.

There are several methods we can use to help us get through tough times without resorting to taking medications. One thing to keep in mind, though, is what can we do to make changes so that the depression lessens. Is it important to look at how we are living our lives and how well we eat and, sleep? And are we having fun. Following are some ways of lessening levels of stress and depression.

Diet:
Raw fruits and vegetables, whole grains, brown rice, seeds and nuts. Meats: Salmon and turkey have tryptophan (calming effect) and protein. Try to avoid caffeine, sodas and pops, saturated fats, sugar and processed foods.

Essential Oils: basil, bergamot, chamomile, clary sage, grapefruit, juniper berry, lavender, melaleuca/tea tree, patchouli, rosewood, sandalwood, spearmint, spruce, tangerine, thyme, ylang ylang

Essential oils can be used in several different ways on the skin, on clothing, in a diffuser, in a bath or in beauty products.

Herbs: Ashwagandha, hawthorn, kelp, lavender, milk thistle, rosemary, wild indigo.

We need to make sure that the herbs we take are safe for us; some medical conditions bring restrictions on what can be used.

Minerals: Calcium and magnesium is another combination that is calming for the nervous system. Many will take this at night before bed for a better sleep. The magnesium helps our muscles to relax and provides a better sleep.

Vitamins:
Vitamins B: Vitamin Bs are excellent for stress, energy, depression and are water soluble. What your bodies does not need will be eliminated. Our bodies are different in what we require and some of us are very sensitive to what we consume. I can go for two to three months without taking the Bs and may need them for two to three weeks the next month. There is now a liquid vitamin B that is quickly absorbed by the body. Vitamin Bs are beneficial for both males and females, from working full-time, being a full-time parent, at school or making a lifestyle change.

** **A caution:** Niacin (B3) may not be recommended if you have a liver disorder, gout or high blood pressure.

Following is a bit on all the vitamin Bs that you will find in Chapter 4.

Vitamin B1 (Thiamin):
One of the coenzymes in the energy producing process. Deficiency of thiamin impairs nerve impulses, lack of appetite and production of cellular antibodies.

Vitamin B2 (Riboflavin):
It aids in weight loss, nerves and thyroid problems (that can be triggered by stress.)

Vitamin B3 (Niacin, Nicotinic acid, Niacinamide):
B3 is used to treat heart disease, mental illness and arthritis. Lack of B3 affects the skin, gastrointestinal tract and nervous system and leads to severe diarrhea. The nervous system is affected by signs of anxiety, fatigue, loss of appetite, headaches, insomnia, depression, hyperactivity, hallucinations and smells and taste are dulled. ** A caution: Niacin (B3) may not be recommended if you have a liver disorder, gout or high blood pressure.

Vitamin B5 (Pantothenic Acid):
Some B complexes will add additional B5 to the formulas for stress. This vitamin helps to produce the adrenal hormones and our antibodies. B5 is found in all of our cells and organs and helps with the production of our neurotransmitters. It has also helped with preventing anemia, depression, anxiety and works with our intestinal tracts. The lack of B5 can be depression, tiredness, tingling in hands, and headaches.

Vitamin B6 (Pyridoxine):
Lack of B6 affects the nervous system. The lack of protein does not allow the brain to develop and function in babies. It affects teeth development and causes teeth decay. Use of oral contraceptives may deplete the B6 and cause depression. B6 has been used to help with arthritis, numbness, burning sensations in extremities, fingers that go to sleep, swollen joints, reduced sensation in joints and leg cramps. B6 has been used in children for anxiety, convulsions and hyperactivity.

Vitamin B12 (Cyanocobalamin)
B12 is also known as Cobalamin. B12 contains a metal called cobalt and is essential to activate folate, for the structure and function of the nervous system. Vegetarians tend to have pallor due to the lack of B12, as meat is one of the greater sources of cobalt is red meat. Without B12 the red blood cells are halted and are not developing right. This can also affect the nervous system, small intestine and eye colour perception. Symptoms of B12 deficiency are irritability, depression, hallucinations and diarrhea. Now doctors at mental institutions and hospitals are requiring that patients are being tested for vitamin levels, mainly for B12.

Remember: You are what you eat. When I eat unhealthy food, my body feels lethargic and my mind is foggy. When I eat the healthy food, my energy is a lot better, and I have a healthier outlook on life.

Disinfectants

Some of the disinfectants are toxic for the kids to be using. The alcohol in them not only kills the bacteria, it harms the lungs and gets absorbed into the skin. There have been reports of kids ending up in the school sick room after using the hand disinfectants. As a mother, I know that the little ones concept of a little is enough does not sink in. The little ones believe the more the better.

What about sending them in with a lotion or a spray with tea tree oil, or creating a spray for their hands with an essential oil that is antibacterial. The kids would love to create their own product. Tea tree oil with lemon, or a citrus mix would be nice too. If we use a base of a natural oil that can be found in some drug stores or health food store and add the essential oils to it. You could use a coconut oil base or a bee's wax base. This way the base is good for the skin and the antibacterial oil will protect the body from the bad bacteria.

FOLLOWING ARE SOME OF THE ESSENTIAL OILS THAT YOU CAN USE:

Basil: antibacterial

Chamomile- Blue: anti-infectious

Cinnamon and Cinnamon Bark: antibacterial

Clary Sage: anti-infectious

Cloves: antibacterial

Cypress: antibacterial, anti-infectious

Eucalyptus: antiviral

Geranium: anti-infectious

Grapefruit: antibacterial

Juniper Berry: anti-infectious

Lavender: anti-infectious

Lemon: anti-infectious, antiviral, disinfectant

Tea Tree Oil: antibacterial, antifungal, anti-infectious, antiviral, disinfectant, fungicide

Myrrh: anti-infectious, antiviral

Myrtle: anti-infectious

Oregano oil: antibacterial, antibiotic, antifungal, anti-infectious, anti- viral

Patchouli: anti-infectious

Peppermint: antibacterial, anti-infectious

Ravensara: antibacterial, anti-infectious, antiviral

Rosemary: antibacterial, anti-infectious

Rosewood: antibacterial, antifungal, anti-infectious, antiviral

Sage: antibacterial, antifungal, antiviral, anti-infectious

Spruce: anti-infectious, disinfectant

Thyme: antibacterial, antifungal, anti-infectious, anti- viral

Dust Mites in Carpets and Mattresses

Dust mites are found in mattresses, pillows, carpets, draperies, fabric furniture and stuffed toys. They burrow into the fabric to escape the light. They thrive in warm, humid conditions, and their main food source is dead human skin flakes and animal dander. This explains why the highest concentrations of mites are found in mattresses and furniture.

Dust mites are the source of one of the most powerful indoor biological allergens. There is a protein from the dust mites that are found in their feces and carcasses are a proven to cause headaches, runny nose, itchy skin, and puffy eyes among sufferers of asthma, rhinitis, related respiratory problems and eczema.

Adult dust mites only live about two to four months. In that time they produce about 200 times their weight in waste product and lay forty to a hundred eggs. One tenth of the weight of a two-year-old pillow, not routinely cleaned, is dust mite feces. (Note: pillows functionally last 3-5 years)

SOME WAYS TO REDUCE DUST MITES BETWEEN CLEANER USES:

- wash all bedding once a week in hot water (mites survive cold water washing)

- vacuum carpets and rugs often

- do routine carpet and drapery cleanings

- put stuffed animals in the dryer on a high heat setting or freeze them for 48 hours

- have good air circulation/filtration in the house and maintain low humidity

- clean surface dust as often as possible

There are products on the market that can be used for dust mites. Again, look at the essential oils and see which ones are good for parasites. Norwex does have a good dust mite formula that is safe to use.

Electrical Pollution

EMF should be considered a harmful invader in your body, just like any other environmental toxin. It interferes with your health at the cellular level because you are an electrical being. Your body is a complex communication device where cells, tissues, organs and organisms all "talk." At each of these levels, the communication includes finely tuned bio-electrical transmitters and receivers, which are tuned like tuning into a radio station.

Two of the more well-known biological impacts from electro-smog are the interruption of your brain wave patterns leading to behaviour issues and the interference with your body's communication system then leading to abnormal neurological functions such as dementia, chronic fatigue syndrome and fibromyalgia. This can have the same effect as heavy metals and toxic chemicals. This causes damage to our DNA that again leads to illnesses like cancer.

THE SIX PRIMARY TYPES OF EMF:

Static Electric Fields: These are made up of static electricity caused by ions released from synthetic materials in your home. The importance of choosing natural materials for your furniture, cabinetry, flooring and other building supplies.

Residual Magnetism: This happens from metal in your bed and can change your magnetic field. This can cause depression, eye strain, fatigue, headaches, hyperactivity, muscle cramps and nightmares.

Power Frequency: This happens with the wiring in your walls, electrical outlets, extension cords, lamps and other electricity sources. When a bedroom is disrupted with power frequency, the cells in our body cannot regenerate properly, leading to insomnia and other diseases.

Power Frequency Magnetic Fields: These are caused by building wiring errors and when power lines to your home run underground near your sleeping area. An electrical panel box located on a wall near your sleeping area or even a refrigerator or TV located on the other side of the wall from where you sleep can also lead to power frequency magnetic fields.

Radiofrequency/Communications: This includes a broad range of cordless phones, wireless devices, cell phones and cell phone towers, all of which can interfere with your health.

Radioactivity (and its by-product radon): Radioactivity enters your home from building materials (such as granite) or radon gas coming up out of the ground.

Light and sound are also part of the EMF spectrum, so if you're near a highway or airport that surrounds your home in artificial light or excessive noise, you can also be impacted by that, although this is less common than the EMF sources listed above.

Ways to reduce EMF in your home:

- Make sure that your bed does not contain any metal.

- Use plug in covers for unused plug ins.

- Reduce the amount of electrical equipment in the sleeping area. Don't have a TV, laptops or cellular phones in your bedroom.

- Reduce the amount of time in front of electronics.

- When buying a home, make sure you don't have cell towers or power stations near the home.

At the time of writing this book the only other thing that came to mind to use around electrical equipment and cell phones is a crystal called aventurine. We can place the Aventurine in the area that we are using electronics or wear the crystal in a necklace.

AVENTURINE

Colour: light to dark mossy green

Good to use by computers, cell phones and electrical equipment.

This crystal is powerful for putting up a shield for those who try to tap into one's energy.

Aventurine is used for stabilizing the heart, lung, throat, insomnia, skin, allergies, adrenal glands and muscular system.

Hair and Skin Products

Sometimes we don't realize the damage that is being done by using hair and skin products that are now on the shelves in the stores. This was one of my first lessons as a mother. My first child had skin sensitivities that were caused by the laundry soap that I was using. We had to find a product that had no scent to it and was gentler on the skin. Thirty years later we have a lot more healthier options available to use.

At the beginning of the chapter there was a list of toxins found in shelf products. We can create our own health care products, and we do need to pay attention to the labels for the ingredients that we are using. Try to make sure they are organic, and I even look for the labels that say the product was cold pressed for the oils. If you can also use products from the area that you are in, you are also helping the environment.

I am going to list a few products that can be safely used for your body and some of them can be used for cleaning, which is another benefit for our bodies and well-being.

ACTIVATED CHARCOAL POWDER

The activated charcoal draws out toxins from the body and skin abrasions and can eliminate harmful bacteria as well.

APPLE CIDER VINEGAR

Apple cider vinegar is starting to become well used in homes for so many different purposes and also becoming known as a super cleaner. It has antiseptic abilities that helps to deter the growth of unwanted bacteria and yeasts.

Animals
Add some apple cider vinegar to shampoos for horse care and pet care.

Hair care
Cradle cap: Use a drop of apple cider vinegar in water for a cradle cap.

Head lice: You can blend a few drops of tea tree oil to some apple cider vinegar and water to rinse the hair. The tea tree oil kills the lice and the vinegar is acidic and detaches the lice from the scalp and hair. With the kids in schools, head lice is becoming common and a concern for parents. From what we understand, head lice loves clean hair and is transmitted from child to child from close contact (working on project together) and by sharing hats, brushes, etc. If your little one is prone to the head lice, you can purchase shampoos that have the tea tree oil in it and use that once a week as a preventative.

Skin
You can wash the skin area with apple cider vinegar to reduce warts.

Stomach
Apple cider vinegar can be used to promote weight loss and provide better digestion when used in cooking.

Yeast infections
Bathing with apple cider vinegar eliminates yeast and other bacteria.

Note: Apple cider vinegar (unpasteurized and unfiltered) is the preferable form to use in cooking and for health benefits.

COCONUT OIL

Coconut oil is an amazing oil to use for the whole body.

Hair:
The oil can be used in your hair to add body to it. When my hair starts to have too much static in it, I will place a bit of oil on my hands and run it through the hair. I found a shampoo with coconut oil in it and the hair got thicker and softer.

Skin:
I place the hardened coconut oil on my hands till it melts and then rub it on the skin to rehydrate it. The coconut oil works faster than any other product that I have used. This oil can be safely used on baby's skin when first born. Please try a wee test spot on the little one first. The coconut oil will be a lot safer than Vaseline, which is a petroleum product. I have added essential oils like lavender to the oil for the relaxing effect.

CALENDULA GEL

Calendula gel is used for abrasions, cuts, burns and infections of the skin. Calendula has the following healing properties:

Vitamins: A, C, E

Minerals: calcium, phosphorous, Coenzyme Q10

Therapeutic action: antispasmodic, astringent (helps the skin tighten, especially for minor cuts), demulcent (relieves skin discomfort), emollient (soothes and softens the skin)

COLLOIDAL SILVER

The liquid can be applied directly to sores and taken internally. Use the colloidal silver to wash the wound and you can soak the gauze in it to apply to a wound. The ointment is great for applying to external wounds on both humans and animals. Colloidal silver can be added in water to use as a household disinfectant.

HONEY: RAW

Raw honey has antiviral properties. You can treat the skin abrasion or infection with a poultice of raw honey, activated charcoal and a few drops of tea tree oil. The raw **honey can be used to make** the charcoal into a paste with the tea tree oil, otherwise the charcoal is just a powdery mess.

VITAMIN E OIL

Vitamin E oil is used for treating skin that has been burnt or for abrasions. Vitamin E oil enhances the skin's healing on a cellular level while the oil helps to hold in the moisture.

Other skin concerns:

DANDRUFF

Dandruff can have several causes and is generally not caused by dry skin. The skin is usually moist, and the dandruff is a result of the skin shedding as the skin cells renew themselves. Those with excessive dandruff may be experiencing an overgrowth of yeast in the skin. Dandruff can also be caused by other factors such as trauma, hormones, sugar, carbohydrates and lack of vitamins and essential oils. There are also hair products that will cause dandruff. Look at the ingredients and compare them to industrial products.

Some of the aids to help decreasing dandruff: coconut oil, essential oils, kelp, vitamin A, B Complex, C and E and selenium. Vitamin A helps to prevent dry skin, and vitamin C helps to strengthen the cells of the scalp.

MAKEUP

There are so many toxic ingredients in makeup and personal scents such as perfumes, deodorants and after shaves. The ingredients that may be used are colour dyes, diazolidinyl urea, dioxins, fragrances, hydantoin, imidazolidinyl, lanolin, lead and more. Some of these ingredients are not even listed on the labels. For example, lead is found in some of the hair dyes. Fragrances can cause headaches affecting the nervous system, and one of the ingredients is a formaldehyde compound. These chemicals are being absorbed into your skin then going to your organs, lungs and nervous system.

I know many people who wear makeup, and swear that they look horrid without the makeup. Have you wondered what your skin tone was like before you started to use makeup? Makeup fills the pores of the skin and does not allow the natural daylight in. This would cause a person to look pale without their makeup. The cover up causes even more damage as the skin cannot heal properly and becomes more toxic.

One of the best things we can do is use plain water on our skin to wash it. If you want to continue to use makeup, there are mineral makeup bases in the market, but I would still check the health foods stores first and ask about the company that is making the product. Still be careful of the ingredients. Some of the products may be only of a partial mineral compound. Make sure it is 100% and talc free. The good products can improve skin and texture. Some brands can stop the growth of bacteria in the skin. The concentration of pigmentation in the mineral makeup can make the colours stronger so that you use less. Do your research.

Herbs: Medicine Found in the Kitchen for Cooking

Even though we have gone over a lot of herbs in Chapter 9, I want to revisit the benefits of the use of herbs in our everyday lives. Herbs are one of Mother Earth's greatest gifts that is underused and taken for granted. Herbs can help us not only heal our body. They help to maintain a good state of health while helping to detox our body daily. The best part is the taste that is added to our food from the herb is what makes us stop and really savour what we are eating. All it takes is a wee sprinkle and the herb can completely change the food experience. Using herbs can help us to enjoy healthier eating without it feeling like it is a chore.

When I recently went travelling, there was only one home that I went into that used herbs in the daily cooking. Everywhere that I stayed at, I was blessed with very healthy and delicious meals. What I did miss was the use of the different herbs whether they were dried or fresh. As I travelled I picked up herbs from the stores and kept them on hand with my camping stuff and even gathered some essential oils on the way, as I needed them. I have over thirty herbs in my cupboard and still buy the fresh ones when I can.

Following are some of the herbs found in my cupboard and their benefits.

Anise seed: This is used in baking and contains methyl ether. Anise seed has a liquorice taste and soothes the stomach

Cinnamon: Great for desserts as it prevents fermentation in the stomach, is a natural antibiotic, lowers sugar cravings as it is a blood sugar regulator. Cinnamon extracts have antibacterial properties and are used to stop and clear fungal strains, candida and a number of intestinal parasites. It is an anti-coagulant and good to eat with meals that have rich foods that are high in oils.

Cloves: The herb is great for desserts, is used for tooth infections, to stop nausea and also used to prevent fermentation.

Fennel: Contains methyl ether which soothes a sore bloated stomach and can be used in cooking, baking and as a tea..

Garlic: Garlic is rich in allyl sulfides, helps to fight bacteria and yeast and tastes amazing and can be added to a lot of dishes. The more you get used to using garlic, the more you add to the dishes.

Horse Radish: This root helps with digestion and is great for the sinuses. This one I make as a sauce in the fall that will last about 6 months in the fridge.

Marjoram: This herb taste good and helps to fight infections.

Nutmeg: Nutmeg, cloves and cinnamon go well together. They help with stomach upset, diarrhea, cold preventative and all of them can be mixed with a bit of honey to eat off a spoon or used in a tea.

Oregano: This powerful herb is one of my favourites for adding to soups and tomato sauces. It offers the highest source of organic phenols, which assist in being antibacterial and antifungal.

Rosemary: Rosemary provides a temporary boost of liver secretions as it helps to emulsify the fats. I use rosemary with my vegetables that are served either raw or steamed.

That is only ten of the herbs that I use in my cooking and baking. This may sound crazy, but I made myself get used to the taste of coriander (cilantro) when I found out how good it was for getting the heavy metals out of our bodies. Now I love it and will add it to a few veggie dishes. This is the same as with raw garlic. At first the garlic felt weird, almost uncomfortable in my stomach. When I started to use it more, my tummy felt better and I started to increase the amount that I was using.

House Cleaning Options

When I had my first apartment I found that I could not handle many of the products on the market and needed to find the ones that did not give me headaches from the fumes or hurt my hands while cleaning. The latex in the cleaning gloves bothered my skin so that I was not able to use them for long. We need to look at what we are using for our cleaning products and how they affect our health. So many of the products on the shelves can cause skin irritations, irritate and damage the lungs and they also affect our neurological system.

I can smell chemical products a mile away, and they are always sure to trigger a bad headache. What about the little ones who don't understand what is happening to them as they get sick in their own home? They are put on inhalers with steroids, getting bad stomach aches, migraines, burns on their skin, weak muscles and not able to concentrate. These effects are from the cleaning products that are being used in the house, and they are absorbed into their lungs and skin. For adults, they have used these cleaning products for so long that they do not realize that the chemicals have damaged their smell or nerve endings.

Following are some ideas that you can use, and again, have fun doing some research, I would love to hear what works for you and is safe.

Apple Cider Vinegar
Apple cider vinegar is starting to become well used in homes for so many different purposes and becoming known as a super cleaner. It has antiseptic abilities that helps to deter the growth of unwanted bacteria and yeasts. This vinegar is also good to use to get rid of the calcium build-up in toilets and sinks. The fumes from the vinegar are not toxic. Add the apple cider vinegar to your wash water with a bit of dish soap or just plain water for cleaning walls, counters, closets, fridge.

Baking Soda
Baking soda can be added to your cleaning water to clean stubborn stains on stoves.

Citrus Peel Cleanser
Fill quart jar with orange, lime and/or lemon peals. Add vinegar to the peels till covered. Store closed for 2 weeks. When using combine 1 cup vinegar cleanser to 2 cup water.

Essential Oils
Essential oils such as tea tree oil, citrus oils and oregano oil can be added to your cleaning water, to wash off surfaces in the home, and they will also add a nice safe aroma to the area that was cleaned. Under the section in this chapter for disinfectants, there is a list of the oils that you can use.

Laundry products
There are now products in the market with no laurel sulfates and are gentler on both our clothing and our body. These products can be found in your local health food stores. You can also get natural soap seeds for washing and use wool balls for the dryer. The dryer sheets that are being used are toxic and again, will irritate the skin and the lungs.

Tea tree oil
Add tea tree oil to your dishwashing solutions as a disinfectant for all areas in your house. Tea tree oil has very strong antifungal and antibacterial properties and should not harm the body. Tea tree oil is an excellent and safe product for using on children's toys. This oil is powerful and can be used in the home and office where you work. I will use the tea tree oil on my cleaning cloth after cutting up meat for both the cutting board, counter in the area I worked and in the sink.

Toothpaste

The toothpaste we use can be harmful. I have tried toothpastes that say they will whiten the teeth, yet they did nothing. On some of the tubes it will say to only use a drop or two of the toothpaste. Children love to put as much as they can on the brush and some of them swallow the toothpaste as the kid's brands taste like a candy. The toothpaste can also be absorbed into the skin. Toothpastes can have fluoride and sodium laureth sulfate in them for the bubbling effect. Neither one of these is all that good for our body.

Look at the ingredients in your toothpaste to see what you are purchasing.

Another option for toothpaste is to use coconut oil with some natural peppermint oil in it for the breath freshener. Cinnamon oil would also be good as it has anti-bacterial properties too. When you are using the essential oils, make sure they are natural and safe to use internally. The coconut oil as a base is very healthy, and there should be no concern if it was accidently swallowed unless the person had an allergy to coconuts.

I used a Neem toothpaste while overseas and noticed that my teeth were getting whiter again, and I did not have that residual taste left in my mouth like other products. Again, do your search and have fun creating your healthy toothpaste without all the chemicals.

In conclusion, I hope that you will have fun creating your healthy home and office. There are so many options and many of them are fun to work with. You will start to see changes when the products with chemicals are taken out and replaced with natural products that are more powerful and healing.

CHAPTER 17

Food Preservation

Learning how we can preserve our locally grown produce by:

Freezing ~ Dehydrating ~ Drying ~ Canning ~ Cold Storage

IT IS TIME FOR HUMAN KIND TO GO BACK TO PRESERVING OUR FOODS FOR THE LEANER times and for the months that the fresh food is not available. Up till about the mid-1960s families on farms, in town and in the small cities had gardens and grew the root vegetables for the winter and the less hardy plants to eat right away or preserve for later use. My mother-in-law shared how there was a truck that would bring fruit to the farms that could not be grown in the area. Now we have the stores and markets.

The preservation methods people used over thousands of years all depended on the area they grew in and what tools were available to cook with. During the thousands of years of human life on planet Earth, a large percentage of people did not have access to cold storage. If you wanted the meat from the hunt to last a longer time, it would get smoked over the fire and/or dried in the sun. Then it was packed away till needed. The herbs, fruits, legumes, meats and vegetables were all used and nothing would have been thrown out. I have a strong feeling that the pot of soup or stew was the last meal to use the leftovers.

The quality of our preserved food depends on how it was preserved and stored. If a person has a freezer that works well, the benefits of what we can store increases immensely. On the other hand, if we have an underground cold storage, that will help to keep the root veggies and some of the fruits for a few months longer.

In Alberta (Canada) our growing season is short in the Calgary – Cochrane area. I have the use of a basement with a cold room, a freezer, places to air dry herbs, canning equipment and a dehydrator. I love to be able to go into the fridge, freezer and cold room to find food from my gardens and from the family farm. I love spending four hours in the kitchen to do one to two batches of canning or baking pies for over the winter for special occasions.

Spoilage of food is due to the microbial action of molds, yeast and bacteria. These are found in the air, water and on counter surfaces. They are also brought home on the food itself. We need to know about what are we preserving and how to do it safely.

Following are some ways of preserving your foods. Your local area should have organizations for food preserving and safety. We do need to make sure we preserve the food properly so that we don't get sick and have the best nutritional meals on the table that we can provide our families.

In the following sections I have greatly decreased the information that I had used in a manual for a workshop that we were teaching in Cochrane Alberta. For the freezing section, the goal was to show some of the fruits and vegetables that we can preserve and many of these can also be processed in other ways. When we grow the foods from our own gardens or buy them from the local farmer, we are greatly reducing the impact on our environment.

FREEZING

Freezing our food makes it easy to use the food later with minimum handling and convenience. Freezing can be superior to refrigeration for some produce like beans. Frozen beans contain more vitamin C than fresh beans stored in a refrigerator for 2 days. If you freeze your own veggies quickly after picking them, they will retain more nutrition than store bought fresh veggies in the winter. Fresh broccoli is an exception; it can stay more nutrient-rich up to nine days after harvesting than when it's promptly frozen.

There are pros and cons to freezing and these are as follows:

Pros:
- A good freezer is expensive to purchase and to keep running but reliable to preserve flavour, colour, texture and nutrients.

- There is flexibility in freezing different food combinations and time can be saved.

- Freezing puts food in a state of quasi suspended animation.

- Quick freezing assists in building small crystal on the tissues versus larger ice crystal on slow freezing which deteriorates the tissues.

- Freezers provide the space to freeze baking such as pies that were baked from the fresh fruit from your yards or the local farmers.

Cons:
- When fruits and veggies contain a high percentage of water, ice crystals can develop in the tissues, making the thawed produce soft or mushy.

- Slow freezing causes some foods to become limper.
- Freezing is not a method of sterilization like heat.
- Chemical compound called enzyme within food causes change in colour, texture and bad odour.
- Blanching destroys many microorganisms but some, notably the molds, continue to grow, although at a slowed down rate.
- Loss of moisture affects appearance and texture.
- Freezer burn: effect of dry air on the surface of food changing colour, flavour and nutrients.
- When food is thawed in a warm room the microorganisms will grow fast and spoil the food before it is cooked.

THEREFORE the key is in the quality of the original produce and that the food is cooked while still frozen.

EQUIPMENT NEEDED FOR FREEZING YOUR PRODUCE:

- A freezer that is big enough for 5 – 6 cu feet per person. A household with two people: 12 cu foot freezer.
- The chest type freezers costs less to buy and operate. Place the freezer it in a well ventilated area.
- You will need moisture, vapour proof packaging.
- Frozen storage packaging options: heavy duty aluminum foil, durable plastic films, freezer bags, glass jars, baking dishes. The headspace in jars should be 1 inch or more for liquid expansion.
- Do not overload your freezer. Put no more unfrozen food into a freezer than will freeze within 24 hours (usually 2 or 3 pounds of food per cubic foods).
- Labels for writing the date when the product was frozen.

METHOD OF FREEZING

- Don't freeze a lot of produce all at once, so that the produce freezes a lot faster. When too much unfrozen food is placed in the freezer at the same time, it will take a lot longer for the food to freeze properly, and the food can get spoilt in the process.

Blanching:
- Blanching kills chemical enzymes which deteriorates veggies during storage. It deepens colour and partially sterilizes it. - You can keep blanched produce from twelve to eighteen months in the freezer, as long as there has been no frost bite or crystalizing of ice.

- You should use soft water or distilled water to do your blanching, as hard water can make vegetables tough.

Method for Blanching:
- Speed is important to hold on to freshness!! Pick young, tender vegetables. Pick in the morning. As a rule, it is better slightly immature than over ripe.

- Large quantity of boiling water (one gallon for each pound of vegetables) or steam. Follow specific time of immersion for each produce in "Preparing Fruits for freezing." Wire-mesh is handy for plunging veggies in boiling water. Start timing when water starts boiling again. At high altitude add ½ minute to time.

- Quick cooling using ice or running water. To avoid losing nutrients, instead of immersing food in cold water, use a pan filled with ice and sandwich food between ice in pan and a bag of ice on top.

- Drain and store.

Under blanching doesn't kill all chemical enzymes **Over blanching** creates a loss in food value.

Alternative to blanching:
- Sauté root vegetables such as carrots and turnips in a little butter or oil until they begin to soften. Then freeze them.

- Roast root vegetables, such as small beets, parsnips, potatoes or sweet potatoes. Coat vegetables with oil and bake until tender at 400 F for potatoes or 375 F for other root vegetables. Freeze.

- Roast sweet and hot peppers before freezing them. Broil each side until the skin chars. Remove from heat, let cool in a paper bag. Peel off the skin, remove seeds and membrane and freeze the flesh.

- Cook and puree any kind of vegetables or fruit to use as a sauce or broth enricher for soups, stews or casseroles then freeze.

Freezing Fruits:
- Freezing fruits preserves colour, flavour, and nutritive values but not always texture (i.e. tomatoes).

- Frozen fruits can be stored for twelve to eighteen months.

- Fruits can be frozen on a tray then placed in bags or containers.

Freezing with no additives: This is the best option as our bodies do not need added sugars. I will freeze my fruit by spreading it out on a cookie sheet. As soon as the fruit is frozen it is placed into a plastic container and back into the freezer. This process ensures that the fruit freezes fast, and is easy to break up when needed later for eating, baking and smoothies.

Freezing using lemon juice: When freezing fruit, you may want to sprinkle the store lemon juice on the fruit so that it does not turn brown. The lemon juice bought in the store has a higher acidic level and is better to use than the fresh lemon juice. Fruits like apples, apricots, bananas and peaches start to oxidize once they have been cut. Fruits can also be frozen directly in orange juice concentrate.

Freezing using absorbic acid: For fruits that oxidize easily, ascorbic acid (vitamin C), an effective anti-darkening agent, is available in crystalline powder. Dissolve ¼ tsp powdered ascorbic acid in ¼ cup of cold water. Sprinkle this amount over each 4 cups of prepared fruit and mix gently. You can also dip your fruit one by one in the solution but ascorbic acid is bitter so use sparingly.

Freezing using a syrup pack: Syrup/sugar packs can be used for fruits. I don't recommend this method as the sugars and syrups are unhealthy for the body. This method has been omitted for this book as we are concentrating on healthy foods for our body.

Please note: There are different ways to freeze fruit, and again, I am not placing the syrup method into the following options.

Apples:
- To freeze in slices, peel, core and slice apples.
- You can place the apple slices in a weak brine with 2 tsp salt to 1 litre water before draining and packing.
- You can add lemon juice or ascorbic acid to any of these to prevent darkening before packing in the freezer.
- For applesauce, core (but leave skins on), either grind whole in a blender or cook until soft in an uncovered heavy pot and put through a food mill. Add a sweetener to taste, if desired.

Apricots:
- Peel apricot skins before freezing because they tend to roughen during freezing.
- Dip a few fruits at a time into boiling water for 15 seconds or until skins loosen. You can also pack with the skin. Chill quickly in ice water and peel. Cut in half and remove pits.
- Slice up the apricot, remove the seed, add lemon juice or ascorbic acid to any of these to prevent darkening.

Bananas:
-Peel and freeze in chunks or as a puree.
- Cut the banana in chunks, sprinkle with the lemon juice or absorbic acid. Place and freeze loose on baking sheets and then bag when frozen.
- For puree, mash with a fork or potato masher or use a food processor, adding lemon juice or ascorbic acid to prevent browning.

Blackberries, Blueberries, Boysenberries, Mulberries and Raspberries:
- Pick out debris and wash. You can measure the amount of berries you need for recipes and freeze them in a freezer bag. Place the bags lying flat in the freezer till frozen.

- Place the berries on a cookie sheet till frozen then put into bags or containers.

Cherries - Sour:
- Wash and chill in ice water before pitting to minimize the loss of juice. Pack dry with lemon juice or ascorbic acid to prevent darkening.

Cherries, Sweet:
- Wash and chill in ice water before pitting to minimize loss of juice. Pack dry with lemon juice or ascorbic acid added to hold colour; light cultivars need more lemon juice or ascorbic acid.

Cranberries:
- Choose deep red, uniform-coloured, firm, glossy-skinned berries. Wash and stem. Pack dry or prepare as a sauce.

Currants:
- Choose the larger cultivars for freezing. Stem and wash. Pack dry and freeze.

Figs:
- Wash, sort, cut off stems, peel and leave whole or slice. Add lemon juice or ascorbic acid to prevent browning and freeze.

- For crushed figs, wash and coarsely grind in blender or food processor. Add lemon juice or ascorbic acid to prevent darkening.

Gooseberries:
- Freeze ripe berries for pies and under ripe berries for preserves. Sort, wash and trim. Pack dry for pies or preserves.

Grapes:
- Wash and stem. Leave seedless grapes whole. Cut in half and remove seeds from others. Pack dry.

- Place seedless frozen grapes on a cookie sheet, freeze and pack in bags or containers for later use. Frozen grapes make a great frozen snack. To peel frozen grapes dip one at a time into cool water while still frozen hard. The skins will slip right off.

Kiwis:
- Peel, slice and pack in syrup. Don't pact dry because kiwis will lose their liquid and become dry. I would suggest that you greatly minimize the amount of sugar you use, as the kiwi needs the moisture and not the sugar.

Lemons and Limes:
- Peel and remove sections from the heavy membrane. Pack dry or add a sweetener to taste.

- If you have whole lemons or limes that you won't use within a few weeks, you can freeze them. The skins will get soft when thawed, but the insides will be fine.

Melons, Cantaloupe:
- Cut flesh in slices, cubes or balls. Add lemon juice or ascorbic acid if desired. The texture of the melon can best be preserved if you serve the fruit before it's entirely thawed.

- You can puree cantaloupes and honeydew melons with ¼ cup lemon juice for each quart, then freeze. Thaw, stir in 2 cups of chopped fruit, top with non-fat yogurt, and you'll have a lovely fruit dessert soup.

Nectarines:
- Freeze like peaches. Their disadvantage is that their skins aren't as easy to peel. You can peel the skin off with a vegetable peeler or small sharp knife.

Oranges and Grapefruit:
- Peel and remove sections from the heavy membrane. Pack dry and freeze.

Peaches:
(The varieties that do not brown readily are Envoy, Harmony, Madison, Redhaven, Sunbeam and Veteran.)

- Use ripe fruit. To avoid darkening, prepare only enough fruit for one container at a time. Wash, skin, pit and freeze in halves or slices. Pack with a small amount of lemon juice or ascorbic acid.

- You can also freeze peaches and nectarines whole. This is good to know when time is short and you want to get the fruit into storage quickly without peeling and slicing it first. Freezing them whole also preserves the colour. Cut up the fruit or place them whole on a cookie sheet after sprinkling them with lemon juice or ascorbic acid. When frozen place in container or bag.

Pears:
- Pears retain better appearance and texture when you can them. If you wish to freeze them, choose ripe but firm (not hard) fruit. Wash, peel and remove cores. sprinkle them with lemon juice or ascorbic acid. To avoid unnecessary darkening, prepare only enough fruit at one time to fill one container.

Plums:
- If freestone plums, wash, peel and pit; half or quarter.

- If clingstone plums, pit and crush slightly, heat just to boiling, cool and puree in a food mill. Alternatively, remove pits and skin then puree in a blender or food processor. Add lemon juice or ascorbic acid to prevent darkening. Freeze.

Pomegranates:
- The tasty seeds of this fruit are what you really eat. Cut halfway into the fruit and then break it apart at this cut. Pop out the seeds, taking care not to bruise them. Once frozen, sprinkle the seeds over fruit salad, cottage cheese or whatever you like. They'll thaw quickly.

Raspberries:
- Clean and remove stems. Pack dry and freeze in bags or container.

- Or clean and remove stems, place on a cookie sheet so that they are not layered, freeze and then pack into containers.

Rhubarb:
- Choose crisp tender red stalks. Remove leaves and discard any woody ends. Wash and cut into 1-inch pieces. Blanch for 1 1/2 minutes in steam or boiling water and pack dry.

- You can also cut up the rhubarb, pack dry and then freeze without blanching.

Strawberries:
- Wash and slice or cut in half. First slice the berries into a bowl, then toss gently with lemon juice if you want, then freeze.

- You also can pack strawberries dry if you are freezing fully ripe berries. To pack dry, freeze whole on baking sheets and bag when frozen.

Tomatoes:
You can freeze tomatoes as a cooked sauce, stewed or they can be put right into the freezer when fresh.

- Freeze whole tomatoes on baking sheets, and when frozen, store them in plastic bags. The skins will conveniently crack during freezing, making it easy to remove them once the tomatoes have thawed. You can simply run them under warm water for fast thawed and easy skin removal.

- To save space and preparation time later, you may also stew tomatoes. Pell and then cut into quarter, and simmer slowly in a covered heavy pot until the tomatoes are soft and release their juices. Then remove the lid and cook as long as you like. You can cook the tomatoes down into a paste but be sure to keep the heat low and stir frequently to prevent burning. Cool and freeze.

- Or you can quick blanch tomatoes, peel and cut into quarters to freeze. To peel tomatoes, submerge them in boiling water for 30 seconds, then plunge into cold water and drain. The skins will slip right off. You can also run the dull side of a knife over the skin until it wrinkles and then peel the skin away. Freeze.

FREEZING VEGETABLES

Once frozen, vegetables cannot be used as if they were fresh. Most vegetables are blanched before freezing. If they are not blanched, they lose colour, vitamins, become tough and change flavour. When using frozen vegetables, it is better to place the frozen vegetables right into boiling water and lightly cook them before freezing them.

Artichokes:
- Select small artichokes or artichoke hearts. Cut off the top of the bud, and trim the thorny end down to a cone. Wash, then blanch in boiling water for seven

minutes or in steam for 8 to 10 minutes. Immerse into cold water till cooled, drain then freeze.

Asparagus:
- Use young, green stalks. Rinse and sort for size. Then cut into convenient equal lengths to fit your containers. Blanch thick spears in boiling water for 4 minutes or thin spears for 2 minutes or in steam for 3 minutes. . Immerse into cold water till cooled, drain then freeze.

Avocados:
- Choose avocados that are ripe with no inside blemishes. Peel, halve and remove pits. Scoop out the pulp and mash it, adding 1 tablespoon of lemon juice per two avocados to prevent browning. Freeze.

Green and Yellow Beans:
- Pick when pods are of desired length but before seeds take a shape that you can see through the pod. Wash in cold water and drain. Snip ends and cut if desired. Blanch in boiling water for 2 to 3 minutes or in steam for 4 minutes. Immerse into cold water till cooled, drain then freeze.

Lima Beans:
- Pick when pods are slightly rounded and bright green. Wash and blanch in boiling water for 1 minute for small beans, 2 minutes for medium beans, and 3 minutes for large beans. Drain and shell. Rinse shelled beans in cold water. Drain and freeze.

- Or in a steam for 3 to 5 minutes. Drain and shell. Rinse shelled beans in cold water. Drain and freeze.

Beets:
- Beets usually taste better canned, but you can freeze them if you cook them thoroughly first. Harvest while tender and mild-flavoured. Wash and leave ½ inch of the tops on. Cook whole until tender (about 25 to 30 minutes for small beets and 45 to 70 minutes for medium or large ones). Immerse in cold water, when cool, remove the skin and cut or leave whole. Freeze. No further blanching is necessary. Immerse into cold water till cooled, drain then freeze.

Broccoli:
If there is a chance the tiny green cabbage worm has invaded the buds, soak in cold salt water (6 tsp salt per gal cold water) for 10 to 15 minutes.

- Select well-formed heads. Buds that show yellow flowers are too mature and should not be frozen. Rinse, peel and trim. Split broccoli lengthwise into pieces and not more than 1 ½ inches across. Then rinse well and pick over. Blanch in boiling water for 2 to 4 minutes or in steam for 3 to 5 minutes depending on the size of the pieces. Immerse into cold water till cooled, drain then freeze.

Brussels sprouts:
- Pick only green buds. Like broccoli, heads that are turning yellow are too mature to process. Rinse and trim, cutting off outer leaves. Blanch in boiling water for 3

minutes for small heads and 4 minutes for medium heads, 5 minutes for large heads, or in steam for 5 to 7 minutes. Immerse into cold water till cooled, drain then freeze.

Cabbage:
Trim off the outer leaves.

- To freeze shredded cabbage, blanch the shredded cabbage in boiling water for 1 ½ minutes or in steam for 2 minutes.

Immerse into cold water till cooled, drain then freeze.

- To freeze cabbage in wedges, blanch wedges in boiling water for 3 minutes or in steam for 4 minutes. Immerse into cold water till cooled, drain then freeze.

Carrots:
Harvest while still tender and mild-flavoured.

- Small carrots: Trim, wash and peel. Freeze small carrots whole. Blanch in boiling water for 2 minutes for small pieces. Immerse into cold water till cooled, drain then freeze.

- Larger carrots: Cut others into ¼ inch cubes or slices. Blanch in boiling water for 2 minutes for small pieces, 3 minutes for larger pieces or in steam for 4 minutes for small pieces and 5 minutes for larger ones. Immerse into cold water till cooled, drain then freeze.

Cauliflower and Broccoflower:
If there is a chance that tiny green cabbage worms have invaded the head, soak in cold salt water (6 tsp salt per gal cold water) for 10 to 15 minutes

- Select well-formed heads free of blemishes. Wash and break into florets. Peel and split stems. Then rinse well and pick over. Blanch in boiling water for 3 – 4 minutes or in steam for 5 minutes. Immerse into cold water till cooled, drain then freeze.

Corn:
Pick ears as soon as they ripen. The natural sugars in corn turn to starch quickly after ripening, so good timing is critical. Corn on the cob is the only vegetable that you should thaw before cooking to get the best flavour and texture. Once thawed, steam or roast.

- Husk, de-silk and wash the ears. If you are freezing whole cobs, choose cultivars that have small ears. Blanch three ears at time in steam or boiling water for 7 to 11 minutes, depending on the ear size. Cool and pack separately or together, grouping enough for one meal. Wrap ears in freezer paper or in plastic freezer bags.

- If you are freezing cut corn, it's still easier to blanch with kernels on the cob first. Blanch in boiling water for 4 minutes or in steam for 6 minutes. Then cool and remove the kernels from the cob with a sharp knife or corn cutter.

Eggplant:
- Eggplant is best frozen when it is partially prepared (sautéed, roasted or breaded and baked) first.
- You can also blanch it in a solution of ascorbic acid (1 tsp ascorbic acid in 2 qt. of water). Peel and cut into slices ½ inches thick.

Garlic:
For best results, store garlic in a cool, dry root cellar.
- You can freeze garlic chopped or in unpeeled cloves or puree garlic, shape into a log, and wrap it in plastic wrap for freezing. Cut off as much as you need at a time while still frozen, and refreeze the rest.

Kale:
See Spinach and other greens

Kohlrabi:
- Cut off tops and roots and wash. Peel. Leave whole or dice into ½ inch cubes. Blanch whole for 4-5 minutes and cubes for 2-3 minutes. Immerse into cold water till cooled, drain then freeze.

Leeks:
Harvest while still tender.
- Wash and trim off outer leaves, tops and base. You don't have to blanch leeks before freezing unless you plan to freeze them for more than nine months. Just slice and freeze.
- For long keeping, blanch in steam for two minutes for sliced leeks and three minutes for whole leeks. Immerse into cold water till cooled, drain then freeze.

Mushrooms:
Select mushrooms free from spots. They may be blanched, sautéed or packed dry.
- To blanch, wash thoroughly and trim off ends of stems. If larger than 1 inch in diameter, slice or cut in quarters. Blanch in a weak solution of ascorbic acid (1 tsp. per 1 pt. of water).
- If sautéed, cool then freeze.
- Mushrooms can be sliced or left whole and frozen fresh.

Okra:
Select tender young pods.
- Wash and cut off stems so as not to rupture seed cells. Blanch in boiling water for 3 minutes for small pods or 4 minutes for large pods, or in steam for 5 minutes. Freeze whole or slice crosswise.

Onions:
- For best results, store onions in a cool, dry root cellar.

Note: The flavour of onions may change after freezing. Be sure to taste and adjust seasonings before serving previously frozen foods that have onions as an ingredient.

- You can freeze onions the same as leeks. Onions need no blanching before freezing them for more than nine months. Just peel, slice if they are regular-size onions and freeze.

- For long keeping, blanch in steam for two minutes for sliced onions and three minutes for small whole onions.

Parsnips:
Root cellaring is the best storage method for parsnips, but you may also freeze them.

- Choose smooth roots; woody roots will be tough and tasteless. Remove the tops, wash and peel. Cut into slices or chunks. Blanch in boiling water for 3 minutes or steam for 5 minutes. Immerse into cold water till cooled, drain then freeze.

Peas: Garden and Black-Eyed:
For garden and black-eyed peas, pick when seeds become plump and pods are rounded. Freeze the same day they are harvested, as sugar is rapidly lost at room temperature.

- Green Peas: shell but don't wash. Discard immature and tough peas. Blanch green peas in boiling water for 1 ½ minutes or in steam for 2 minutes. Immerse into cold water till cooled, drain then freeze.

- Black Eyes Peas: Blanch black-eyed peas in boiling water for 2 minutes or in steam for 3 minutes. Immerse into cold water till cooled, drain then freeze.

Peas: Snap or Snow:
You can harvest snap or snow peas any time before the pods fill out.

- Wash, trim off the flower end and pull out the string. Blanch in boiling water for 2 minutes or in steam for 3 minutes. Immerse into cold water till cooled, drain then freeze.

Peppers, Sweet and Hot:
Select when fully ripe. You can freeze green, red or yellow peppers. The skin should be glossy and thick.

- Wash, halve and remove the seeds and whitish membrane. Freeze.

- Peppers do not require blanching, but you may blanch for 2 minutes in boiling water or steam for easier packing.

- Or roast peppers under the broiler until the skin chars and loosens. Peel the skin off, remove the seed and membrane and freeze.

Potatoes:
Store potatoes in a root cellar; they don't freeze well with just a couple of exceptions. Potatoes can be kept in a root cellar or cold storage for many months. They can be cooked first but the texture and taste really changes.

Pumpkins and Winter Squash:
Harvest when fully coloured and hard-shelled.

- Wash, pare and cut into small pieces. Bake at 375 F, microwave or steam until soft and completely cooked. Then freeze in bags or containers.

Rutabagas:
Harvest while tender and mild-flavoured. Avoid any that are over mature.

- Wash and trim off the leaves. Peel and slice or dice into ½ inch or smaller pieces. Blanch in boiling water for 1 minute or in steam for 2 minutes. Immerse into cold water till cooled, drain then freeze.

Spinach and Other Greens:
Harvest while still small and tender, leaf by leaf or plant by plant. Harvest entire spinach plant as long as it is not overly mature.

- Select beet, Swiss chard and turnip leaves from young plants. Rinse well and trim off large midribs and leaf stems. Blanch in boiling water for 1 - 3 minutes or steam for 3 minutes. Immerse into cold water till cooled, drain then freeze.

- Use only tender centre leaves from mustard and kale plants. Blanch beet, kale, mustard, turnip: 1-2 minutes. Immerse into cold water till cooled, drain then freeze.

- Collards, dandelion, fiddleheads and spinach for 3 minutes. Stir a few times to prevent leaves from matting. Immerse into cold water till cooled, drain then freeze.

Sweet Potatoes:
Use smooth, firm sweet potatoes.

- Wash and microwave, steam or bake at 350° F until soft. Cool and remove skins if you wish. Pack whole, sliced or mashed. To retain bright colour, mix 2 tablespoons lemon or orange juice into each 3 cups of pulp or dip potatoes in solution of 1/2 cup lemon juice per quart of water.

Zucchini and Summer Squash:
- You can shred zucchini before you freeze it. Quick blanch it in boiling water. Immerse into cold water till cooled, drain then freeze.

- Slice or cube summer squash into ½ inch pieces and blanch for 1 to 2 minutes or until translucent.

- Here is a great way to deal with gargantuan zucchini crops. Turn your vegetables into instant soup stock. Puree the zucchini with herbs and onions in a blender, and then freeze until needed to make a thick flavourful soup base.

FREEZING HERBS

Harvesting your herbs:

Herbs should be harvested in the morning before the sun starts to warm them.

You can add frozen herbs in your cooking. Herbs will get a stronger taste after being frozen.

- With chervil, parsley and savoury only the young leaves should be harvested. Just pinch or cut the leaf off and leave the plant and stem as it will continue to grow and produce more new leaves. Wash your herbs well. Dry on a clean towel. Place in container and put in freezer.

- These are safe to freeze for about a year: Basil – Chervil - Chives – Dill – Parsley - Oregano - Rosemary - Sage – Thyme.

- You can also freeze herbs in ice cubes. Herb ice cubes are particularly good if you make a lot of soups and stews. Pack 1 or 2 teaspoons into ice cube trays, cover with water and pop into freezer. Then put frozen cubes into a bag.

FREEZING MEAT & DAIRY

It is best to use a commercial blast freezer (-10 F.) for quick freeze. If you don't have access to one, only freeze so much at a time. If too much is placed in the freezer the meat will not freeze properly and the meat will spoil.

- A quick freeze is better than slow freeze.

Meat:

The storage time for meat vary according to type, for example: ground meat shouldn't be stored as long as roast.

Leave the package wrapped until ready to cook.

- The refrigerator is the best place to thaw meats. Slow thawing allows the meat to absorb the thawed ice crystals.

- You can place the meat frozen in a sealed bag in cold water for a quick thaw.

- **Never thaw meat and allow it to return to room temperature.** It is best to cook meat while it still contains a few ice crystals.

Dairy products:

You can freeze butter, cheese (hard, semi-hard, soft and cottage cheese), cream (only heavy cream), ice cream and mild.

- For thawing, place the frozen product in the refrigerator to thaw, then use as if it was fresh.

FREEZING POULTRY

- Thaw wrapped poultry in the refrigerator or submerge it in cold water.

Caution:
Do not freeze stuffed poultry.

Never thaw poultry at room temperature.

FREEZING EGGS

- Select eggs as fresh as possible. Wash eggs and break each one separately in a bowl and examine eggs by smell and appearance before mixing with other eggs.

Whole Egg: Gently mix the whites and yolks without forming air bubbles by putting them through a sieve or colander. Pack eggs into plastic freezer jars leaving ½ inch headspace Yolks: gently mix the yolks without forming air bubbles. To each 6 yolks add 1 tsp of sugar or ½ tsp of salt to reduce coagulation. Pack same as eggs.

Egg Whites: gently mix the whites without forming air bubbles, pack same as whole eggs.

Use these measurements for frozen eggs:

3 tablespoons whole egg: 1 egg

2 tablespoons egg white: 1 egg white

1 tablespoon egg yolk: 1 egg yolk

CAUTION -

Not recommended for freezing:

- green onions

- radishes

- cooked eggs

- potato salad

- cucumbers

Dehydrating

North American tribes used methods of drying meat that they called charqui, which later became known as jerky. Pemmican is made by pounding the dried meat with a rock, then gradually pound in fat, dried fruits and vegetables. This was packed away to use during the fall and winter time.

Historically, food would be harvested then spread out to dry outside. This has been done in many cultures over the years. After a few days, it would be brought indoors to store. The results weren't always perfect. Sometimes food would spoil, fruits would turn brown and hard, veggies would be stringy and tough and meat would be like shoe leather. After it is refreshed and cooked, it would be acceptable. Some of the herbs and veggies were dried inside of the farm houses or homes in towns, hanging down from the rafters.

Our tastes have changed and people want food that looks perfect and the same colour it was when fresh. Hopefully this will change again and people start to realize that preserving our fresh organic food is healthier than buying it from the grocery stores.

PROS AND CONS OF DEHYDRATING:

Pros: Dehydrating can easily involve the whole family. Heat of electrical dehydrators do not present a hazard for children. The equipment is user friendly. There are few rules to follow, and you can create a lot of dried fruit and raw food combinations.

Cons: Dehydrating takes up electricity but once it's dry, it doesn't need to keep going and can be stored in air tight containers in your cupboard.

RESULTS OF DEHYDRATING

-Vitamin C is an air-soluble and a nutrient that can be lost in the dry air process when cells are cut and exposed to air. - The fibre, carbohydrates, minerals, caloric value of dried food is exactly the same as fresh.

- Any food that contains sugar will taste sweeter because of the concentration of the natural sugar.

- Vitamin A is retained during drying process.

OUTDOOR DRYING:

Outdoor drying requires a minimum of 90° C, a low humidity, little air pollution and control of insects and birds. You would require drying racks and netting to keep out the birds and other critters in the area.

INDOOR DRYING:

Dehydrators:
There are a few dehydrators on the market, two common ones are Nesco American Harvest, and the Excalibur. The electric dehydrators provide consistent temperature and air circulation for a quick and even drying process. The electric dehydrators only require cleanliness and handling electrical device. Keep it in well ventilated area. Air needs to flow in and around the dehydrator and away from the source of heat (plastic melts easily).

Drying Racks:
A person can still use drying racks inside, but then you must be careful that your product does not get a lot of dust on it and is not bothered by the bugs.

Oven Drying:
This is limited because the cost is higher than an electrical dehydrator and because it is not designed to carry away the moisture.

To use oven for drying the requirement are heating element with sufficient voltage for drying area, Fan to blow air evenly over all the food, thermostat, drying trays, made of safe, food-grade material, such as stainless steel, nylon, Teflon-coated fibreglass or plastic. Do not use copper, cadmium and zinc galvanized plated metal.

METHOD OF DEHYDRATING

1. Select the best quality product at the peak of ripeness and flavour. Wash carefully to remove debris, dust and insects. Cut away bruised or damaged sections.

2. Pre-treatments for dehydrating: blanching and dipping in antioxidants solution such as lemon, lime, ascorbic acid or a blend of ascorbic and citric acid.

3. Lay food pieces evenly on trays. Don't overlap.

* Do not turn off your dehydrator or leave partially dried food on the trays as it may spoil.

4. Testing for dryness: During final stage, let a few pieces cool and feel for dryness. Fruits are pliable and leathery with no spots of moisture. Tear in half, pinch and watch for moisture drops along tear. If no moisture, then it is sufficiently dry for long term storage.

Fruit rolls should be leathery with no sticky spots

Jerky should be tough but not brittle

Dried fish should be tough but not brittle

Vegetables should be tough or crisp

** Store dried food in small batches. Check for moisture build-up within two weeks of storage, if so, re-dry making sure there is no mold and then store in fridge or freezer.

PRODUCE THAT DEHYDRATES WELL:

Apples	Apricots	
Bananas	Beans (green)	Blueberries
Cranberries	Cherries	
Grapes: Green	Grapes (Red)	
Kale (Curly * sprayed with Bragg Sauce)		
Mangoes	Mushrooms	
Raspberries		

Saskatoon berries   Strawberries

Tomatoes

OTHER IDEAS & COMBOS:

Jerky: ground beef or filet beef jerky

Leather: fruit (apples and raspberries) or (cantaloupe and blueberries)

Leather: vegetable (sweet potatoes and peppers)

FRUITS

Fruits and roll ups 130 F to 140F (55 C to 60C). This helps to minimize loss of vitamin A and C. All food sweat at the beginning of dehydration, can have the temperature higher for the first couple of hours (140 F).

Fruits are ideal. They are high in sugar and high in acid, so less prone to spoilage by microorganism. You can dry fruits with edible skin on or off.

- Halve or slice in ¼ or ½ inch.

- To make the skin more porous and speed up drying time for figs, prunes, grapes, blueberries, cranberries, dip into boiling water for 1 to 2 minutes.

- To prevent oxidation, and have a superior product, pre-treat into a solution of ascorbic acid (or citrus juice) the following: apples, pears, peaches and apricots.

- Dried tomatoes can be powdered.

- Fruits are often dried for snack. They are so concentrated that one has to ensure not to eat too much.

- The natural sugar in fruits acts as a preservative, so fruits don't have to be dried as fully as less sweet food.

Fruit Rolls
Almost any fruit will make an excellent fruit roll. Apples are high in pectin and fibre and have an excellent texture when dried. Fruit rolls don't need sugar. If sugar is added, the rolls tend to become brittle during storage.

HERBS & SPICES

Fresh herbs and spices do have a stronger aroma than commercial bought herbs. Dried herbs are usually three to four times stronger than the fresh herbs.

Most leaves should be harvested before they start to blossom. The herbs should be gathered early in the morning before heat dissipates the flavouring oils.

- Heat is the lower setting 90°F to 100°F (30°C to 40°C) because their aromatic oils are sensitive.

- Basil takes a long time to dry. Cut leaves in half.

- Herbs are dry when they snap and crumble easily. To be certain that herbs are sufficiently dry, place in an airtight container for several days. If condensation appears on the inside of the container, they need further drying.

- Glass jars are the best for storing herbs.

- To dry herbs without a dehydrator, hang inside a perforated paper bag, to limit the dust and effect of light.

MEAT

Should be dried at higher setting (160° F, 71° C). That temperature destroys some bacteria and other microorganisms. Homemade jerky is much less expensive. Most lean meat will yield about one pound of jerky per three pounds of fresh meat. It is the fat portion that soon turns rancid.

Jerky meat must be brought to an internal temperature of 160° F. You can do this before drying by boiling the marinated meat for 5 minutes or after drying by putting in oven for 10 minutes at 275° F.

Steaks to use: lean, minimal marbling (fat) filet, flank steak, round steak, sirloin

Jerky from pork, chicken, turkey use precooked and processed meat. Dry at highest temperature setting. As an additional precaution, put in your oven at a minimal setting (165° F for at least 30 minutes)

- Jerky from game meat, freeze the meat for at least 60 days before drying.

- Pat jerky with paper towel several times as it dries to remove oils.

- Store jerky in refrigerator or freezer. If dried properly, it will last several weeks at room temperature while travelling or camping. If ice crystals form inside the bags, repackage in a dry container.

Lean fish can be used for jerky. Fat fish will not keep at room temperature more than a week.

VEGETABLES

Some vegetables are quite good dried, other ones lose their appeal and are better frozen.

- Most vegetables must be blanched to slow down enzyme action during drying and storage. Blanching helps to soften the cell structure, allowing the moisture to escape more easily and also allows vegetables to rehydrate faster.

- There is no need to blanch onions, garlic, peppers and mushrooms. They can be placed right into the dehydrator after being washed off and trimmed down.

STORING OF DEHYDRATED FOOD

Store in airtight, moisture proof container to prevent contamination and rehydration caused by humidity. The home vacuum packaging device is an ideal method. Store separately because flavour can transfer.

- Tomatoes and onions are prone to absorb moisture from air, so package immediately.

Storage area needs to be cool, dry and dark. The freezer or refrigerator is ideal, particularly for low acid foods such as meat, fish and vegetables.

Drying

We can preserve our herbs and flowers by air drying them. You would want to pick a place where there is not much dust circulating.

First I gently wash the garden dirt off the herbs and lightly shake off the water.

Methods of air drying:
- Tightly tie up the ends of the stalks and hang upside down to dry.

- Pick off the leaves and place in a hanging wire basket. May need a thin cloth to hold in the leaves.

- You can also place your herbs in a nylon / plastic netting to dry. This method is great for onions and garlic.

Canning

Canning our fruit and vegetables can be fun as there are so many ways of canning it. Fruits can be turned into fruit butters, jams, jellies, marmalade, preserves (made with chunks for fruit), conserves (made with fresh fruit, dried fruit and nuts). We can also make amazing pickles with dill and garlic, hot pickles and sweet pickles. Salsas, relishes, spread and ketchups are fun to make.

Even though I prefer my fresh vegetables and very rarely buy anything that has been processed, I love canning carrots, beans and beets for the winter to use as a garnish for meals. When it comes to canning season, I make sure that I have a four hour time period to get at least one big batch of canning done. Nothing tickles my heart more than to see the pickles and jellies lined up on the shelf in the cold room.

There are different methods of canning and a few rules that you need to follow. After a lot of thinking on how to proceed with this chapter I am going to leave this up to the experts. I will share some of the different methods, but I highly recommend that if you are really interested one of the best books that I found is the Bernardine Processing book. This is where my friend and I gathered most of our information for the workshops we held. There are also different processing times that are required for the altitude that you are living in.

TYPES OF CANNING:

Boiling Water Canner:
The boiling water canner can be used for tomatoes.

Pressure Canner:
Recommended for recipes that call for tomatoes mixed with other vegetables, meat or fish: as the acidity of the other ingredients are too low to be safe for regular processing.

Low acid foods such as meat, poultry, seafood and vegetables need to be processed in a pressure cooker to destroy the toxins that causes bacterial spores to grow. Recipes such fruits and pickled foods have the higher acid levels can be processing with the boiling water method because of the added vinegars, citric acid and lemon juices.

You need to process low acid foods at 240° or 160° Celsius to destroy the harmful bacteria.

The pressure canning has a locking lid that provides a vessel for the water and the steam to produce faster than it can escape. The temperate gets hotter in the canner and heats the food in the jars to 240 degrees.

Make sure you are using up to date canning books, as the older versions have the older unsafe methods.

You want to use the correct processing times and temperatures to avoid any unwanted and unsafe bacterial growth. www.homecanning.ca will provide many more recipes and information for the safe home canner. Once we understand the methods and follow the procedures, we can do our canning and preserving with ease and fun.

You cannot use a pressure cooker or sauce pan for canning low acid foods. The function of the cooker is different from the canner. The pressure canner is taller with a lid that locks into place and it also has a pressure regulating device. The Bernardin book asks for a WEIGHTED GAUGE pressure canner, as this one is specifically made for home canning and has weights to add that are required for the different required pressure levels.

The Bernardin book has all the required methods for proper processing times and methods. Once we have taken the time to read the instructions properly, done a batch or two of canning, the process becomes very fulfilling.

We can provide our family with food over the winter as treats such as jams and pickles. We can also preserve the foods such as tomatoes, vegetables, seafood and more for the nutrients that we require that are not in season. When we have an abundance of produce, fruits and meats, and don't have the freezer space, we can keep this abundance for later on. This not only provides our families with food that comes from our gardens, local farms and orchards. We are reducing the cost of transportation of our food and having a positive impact on our environment. We in Canada are blessed with such a huge variety of food to keep us healthy all year around.

LINKS THAT YOU MAY FIND BENEFICIAL:

Bernardin: www.bernardin.ca

Home canning safety: www.homecanning.ca

Home canning supplies: http://www.canningsupply.com/product/Steam_Canner/canners

Preparing your vegetables for freezing from "Preserving summer's bounty" by Rodale Food Centre.

Cold Storage

With the cold storage we need to consider the location that we live in. An example is Alberta and British Columbia in Canada.

In Alberta it is easier to have a cold room in the basement of our house or to build a root cellar just outside the house. In British Columbia I saw a doorway going into a root cellar by a farm house. In Australia, I have not yet been in a house that has a basement. So this option may not be as available there.

REASONS FOR COLD ROOM STORAGE:

- Convenience

- Food Security

- Globally responsible: Every time we have food imported it has an impact on the environment whether is it using boats, planes, planes or trains.

- Less packaging

- Quality of Food

Cold room storage is considered as a cool, dark, usually humid places suited to storing vegetables, fruits, nuts and other foods, preserving them for weeks or even months, without the use of additives. In Canada many houses have a cold room in the design of the building. Some modifications can be necessary, so it operates as it should. A basic cold room has at least two walls of undeveloped cement and a cement floor. This helps the room to contain the cooler temperatures of the earth.

Outdoor root cellars can be created with an organic blanket, a trench silo, hole in the ground cellar pit or even a garbage can cellar.

Again, I am going to encourage you to seek out what methods of cold storage would work best for you. Take the time to do your research and make sure you are ensuring the safety of your produce over the colder and leaner months.

CHAPTER 18

Gardening for Health

WHAT ARE THE BENEFITS OF HAVING YOUR OWN GARDEN?

Why garden when we have so many grocery outlets and now more markets with fresh foods?

IN THE EARLY 1960S THE GROCERY STORES STARTED TO CARRY A LOT MORE FRUITS AND vegetables year round. At this time the population, especially in the United States and Canada, was influenced by social status. Being able to buy your groceries in the store was a sign the you had money. The interest in gardens started to decrease. Less people were growing their food and preserving it for the winter.

During this same time there were companies that were putting together chemical mixtures and were employed by some of the governments to create bigger yields and bug resistant crops. The bigger the crop, the bigger the profits. Food was being preserved with chemicals, and sugars and excessive amounts of salt was being added to the food for longer shelf time. The chemicals were additives to enhance the colour and taste of the products.

Unknowingly farmers were being talked into using the poisonous products that not only started to contaminate our food but also the health of the farmers and their families. As a helper on a family farm, I heard several stories of how people who are now adults, have to go through tremendous whole body detoxing and healing as they were getting older. These people had lived on farms and went out to the field to pick the harvest or pick rocks out of the gardens. Their bodies come into contact with the chemicals that were quickly absorbed into their skin and affected their organs. Neither the farmers nor their children knew what was going on.

Today, 2016, so many people are looking for organic food and finding ways to grow their own crops. It is amazing how much we can grow in so little space. If you have an apartment you can grow herbs and veggies in pots on the balcony or in your kitchen. There are grow towers for those who don't have the proper sun or soil for good growing conditions. There are workshops for organic growing, permaculture and safe food preservation methods.

I had an amazing opportunity to not only have a huge yard to garden in but also a family farm to work on during the summer when I had the extra time. We did not use chemicals or pesticides on the gardens and found natural ways to deter the bugs. During the twenty years of being so blessed with the opportunity to grow my vegetables and fruit, I had realized that I could have grown a lot more. Though each year I had amazing harvests and thanked Mother Earth and Mother Nature for providing the right conditions to fill my freezer and pantry shelves.

Following is what I enjoyed during the last ten years as the plants matured:

- Raspberries, Rhubarb and Saskatoon berries for my fruit.

- Garlic, horseradish, parsley and sage were the herbs that I grew and being perennials made it easier to regrow each year.

- Plants started from seed were beans, beets, peas, kale, lettuce, potatoes, radishes and spinach. The carrots and potatoes did not really grow well in my garden, so I would get them from the farm garden.

What is Organic Gardening?

Organic gardening is a process of growing your produce without the use of any of the chemicals sprays and fertilizers, known as herbicides and pesticides, produced to get rid of weeds and pests. When these chemicals are applied to the produce, they coat the produce to protect it from bugs and get absorbed in the plant and the weeds around it. When the chemicals are sprayed or applied, the residue also goes into the soil and will remain there for up to three years or more.

I always know when something has been sprayed in the area, as the smell is in the air, and I will get a headache. If I was at the family farm, they would let me know if the neighbours were going to be spraying so that I could go inside the farm house or stay home that day.

Strawberries and peppers (Capsicum) are known to be the heaviest sprayed. At the farm we tried for about six years to grow thousands of strawberry plants without using the herbicides, and it was almost impossible to stay on top of the weeds that kept on spreading. The weeds seemed to be worse in that area. I have heard about people who cannot cut up peppers as their skin will break out in a severe rash, but they can eat the pepper after being cut and cooked. The chemicals from the herbicides and pesticides have an effect on our organs and health. At the time of writing this book, there is an epidemic in South America where the babies are being born deformed and females are being warned not to get pregnant nor go to that area. I truly believe this is connected to the chemicals that are being sprayed on the farms crops down there.

We are becoming more aware of how our bodies are reacting to what we consume. This even overlaps to the dairy and meat products on the shelves. The farm animals are being feed hormones and antibiotics for faster growing poultry and cattle. So many people are having problems with the wheat products. My body will tell me when a meat has a lot of chemicals in it. This is disgusting, but I can smell the chemicals as they leave my body. When it is that high, I will throw out the rest of the meat. Over the years I have learned to consume a lot more vegetables and much less meat, as I personally feel a lot better.

A lot of stores are starting to carry organic products, and in Canada there are a lot of strict guidelines about what is organic and the process the farmer went through to obtain the status. As I travel I see a lot more small farmers going the organic route for their crops and meat products. More and more people are slowly converting to a healthier lifestyle as we become aware of what is on the shelves.

Many of us cannot afford to buy all organic, so what I do is to see where the product was grown or processed. I will not personally buy vegetables that come from overseas. When I am in Canada, I will buy garlic that was grown in the United States if I cannot find the organic garlic from the local area. We don't want to live in fear of where the food came from, but we want to empower ourselves to search for healthier and more local products.

Here is a link for the area that I live in and with research you will be amazed who is now getting involved in organics and their journey to get there.

Alberta Farm Fresh Producers:
www.albertafarmfresh.com Alberta Farm Fresh Producers has a listing of farmers who grow products that a person can pick for themselves. Fruit, herb and vegetable growers. Great for an outing to the country to experience the quiet of the farm. Some farms have organic gardens.

Gardening Preparation and Permaculture

After years of gardening, I did not realize how little I knew. I will be going to the experts to learn a lot more about soil conditions and placement for plants that grow well together, and I would love to see you do the same. At this point of the book, there are workshops being held in Brisbane Australia that I want to attend. In Alberta, Canada I know there have been many workshops advertised over the last three years, and I am hoping to take in some of those too. When we get to take the workshops there is a lot of interaction, sharing of knowledge and gardening requirements for the area you are residing in and soil that you are working with.

In Alberta the ultimate time to add extra peat moss and manure to your gardens is in the fall time. That way the soil gets a better chance to absorb the nutrients and the peat moss is not too acidic for the plants. This would also be a good time to add the mulch and straw for better moisture absorption during the next growing season. During the months from September to April the soil has the chance to rest and absorb the above with the rain and snow. Again, this all depends on how long your growing seasons are and the soil requirements.

While working at the farm, we got to see what works and what does not work. When Mother Nature provided the perfect weather and no severe rainstorms the harvest was amazing. We boasted about bumper crops of zucchini, carrots that would break the records for size and taste. When the weather was harsh, the gardens did not do well. As I travel I get to see what the other farmers are doing and how some of our troubles could be lessened. This is why I am starting to see why we should not disturb the soil as much. When we compost of fallen leaves of the trees on top of the soil till the spring, we provide a home for the ladybugs and other bugs that help our gardens out.

Compost from your bin can be added at this time to the soil and dug in along with the peat moss and manure. I just dig out the compost from the bottom of the bin and spread the mixture on top of the soil / garden. You can use a rake to even out the mixture for a better coverage. As you dig out the compost, it helps to add back a few shovels of soil from the garden to the top of the compost bin to aid in the decomposition of the recently added fruits, coffee grounds, egg shells and veggie scraps. You can also add leaves to the bins.

PERMACULTURE:

Permaculture is the process of maximizing your garden space and using the land to produce more with less energy being added. The garden space that provides the ideal growing conditions for all of the plants. For example, beans like hotter weather and the peas like the cooler air and shade. Placing plants together so that they assist each other with their growth, pollination and even as a pesticide for the surrounding plants. This would also include drainage for the rains, compost and mulch to hold the water in the soil for plant compatibility.

I had a yard that had in the front yard some comfrey, horseradish and Saskatoon bushes. These plants seemed to thrive there and grew faster that the plants in the back. There is a section of the front garden that offered heat in the morning and shade in the afternoon. Again, there were plants that grew really well yet there were some plants that just died there. In the backyard along the garage I planted raspberry canes and they thrived there as they loved the heat from the garage wall and fence.

Social media has a lot of permaculture and organic growing pages. I like finding information on holistic healing and get to meet and see some wonderful permaculture ideas and websites. In Calgary I met some fellows that were using the backyards of a friend to grow organic gardens and they offered permaculture workshops. The motto around the world is becoming, don't grow lawns, grow your food and medicines. Be GMO free, grow organic and be much healthier and wiser for it. With the use of permaculture for your region you can have both your grocery store and pharmacy right outside your door.

Seeds

GMO SEEDS

GMO seeds have been developed and treated. These seeds have been treated with chemicals to produce crops that are bigger, to withstand harsh growing conditions and the seeds from those crops are known not to resprout. Does one wonder what this food is really doing to their body? Check out the resources on the internet and supporting books that show which seeds not to buy for your garden.

NON-GMO SEEDS

Organic gardening involves trying to use the heirloom seeds or certified non-GMO seeds that have not been treated. The heirloom seeds are the seeds that were tried and true for the region. They have not been altered, and the value of your produce will be better. Each year I find more non-GMO seeds being sold and the prices for them are getting a lot better so that you and I can afford to plant more. When we save the seeds from our crops, the value will go even further.

Farmers have been forced to plant GMO seeds and can still end up with failing crops. The produce from the seeds are causing toxic effects on humans and animals. There has been an uprising worldwide trying to put an end to a huge company that has tried to take over the produce industries, including developing toxic fertilizers and pesticides. This company also has their hand in many products on the grocery shelves.

What can we do? We can order seeds from companies that have had their seeds tested and have taken the pledge to provide non-GMO seeds.

Have fun researching for your seeds and create a vision board for your gardens for your next gardening season. Start a seed share and get a group started in your own community. It won't take long before we are back on track again with our food that is our medicine.

Natural Herbicides and Pesticides

HERBICIDES: WEED DETERRENTS

There are many natural ways of deterring weeds from our gardens. Even though we can eat many of the weeds, their growth can cause trouble and interfere with the growth of our vegetables and fruits. When using permaculture techniques, we can utilize ways to keep the weeds down. I have tried many ways to minimize thistles and the weeds that are tubular. Some work really well, and we need to be patient. Over the years of providing newsletters I was able to gather information for this to share.

Here is a homemade weed killer recipe. Excellent eco-friendly alternatives to chemical products.

NATURAL WEED KILLER

What you need:
1 gallon white vinegar

1 cup table salt (one could probably cut down on the salt)

1 tablespoon dishwashing liquid

What to do:
Remove approximately 2 cups of vinegar from the jug, pour in the salt and dishwashing liquid.

Return the 2 cups of vinegar to the jug. Close the lid and shake to mix.

Transfer to a spray bottle (after shaking to mix the ingredients) as needed.

Label the mixture, if any is left over, to identify for further use.

It works as well, if not better, than chemicals but is much cheaper. Be careful, it will kill whatever you spray it on! When you purchase the vinegar, 10% acidity, 20% acid is best, and spray it on the weeds in the heat of the full sun. You will have an effective weed killer without harming the environment

HOT WATER is now being used in Australia along the roadways. The intense heat kills the plant. Another thing to keep in mind is that we want to tackle the weeds while they are still young and before they go to seed.

PESTICIDES: ANIMAL DETERRENTS

Some of the local wild animals love our gardens. The deer love to nibble on tulips and eat the flower bulbs before they bloom. Birds love to eat the tips of the fresh pea plants and stunt the growth of the peas. Squirrels love to dig into planters that are just starting so that they can hide the peanuts that the neighbours feed them. Possums love to eat the garden plants. Again, squirrels love to eat the top of the poppy plants before you get the seeds from the pods. We need to be faster than the squirrels.

Here is something that we can work on during the winter to prepare for the spring for when we are planting again. Take the time to figure out what the animals love to get into over the summer. Netting can be purchased to be placed around the vulnerable plants. Your favourite tulip bulbs planted where the deer don't normally go. Placing coffee grounds in the gardens where the cats think they should void. Take the time to figure out what the animals love to get into over the summer. At the end of the summer, I love to share with the animals, but in the meantime, we need to protect the gardens so that there is an abundance of plants, fruits and vegetables for everyone, humans and animal friends.

Following are some safe pesticides that will not harm the plants or the land:

Ants:
ants don't like peppermint or spearmint. We can make a spray to deter them from the plants or from coming into our homes.

Essential oil mix: 4 – 8 drops of each oil to one gallon of water: garlic, peppermint, pennyroyal, spearmint.

Aphids:
Essential oil mix: 4 – 8 drops of each oil to one gallon of water: cedarwood, hyssop, peppermint, spearmint

Garlic oil sprays (see below for mixture)

Bean Beetle
Essential oil mix: 4 – 8 drops of each oil to one gallon of water: garlic, peppermint, thyme

Cabbage Loopers:
Garlic oil spray (see below for mixture)

Cabbage root fly
Essential oil mix: 4 – 8 drops of each oil to one gallon of water: sage, thyme

Caterpillars
Essential oil mix: 4 – 8 drops of each oil to one gallon of water: pennyroyal, peppermint, spearmint

Cats:
Cats do not like getting coffee grounds between their toes and will avoid the gardens with the grounds. The coffee grounds can be spread along the areas that the cats frequent and where the soil is good.

Cutworm
Essential oil mix: 4 – 8 drops of each oil to one gallon of water: sage, thyme

Earwigs:
Garlic oil spray (see below for mixture)

Gnats
Essential oil mix: 4 – 8 drops of each oil to one gallon of water: patchouli, spearmint

June Bugs:
Garlic oil spray (see below for mixture)

Leafhoppers:
Garlic oil spray (see below for mixture)

Mice:
Plant peppermint, mint and spearmint plants by doors and windows to help keep out mice. Keeping fresh spearmint in cupboards will help to keep mice out of food products. Putting dried food in storage containers such as glass jars will also be a good deterrent from both the mice and other food bugs.

Moths:
Plant parsley with the tomatoes to keep moths away from the tomato plants. This could be done for the lettuce plants too.

Essential oil mix: 4 – 8 drops of each oil to one gallon of water: hyssop, lavender, peppermint, spearmint

Rats:
Planting catnip in yards will keep rats away. You would also want to keep your compost pile away from the house as the food is a magnet for the rats.

Squash Bugs:
Garlic oil spray (see below for mixture)

Squirrels:
Blood meal is used to help keep the squirrels out of your favourite plants and gardens. Flower pots are the favourite hiding spots for the squirrels, and this can contribute to losing all that you planted. The squirrels love to dig in the soil, dig out your seeds and little plants. This summer one of the bigger pots was covered with a metal screen until the plants got big enough to deter my little friends. Blood meal added to the soil or on the top is another good deterrent.

Weevils
Essential oil mix: 4 – 8 drops of each oil to one gallon of water: cedarwood, patchouli

White Fly
Essential oil mix: 4 – 8 drops of each oil to one gallon of water: lavender, sage

Garlic oil spray (see below for mixture)

Garlic oil spray:

How to Make:
Soak 3 ounces of finely minced garlic cloves in 2 teaspoons of mineral oil for at least twenty-four hours. Slowly add 1 pint of water that has 1/4 ounce liquid soap or commercial insecticide soap mixed into it. Stir thoroughly and strain into a

glass jar for storage. Use at a rate of 1 to 2 tablespoons of mixture to a pint of water. If this is effective, try a more dilute solution in order to use as little as possible.

How to Use: S

pray plants carefully to ensure thorough coverage. To check for possible leaf damage to sensitive ornamentals from the oil and soap in the spray, do a test spray on a few leaves or plants first. If no leaf damage occurs in two or three days, go ahead and spray more.

PLANT MOLDS AND FUNGUS

Plant molds and fungus can create problems with the growth and quality of your produce. When we use the natural ways for the molds and fungus, it will also help the soil and plants in the area. The essential oils from our plants have very powerful properties that work on a cellular level for all the organs within the body.

Ten drops of essential oil to one gallon of water: cinnamon, niaouli, patchouli, tea tree oil.

Some studies also suggest that a garlic oil spray has fungicidal properties.

Nettle mixture:

How to Make:
Pick fresh nettle and preferably with gloves on. (There are two varieties of nettle and one can sting the skin.) After you have picked quite a bit of it, place it in a pot and bring it to a boil. Once the nettle comes to a boil, bring to a simmer and keep the lid on the pot. Simmer for about an hour, turn off the heat and let it cool overnight. Strain the leaves from the water and put the nettle into a spray bottle for use.

Indoor growing options

In Canada and the United States of America we have access to purchasing indoor growing system for vegetables over the cooler months. These are called garden towers. One friend shared that her tower supplied enough vegetables and herbs for a wedding dinner. You can grow herbs, tomatoes, cucumbers, peppers, lettuces and more. These garden towers use little space and have a grow lamp if there is not enough light and heat for the plants.

This would also be a wonderful system to have if you live in an apartment or basement suite and don't have the use of a garden in your yard or a community garden. Again, here is where using the internet and social media we can find some amazing ways to grow our food in our own home.

CHAPTER 19

A Recipe or Two, Tasty and Healthy

EATING HEALTHY AND TO SATISFY THE TASTE BUDS TAKES PRACTICE AND A LITTLE BIT OF time, yet it is worth it. My meals are mostly vegetarian, but I do have those moments when I crave beef but that does not happen often. When we get the right proteins, oils and enzymes into us, there seems to be a smaller craving for meat or dairy products.

It is fun to eat healthy, and yes, I can be obnoxious when I share some of the nutrients that we are eating at the table and what healing properties are in the food. Doing this I hope to plant a seed of knowledge in those who listen. A journey to my table is an adventure and not what you would normally see in a four course meal or several dishes. As I cook for one person, I find dishes that everything can go into and taste amazing. The herbs make a huge difference in the taste and can be healing at the same time. If it is a big dinner, you would be surprised to see what was processed right from the garden, or the herbs that were dried or frozen, and fruit that was frozen to prolong the nutrient value.

Each meal has herbs, veggies, protein and oils in them. When I don't consume all of them, I seem to get tired and know exactly when I need to change what I am consuming. There are so many recipe books out there now, vegan, protein, vegetarian and many more culinary adventures. Recipes can be found in bookstores, on the internet and at the markets. I gather ideas and put them together, and I encourage you to do this too. Find your favourite ingredients, add what your body is craving, and have fun putting together your healthy meal with supporting nutrients that our bodies crave.

Each recipe will have notes of the healthy ingredients in them to show you what you are eating and how we can heal the body at the same time.

BLACK BEAN DIP

2 cups cooked black beans (antioxidant, protein, B5)

4 tsp tomato paste or fresh tomato (cardio vascular, bone health, anti-cancer)

3 tbls water   (clean water can help to hydrate our muscles and flush out toxins)

2 cloves garlic   (powerful antioxidant, antiseptic, antispasmodic, diaphoretic, diuretic)

2 tsp lime juice   (very high in vitamin C)

½ tsp cumin   (anemia, asthma, bronchitis, digestion, insomnia, skin disorders)

½ tsp salt(sea salt is packed with minerals)

1/8 tsp cayenne pepper (one of the best stimulants for circulation and cleanses the blood)

2 green onions   (antibacterial, antifungal and expectorant, colon cancer preventative properties)

Hot peppers

Cilantro: handful (releases heavy metals, for anti-anxiety, antiseptic, antifungal, antioxidant, anti-parasitic)

- The above ingredients can be either blended together to make a smoother dip, or served unblended and served like a salad.

COCONUT OIL TREAT

Coconut oil ½ to one cup (antibacterial, anti-inflammatory, antiviral, astringent, vermicide)

Cocoa 1 tablespoon (antioxidant, blood sugar regulator, heart health, reduces effects of high fat diet)

Honey 1 teaspoon (antibacterial, antifungal, antioxidant)

Mixuture of seeds and nuts (Chapter 11. This is your fun to have, lots of protein and omega oils.)

Melt the coconut oil on the stove at low temperature. Add the cocoa and honey. Mix well. Turn off the stove, add your choice of seeds and nuts. Pour into a glass pie plate or baking pan. Let sit in the fridge to harden. Cut up and enjoy. This treat must be kept in the fridge if the weather is warm, as the oil will melt.

LEMON DRINK
(FOR THE EVENING OR MORNING, I PREFER MINE IN THE EVENING)

Juice from ½ of a lemon (lemon juice helps to cleanse the liver, is high in vitamin C)

Grated ginger 1 teas or less (antibacterial, anti-inflammatory, antioxidant, thermogenic

Honey 1/2 teaspoon (honey with lemon juice or cinnamon help in reducing weight).

Cinnamon: add to taste (antibacterial, antifungal, antioxidant, blood sugar regulator)

ASIAN CUCUMBER SESAME SALAD

2 large carrots (antioxidant, colon support, eye health, heart (cardiovascular support), stomach (digestion).

2 tbsp cilantro (release heavy metals, for anti-anxiety, antiseptic, antifungal, antioxidant, anti-parasitic)

1 tsp ginger (antibacterial, anti-inflammatory, antimicrobial, antioxidant, antispasmodic, anti-pyretic, carminative, diaphoretic (if taken hot), thermogenic

1 green onion (antibacterial, antifungal, anti-inflammatory, antiviral, expectorant0

2 large cucumbers (anti-inflammatory, antioxidant, estrogen balancing, intestinal tract, muscle inflammation)

1 sweet pepper (blood cholesterol, blood support, cataract prevention, diabetes: regulate, eyes, heart, immune, system, liver, muscle: cramps, muscle: spasm.)

1 tblsp lime juice freshly squeezed. (ant-oxidant, antiscorbutic, blood cleanser, immune system, liver cleanser, scurvy.)

1 tsp salt

1 pinch red pepper flakes

1 tsp sesame seeds (arthritis, asthma, blood: cholesterol, blood: support, blood pressure (too high), bone support, cholesterol (lower), colon support, diabetes, liver, lungs, menopause, menstruation cramping, migraines, osteoporosis, rheumatoid arthritis, sleep, stroke prevention).

2 tbls rice vinegar

1 tbls sesame oil (anti-inflammatory, antioxidants, Alzheimer's, arteries, blood (decrease LDL), blood (increase HDL), bone support, brain, cancer prevention, coronary artery disease, coronary support, diabetes, heart (cardiovascular support), heart (support, inflammation), nerve (support), skin care)

1 tbls maple syrup for taste

- Slice the vegetables and mix together with the seasonings and oil.

BEET SALAD

3 beets, medium or bigger   (anti-inflammatory, antioxidant, hepatic, anemia, blood cleanser, fetus development, heart (cardiovascular support), liver cleanser.)

½ cup chives

1 lime with zest (antioxidant, antiscorbutic, blood cleanser, immune system, liver cleanser, scurvy.)

1 orange & zest (anti-cancer, antioxidant, blood cleanser, cholesterol (lower), colds, colon cancer, heart (support), immune system, kidney: stone, liver.)

1 dash salt (sea salt)

2 tablespoon Olive oil (anti-inflammatory, antioxidant, blood (HDL, LDL), breast support, depression, DNA protection, heart (cardiovascular support), heart (support), hypertension, inflammation, metabolism, stroke prevention, tumour (reduce))

IN CONCLUSION:

I really enjoyed this last chapter. This is how I think when I eat my food:

What is in the ingredients?

Will it hurt my stomach?

Will I feel energized after?

What can I eat that will heal my body?

What can I eat to support my body?

When we eat for our health, we create an amazing healthy body and lifestyle that we truly deserve to have and enjoy.

I hope this book has helped you see all the amazing ways we have for healing:

- Different natural healing techniques.

- What nutrients are in our food and how they assist our organs.

- How the food, herbs and essential oils can heal our bodies energetically and on a cellular level.

The best part that I truly love is that I can eat very well and know that as I fill my body not only do my taste buds love all the herbs and food that I prepare, my body is also doing a happy dance.

I know that there is a lot more that I could have added for the gardening and in some of the other areas, but that is where we can have more fun researching and sharing with our family and friends.

Blessings for your journeys to an amazing healthy lifestyle! Remember to have fun!

We are energetic beings that require the proper nutrients for our bodies:

Physically, Mentally, Emotionally and Spiritually.

You are a beautiful amazing soul that just needed to be recognized by you!

Sending lots of love, light and blessings for all your journeys.

PS: Thank you for joining me on this journey of health and well-being.

~~~

REFERENCES

Authority Nutrition: https://authoritynutrition.com/foods/pork/

"Ball Blue Book guide to preserving": 100th year anniversary first published in 1909

BBC Good Food: https://www.bbcgoodfood.com/howto/guide/health-benefits-figs

Canadian Housing and Mortgage Association: http://www.cmhc-schl.gc.ca/en/co/maho/yohoyohe/momo/

Encyclopedia of Natural Healing: http://infoonnaturalhealing.com/nutritional-supplements/

Everything about Health: http://nutrition.about.com/od/nutritionalinfoveggies/

Growing and Using Healing Herbs: by Gaea and Shandor Weiss

Health Benefits: https://www.healthbenefitstimes.com/health-benefits-of-green-onions/

Herbs are Special: www.herbsarespecial.com.au/free-herb-information/comfrey.html

Herb Wisdom: www.herbwisdom.com/herb-goldenseal.html

Holy Basil: www.holy-basil.com

International Highlife: information on Cannabis

Mango: http://www.mango.org/en/About-Mangos/Mango-Nutrition

Medical News Today: http://www.medicalnewstoday.com/articles/275921.php

Medicine Hunter: www.medicinehunter.com/arnica

Mercola: http://foodfacts.mercola.com/pumpkins.html

Merrilyn Hope: www.merrilynhope.com/comfrey-the-miracle-healing-herb/

Nutrition and You: www.nutrition-and-you.com

Nutritional Healing: by Phyllis A. Balch CNC, James F. Balch MD.

Organic Facts: www.organicfacts.net

"Preserving Summer's Bounty": A Rodale Garden Book, Rodale Press Emmaus

Pure Healing Foods: http://www.purehealingfoods.com/chiaInfo.php

Pyroenergen: http://www.pyroenergen.com/articles09/green-onions-scallion.htm

Right Health: http://www.righthealth.com

Self Nutrition Diet: http://nutritiondata.self.com/facts/dairy-and-egg-products/106/2

Skin Deep: www.skindeep.ca

Today's Herbal Health: by Louise Tenney, M.H.

ToxicFree R Foundation Information taken from The Toxin Alarm TM Guide

USDA National Nutrient Database for Standard Reference

Web MD: http://www.webmd.com/diet/features/summer-corn-more-than-delicious

Whole Foods: http://www.whfoods.com/genpage.php?tname=foodspice&dbid=44

In Conclusion:

We are being led to look how we are truly living our lives and how we feed our body, mind and soul. Human beings went from eating the bounty of Mother Earth to eating manufactured products filled with chemicals and food colorings that have created illness within and without.

It is time to really look at how we are nurturing our body: physically, emotionally and spiritually. Mother Earth has so many medicines to offer:

Dairy, Essential Oils, Fruit, Grains, Herbs, Legumes, Meat, Nuts, Oils, Seeds and Vegetables.

We also have methods of healing through energy work and supportive spiritual practices that help us to release energy blocks and old world thinking that no longer serves mankind.

Kimberley has been gathering information since the mid 1990's and was looking for a way to share it. Her passion for eating healthy, learning about energy work and how the medicines of Mother Earth can heal on a cellular level brought forth her 2nd book.

Blessings for your journey to an abundance of good health and a joyful well being!

CPSIA information can be obtained
at www.ICGtesting.com
Printed in the USA
LVOW08s0417141017
552390LV00001B/1/P